Thinking and Seeing

Thinking and Seeing

Visual Metacognition in Adults and Children

edited by Daniel T. Levin

A Bradford Book
The MIT Press
Cambridge, Massachusetts
London, England

This book was set in Palatino by SNP Best-set Typesetter Ltd., Hong Kong and was printed and bound in the United States of America.

Library of Congress Cataloging-in-Publication Data

Thinking and seeing : visual metacognition in adults and children / edited by Daniel T. Levin.
     p. cm.
  "A Bradford book."
  Includes bibliographical references and index.
  ISBN 0-262-12262-6 (hc. : alk. paper)—ISBN 0-262-62181-9 (pbk. : alk. paper)
  1. Visual perception—Congresses. 2. Metacognition—Congresses. I. Levin, Daniel T.
BF241.T48 2004
152.14—dc22

2003064194

10 9 8 7 6 5 4 3 2 1

Contents

Acknowledgments

I would like to thank Katherine Floody for her invaluable assistance in organizing the Kent Forum on Visual Metacognition and this volume; the Kent State University Applied Psychology Center and its director, Stevan Hobfoll, for underwriting the forum; and The Inn at Honey Run in Millersburg, Ohio, for providing us with a home for the forum.

Preparation of this book was supported in part by NSF grant SES-0214969 to Daniel Levin.

Thinking and Seeing

Introduction

Daniel T. Levin

Several times during my career, I have noticed that the most exciting moments often occur when an experiment I have had no hope for actually works. This is particularly true of the risky ones that have only one good outcome. Experiments carefully designed to produce an interesting result no matter how they come out are also satisfying, but ultimately the satisfaction is in the incremental process of coming up with them in the first place. In contrast, setting up a risky experiment often involves a sense of tension that borders on dread, which, however, is sometimes richly rewarded.

I distinctly recall one evening when Dan Simons and I were setting up the second in a series of change blindness experiments. We had previously shown that subjects miss between-view changes that occur across the cuts in a motion picture. So, subjects saw a brief film depicting a conversation between two actors and as the view cut from one actor to the other, we purposely made the kind of "continuity errors" despised by professional filmmakers. For example, across one cut, one of the actors was clearly wearing a large colorful scarf, which disappeared in the next shot. We inserted nine of these visual discontinuities (intentionally—we also put in a few by mistake). We found that subjects missed every one of the between-view changes. This suggested that the visual system does not consistently represent and compare a large number of visual details to verify between-view consistency. Similar failures, collectively referred to as "change blindness," have recently been documented using a wide variety of methodologies (see Rensink, 2002, for recent review). Change blindness is also consistent with some turn-of-the-century discoveries by filmmakers that between-view inconsistencies in detail often escaped the audience's notice (For review see Levin and Simons, 2000). Moreover, it is consistent with findings by psychologists that people cannot integrate complementary patterns across views (for review see Irwin, 1991) and with their comments on the "sketchy" nature of visual memory (Hochberg, 1968, 1986).

Although these observations should have made our initial finding unsurprising, we found ourselves shocked at the degree to which people missed continuity errors that seemed to jump right out at us.

These observations, combined with recent research on object tracking in infants (Xu and Carey, 1996), led us to predict that people would miss changes even when they were looking right at the changing object. Thus, for our second change blindness experiment, we created brief videos depicting a "single" actor who completed a simple action such as sitting down or answering the phone. However, the "single" actor was actually two different people, one transforming into another across a cut. We predicted that these changes would go unnoticed. Indeed, when we had shown a demonstration video in which I changed into Simons to a roomful of psychologists, only about half of the viewers noticed the change, even though Simons and I were sitting right in front of them on either side of the video monitor. Thus we had both a theoretical reason to predict change blindness and a pilot experiment demonstrating the effect for exactly the kind of actor-swap our second experiment was designed to explore. Nevertheless, as we sat there that evening reviewing our videos, we were completely convinced that at most perhaps a few subjects would miss our actor swaps, thus contradicting our dramatic anecdotal demonstration and severely limiting the significance of our first experiment.

Despite our conviction the second experiment would be a flop, we ran it anyway. Once again we were shocked to see subjects miss plainly visible transformations in central objects (Levin and Simons, 1997). We experienced essentially the same shock when we set up the real-world version of the same experiment, and found that subjects missed changes to their conversation partner (Simons and Levin, 1998). Anecdotal evidence from our own and other laboratories doing similar research confirms that experimenters are not only ones who are incredulous at change blindness. I have heard numerous reports that subjects do not believe that the changes or other events they missed actually occurred, and in some cases insist on reviewing the stimuli.

Clearly, something about these experiments, and related ones exploring other visual limits (see, for example, Mack and Rock, 1998), runs strongly afoul of nearly everyone's expectations about what should be visible. Although this kind of conflict between actual and presumed cognitive functioning has been explored to some degree by researchers in metamemory and even in social psychology, it remains almost completely unexamined for vision. More generally, there is a large field of research exploring metacognition, but this research has almost exclusively explored issues in metacognitive control such as study time allocation, judgments of learning, and correlations between metacognitive measures and memory performance. Much less research has explored people's explicit or implicit beliefs about their own capabilities, even though many influential models of metacognition include something akin to a metacognitive model of the cognitive system. Moreover, although a large literature on executive function makes use of visual tasks, there is still no systematic account of metacognitive control for vision.

The striking paucity of research on visual metacognition was one of the primary motivations for organizing the Kent Forum on Visual Metacognition in June of 2002, which was an attempt to start a dialogue about visual metacognition by bringing together researchers from a number of different areas. Although many areas of research are directly relevant to understanding visual metacognition, few have focused on it, so there was no distinction between experts and beginners among forum participants. Instead, everyone had something to contribute, and the freewheeling discussion started approximately five minutes after the beginning of each talk, and continued late into the evening.

I hope this volume, based largely on papers presented at the forum, will serve as an open invitation to do research on visual metacognition, a field with much to discover and without the sometimes oppressive weight of a long scientific tradition. However, I suspect that this research will not be long isolated; it will make important connections between diverse areas of cognitive psychology now being actively investigated. Below I briefly summarize how each of these areas might serve to improve our understanding of visual metacognition. Most, but not all, of this diverse research is represented in this volume.

Cognitive Development: The Emerging Understanding of Seeing

One of the richest and most compelling bodies of work on which to base research into visual metacognition in adults is that on the developing theory of mind and understanding of perspective taking. No researcher has been more prominent in this tradition than John Flavell, and we were honored to have him at the conference. As reviewed in Flavell's chapter, this developmental research asks how children come to realize that representations are not simply copies of the real world, but instead are filtered, reduced, and interpreted versions of that world. One of the most important insights from this literature is that even young children can, in many cases, reason effectively about visual representations. This immediately raises the question, where do adults go astray when reasoning about representational failures such as change blindness? With the developmental research as a foundation for understanding metacognition in adults, we may find either that these early-developing explanations of cognitive capacity simply run out at the specific situations used to demonstrate metacognitive errors in adults, or that they are automatically applied as heuristics for situations where they are not really effective.

One of the most important tests of this understanding is whether children can reason about representations that are false, especially when they know the true state of affairs. This capability has been extensively explored using many different versions of the false-belief task. The point of this task is to test children's understanding about the difference between representation and reality in a situation where the two diverge. In the typical paradigm, a child witnesses an event along with another agent (usually a puppet). The puppet then leaves the room, providing the opportunity for the child alone to witness a change (for example, a hidden object is switched to a new hiding place). Will the child realize that the puppet has not witnessed the change and cannot be expected to know where the new hiding place is? By age 4 (and perhaps much earlier), children can reason effectively about this situation. A closely related line of research explores the degree to which children understand that representations arise from specific opportunities that may not be universally shared. This research was inspired by Piagetian tasks demonstrating that children tend to hold an egocentric conception about people's understanding of the world: failing to realize that others may not see what they see, or know what they know, they ascribe their own knowledge and point of view to others who plainly cannot share them. Although Piaget argued for a fairly radical shift in understanding of the impact of these differences in opportunity, subsequent research, much of it reviewed in chapter 1, has emphasized a more gradual shift from an entirely egocentric point of view to one that effectively tracks the effect of perspectives on representations.

One implication of research on perspective taking and the false-belief task is that the basis of children's understanding of representation might be heavily based on vision (and perhaps the other senses as well). A number of authors have pointed this out, arguing that children first focus on visual cues for potential targets of attention by tracking the target of others' gaze (for example, Gopnik, Slaughter, and Meltzoff, 1994). An understanding of these cues might then allow children to bootstrap the insight that people look at things because they are interested in them. The details of this bootstrapping process remain relatively unexplored, and few links have been established between gaze perception and the more general understanding of events that express an actor's intentions. This latter understanding may be the critical thread that unites what would otherwise be a complex set of incoherent actions into a coherent expression of some actor's beliefs, desires, and goals. For example, consider an infant who sees someone look at a fork, then grab it, then use it to stab a noodle, then lift the noodle to their mouth. To understand this series of movements, it is necessary to correctly parse each of the actions and relate them coherently to an overarching goal. Megan Saylor and Dare Baldwin (chapter 2) describe research demonstrating that young infants are sensitive to interruptions that occur in the midst of intentional actions. Accordingly, this research begins the process of uncovering the foundations of an intentional theory of mind, and expands on the gaze perception findings by elaborating on the possibility that observers of action use a correlated set of intention-relevant cues (including gaze and changes in body direction) to interpret human action in intentional terms. Saylor and Baldwin also use recent research on adults' and infants' action-parsing tendencies (and some possible changes in such tendencies across development) to make predictions about change blindness occurring during the processing of everyday action scenarios.

One situation where a metacognitive understanding of self and others is critical is language learning. Children need not only to understand the referent for a word, but also to monitor their own knowledge about words and about the world in general. This latter skill is explored by William Merriman and John Marazita (chapter 3) who begin with a discussion of the importance of word- and meaning-cued awareness of lexical ignorance. According to their recent research, children need to successfully monitor their own knowledge of word meanings in order to realize that there is a gap in their lexicon (either because they have encountered a word they do not know or because they have encountered an object or event they do not know the word for). Merriman and Marazita argue that such monitoring may be part of children's more general monitoring of their efficiency in recognizing previously seen stimuli. As a measure of this process, Merriman and Marazita measured children's success in a picture recognition task and found it to be correlated with awareness of lexical ignorance. Their findings suggest that a broad awareness of cognitive and perceptual fluency may develop in the service both of word learning (in which case, fluency may be associated with a known lexical item, and therefore indicate that a lexical search would be warranted), and visual memory more generally (in which case, recognition may induce a broad sense of familiarity with a visual stimulus).

Not only might visual metacognition rest on the more general foundations of theory of mind and knowledge monitoring, but it is also possible that more specific kinds of perceptual development are closely related to verbalizable under-standings of the perceptual process. Research reported by Carl Granrud (chapter 4) demonstrates a compelling link between children's understanding that distant objects falsely appear small and size constancy. One of the most interesting things about this research is that an apparently seamless perceptual process may be rooted in a metacognitive insight that occurs during middle childhood. Although it may initially involve a conscious correction of perceptual experience, later, in more practiced adults, this process may be automatic in all but the most unusual circumstances (thus the nearly universal observation that people and cars look like miniatures when viewed from a skyscraper). The important point here is that verbalizable metaknowledge is closely related to perceptual performance in children.

Thinking and Seeing in Adults: Extramission and Change Blindness Blindness

One of the few exceptions to the general lack of research on visual metacognition in adults is a fascinating set of studies reported by Gerald Winer, Jane Cottrell, and their colleagues over the past ten years. It is fitting that this work, reviewed by Winer and Cottrell (chapter 5), got its start as developmental research. These experiments demonstrate that people seem to believe that seeing some-how requires that something leave the eyes, a position characteristic of pre-Enlightenment science. Referred to as "extramission," the notion that, in order to see, something (for example, rays) must be emitted from the eyes runs strongly counter to the seemingly obvious insight that the eyes have nothing in them to produces that something. As described by Winer and Cottrell in chapter 5, this research first tested the hypothesis that children would endorse extramissionist beliefs, while adults clearly would not. If this were so, researchers could then explore the developmental milestones associated with a correct understanding of vision. However, much to Winer and Cottrell's surprise, even their adult control groups endorsed extramissionist beliefs a distressingly high percentage of the time. This misconception proved robust over a wide variety of situations, and was even resistant to some (but fortunately not all) educational interventions.

In our own research, my colleagues and I began with the straightforward insight that because change blindness findings are surprising, people might hold some set of incorrect beliefs about seeing that leads them to falsely predict that they would detect changes. When we asked subjects to judge whether they would succeed in the same situations for which we had already demonstrated change blindness, we found that people did indeed massively overestimate their ability to see changes. In following up on these findings, we have found that these over-predictions are robust, and that they appear to be linked to misconstruals about visual attention similar to those documented in children (Flavell, Green, and Flavell, 1995). Finally, according to research reviewed by myself and Melissa Beck (chapter 6), overestimates of change detection appear to be caused, at least in part, by the use of heuristics deriving from a theory of mind. In a similar vein, Brian Scholl, Daniel Simons, and I (chapter 7) review research stemming from observations that Scholl made while running change detection experiments using Rensink's well-known flicker paradigm, in which different versions of a scene (one original and one with some visual change) are alternated back and forth. In Scholl's task, subjects actively searched for changes and simply reported when they saw the difference between the two scenes. Scholl found that subjects were incredulous when told of their inability to detect changes. Some even insisted that the changes they finally detected after a prolonged search must have been added to the scene just before they actually saw them; otherwise, they would surely have seen them before. Scholl suspected that, though all changes had of course occurred right from the start, the intuition that they had not might stem directly from false beliefs about the detectability of changes. The subjects' reports might therefore be used as an indirect measure of their metacognitive error, which would avoid some of the demand characteristics inherent to actually asking subjects about the perceptibility of visual changes.

What is perhaps most significant for our purposes, Scholl's task illustrates the potentially close relationship between metacognition and performance. If incorrect beliefs about seeing affect on-line judgments about the specific nature of an ongoing task, these same beliefs might lead subjects to be negligent in searching for targets they have few opportunities to observe. Heather Pringle, Arthur Kramer, and David Irwin (chapter 8) describe Pringle's research on individual differences as predictors of change detection for driving-related scenes, focusing on the relationship between working memory capacity and attentional span, on the one hand, and change detection, on the other. Following up on Pringle's previous finding that subjects scoring high in attentional breadth are better able to detect changes in a flicker task, they observed that good attentional breadth allows individuals performing a flicker task to effectively search scenes with long saccades and fewer dwells on a given location. Such individual difference studies, sorely lacking in the visual search literature (with some exceptions in the broader executive functioning literature) are clearly important for understanding change detection, as are the responses to Pringle, Kramer, and Irwin's self-report questionnaire, in which subjects were asked how effective they thought they were in detecting changes, and to what degree they thought factors such as visual salience and task relevance affected their search for changes. These responses have the potential to help isolate situations where metacognitions about a just-completed task diverge from actual performance. Pringle, Kramer, and Irwin's results suggest some divergence, and more generally, illustrate the potential of integrating research in executive functioning and in metacognition (see also Fernandez-Duque, Baird, and Posner, 2000).

The Metacognitive Tradition

Although there is, as yet, little research exploring visual metacognition, extensive research has explored metacognition more generally, most of it focused on metacognitive control over ongoing cognitive tasks. For example, many experiments have explored how individuals monitor the degree to which they have learned text-based information. If people are unable to figure out when they have effectively learned something, they may stop studying information prematurely or waste time studying information they have already learned. One important consideration here is whether the predominantly verbal materials used in this research limit its generalizability with respect to visual metacognition. Rachel Diana and Lynne Reder (chapter 9) explore the degree to which contextual information controls strategy selection in problem solving, and argue for a commonality between the visual and verbal learning that might facilitate this kind of interchange. A key insight from this kind of research is that people need not be aware of metacognitive monitoring, even where it contributes to relatively complex problem solving. Accordingly, there is a sense in which visual behavior may be particularly saturated with metacognition, especially when the visual system must select from the broad array of information available in real-world scenes.

In addition to scientific research on metacognition, there is a considerable philosophical literature exploring misconstruals of visual consciousness, much of it focused on the hypothesis that people fall prey to the "grand illusion" that visual experience is richer than it actually is (see Noë, 2002, for review), or that a rich visual experience arises from a detailed representation of the visual world (see, for example, Rensink, 2000). Although, we were unable, because of a schedule conflict, to have any philosophical representation at the forum, Jonathan Schooler, Erie Reichle, and David Halpern's discussion of "zoning out" while reading (chapter 10) reflects this tradition nicely. Their novel paradigm attempts to measure the degree to which subjects can read without awareness of the contents of the text (or even of reading at all). Thus, while their subjects were reading a text, they were occasionally prompted to indicate if they were attending to the text or were zoning out at the time of the cue. Their basic finding is that subjects zoned out a good deal of the time. It is therefore possible to argue that we are sometimes unaware of the contents of our conscious experience: if we were always aware of our conscious experience, then surely we would be able to stop these nonproductive lapses dead in their tracks. Instead, we can spend a considerable amount of time engaged in a completely different task than the one we intended to perform. Schooler, Reichle, and Halpern discuss these findings in the context of Schooler's previous distinction between consciousness and metaconsciousness. This point of this distinction is that metaconsciousness represents reflective processes necessary to monitor conscious processes. Because we are sometimes aware of something even when we do not engage metaconscious processing, the contents of awareness may be only inconsistently related to ongoing goals.

The consciousness-metaconsciousness distinction has a number of important implications for understanding visual metacognition more generally. For example, Schooler (2001) argues that people are metaconscious less often than they think they are. Therefore, if people's beliefs about vision do not account for the possibility that they may be aware of something, but fail to monitor the contents of awareness, they may overestimate the degree to which they truly track visual information over time. On this account, overoptimism about change detection may result, at least in part, from a misconstrual of the degree of processing and reflection that visual information receives. This may be particularly true of situations where apparently complex information can be processed efficiently: people may think that seeing a well organized real-world scene is associated with awareness and reflection when it actually is not.

Concepts and Folk Psychology

Another source of inspiration for understanding visual metacognition is from the concept literature. Not only is research exploring folk psychological concepts relevant (see, for example, Schwanenflugel, Martin, and Takahashi, 1999), but the more general theory-based approach to concepts (see Medin, 1989, for review) can help us understand the degree to which people really draw on systematic explanations when they respond to questions about visual limits. People may rummage through past exemplars of experience and respond based on the most similar one. Alternatively, they may use some more organized theory to respond, perhaps borrowing from early-developing foundational understandings of intentional behavior and theory of mind.

There is some evidence to support both hypotheses (Levin, 2002), but a more basic point is that when people engage mental explanations, they may fall victim to a fundamental cognitive illusion that their explanations are more detailed than they actually are. Frank Keil, Leonid Rosenblit, and Cardice Mills (chapter 11) describe research exploring this phenomenon, which they refer to as the "illusion of explanatory depth" (IOED). The IOED might be compared to the hypothesis that people think they will see changes because they overestimate the completeness of their visual representations. Keil, Rosenblit, and Mills explored the IOED by asking subjects to rate how fully they understood the principles behind the operation of complex artifacts such as crossbows and refrigerators. Subjects were then given a detailed explanation of how each object worked, and asked to rerate their knowledge in light of the real explanation. Across an extensive series of experiments, these ratings were considerably less optimistic than the first ratings, demonstrating subjects' realization that they did not know as much as they initially thought.

The illusion of explanatory depth presents a particularly rich source of inspiration, in part because it is closely linked to the presence of visible parts. Thus the more people see of a mechanism, the more they are overconfident that they understand it. As Keil, Rosenblit, and Mills point out, this might reflect a similarity between the IOED and visual overconfidence. In both cases, perceptual fluency is presumed to have a deep representational basis. It is interesting to note here that in the case of change detection, people do think they can see changes, but they do not appear to directly consider the need for representations to do this. Instead, it appears as though they are more focused on the organization inherent to real-world scenes, and presume this will allow them to be aware of all of the information they contain (Levin et al., 2002). The IOED might be similar in that subjects also focus on a level of meaningful organization while neglecting the plausible presence or absence of its representational foundation.

Thinking and Seeing in the Real World: Looking Ahead to the Impact of Metacognitive Errors

Research on thinking has important applications that go far beyond the impact of cognition on perception. One of my goals in arranging this forum was to include discussion of those applications. Clearly, it is important to understand how metacognitions impact task performance, and in the case of visual metacognition, they probably do. If people misunderstand the salience of some kinds of visual information, they may fail to put forth sufficient effort, especially in novel situations for which they have had little opportunity to calibrate themselves empirically. However, people's beliefs about cognition affect not only their own performance, but also their judgments about other people's experience. As philosophers, developmental psychologists, and social psychologists have been emphasizing for years, causal attributions about others' behavior are central to an extraordinarily wide array of judgments. Similarly, judgments about others' cognitive limits have immense potential for error, especially where people make predictions about others without an opportunity to test those predictions empirically.

How many times have computer programmers assumed that their users can detect some visual cue that is actually impossible to see? (For a fascinating example, see Benway and Lane, 1998.)

Another setting where cognitive misestimates are potentially important is in how jurors consider legal testimony. In this case, people must rely on their understanding of cognition not only to accurately weigh the reliability of reports about long past events, but also to accurately determine who is to blame for the failures that lead to accidents. In the former case, misunderstandings of memory have already been implicated as a cause for false convictions in criminal cases (Wells, Small Penrod, Malpass Fulero, and Brimacombe, 1998). In the latter case, visual metacognitions may be equally important to the large number of legal cases in which jurors must determine who should be blamed for what, given their putative cognitive limits. Although criminal cases relying on eyewitness testimony are dramatic, they are relatively uncommon and account for only a small proportion of legal testimony, in part because legal fact finders are well aware of the unreliability of this kind of testimony. In contrast, tort cases (that is, cases in which blame is assessed for some injury) are quite common and rest on a whole series of assumptions about the average person's capabilities. Jeffrey Rachlinski (chapter 12) describes the potential impact of metacognitive errors on evaluations of this kind of testimony, and gives a fascinating guide to the legal system's attempts to design a normative standard of human capability. As he points out, the legal system has at least implicitly recognized how hard it is to understand who should have seen or known something in hindsight, and has been struggling with this limit for many years. Thus, while research on visual metacognition may inform legal practice, the reverse may well be true: psychologists may find a fascinating source of folk knowledge embodied in legal practice as it has evolved over the past few centuries.

Conclusion

The study of visual metacognition is wide open to new approaches, new investigators, and a truly creative interdisciplinary research agenda. The research discussed in this volume can serve as a starting point for a new line of inquiry about how people think about seeing. Thus research on the developing theory of mind asks how children bootstrap an intentional interpretation of complex visual actions via a more basic understanding of the mechanisms of seeing and visual attention. More traditional metacognition research asks how people decide to stop exploring a stimulus, and how they select strategies, often based on visually presented information. Research in concepts provides a framework to ask how systematic our understanding of seeing is, and even research on social cognition may be critical for understanding how we interpret and perhaps misunderstand our own visual experience via biased reasoning and entrenched attributional processes. Combined with insights from philosophy and the neurosciences, research into visual metacognition may help us develop a systematic understanding of how people construe their own perceptual experience, not only when they talk about it, but also when they navigate complex tasks both in the laboratory and in the real world.

References

Benway, J. P., and Lane, D. M. (1998). Banner blindness: Web searchers often miss "obvious" links. *Internetworking: ITG Newsletter, 1(3)*.

Fernandez-Duque, D., Baird, J. A., and Posner, M. I. (2000). Executive attention and metacognitive regulation. *Consciousness and Cognition, 9*, 288–307.

Flavell, J. H., Green, F. L., and Flavell, E. R. (1995). The development of children's knowledge about attentional focus. *Developmental Psychology, 31*, 706–712.

Gopnik, A., Slaughter, V., and Meltzoff, A. (1994). Changing your views: How understanding visual perception can lead to a new theory of the mind. In C. Lewis and P. Mitchell (Eds.), *Origins of an understanding of mind* (pp. 157–181). Hillsdale, NJ: Erlbaum.

Hochberg, J. (1968). In the mind's eye. In R. N. Haber (Ed.), *Contemporary theory and research in visual perception* (pp. 309–331). New York: Holt, Rinehart and Winston.

Hochberg, J. (1986). Representation of motion and space in video and cinematic displays. In K. R. Boff, L. Kaufman, and J. P. Thomas (Eds.), *Handbook of perception and human performance*. Vol. 1: *Sensory processes and perception* (pp. 22.1–22.84). New York: Wiley.

Irwin, D. E. (1991). Information integration across saccadic eye movements. *Cognitive Psychology, 23*, 420–456.

Levin, D. T. (2002). Change blindness blindness as visual metacognition. *Journal of Consciousness Studies, 5–6*, 111–130.

Levin, D. T., Drivdahl, S. B., Momen, N., and Beck, M. R. (2002). False predictions about the detectability of unexpected visual changes: The role of beliefs about attention, memory, and the continuity of attended objects in causing change blindness blindness. *Consciousness and Cognition, 11*, 507–527.

Levin, D. T., and Simons, D. J. (1997). Failure to detect changes to attended objects in motion pictures. *Psychonomic Bulletin and Review, 4*, 501–506.

Levin, D. T., and Simons, D. J. (2000). Fragmentation and continuity in motion pictures and the real world. *Medici Psychology, 2*, 357–380.

Mack, A., and Rock, I. (1998). *Inattentional blindness*. Cambridge, MA: MIT Press.

Medin, D. L. (1989). Concepts and conceptual structure. *American Psychologist, 44*, 1469–1481.

Noë, A. (2002). Is the visual world a grand illusion? *Journal of Consciousness Studies, 9*, 1–12.

Rensink, R. A. (2000). The dynamic representation of scenes. *Visual Cognition, 7*, 17–42.

Rensink, R. A. (2002). Change detection. *Annual Review of Psychology, 53*, 245–277.

Schooler, J. W. (2001). Discovering memories in the light of meta—awareness. *Journal of aggression, maltreatment and Trauma, 4*, 105–134.

Schwanenflugel, P. J., Martin, M., and Takahashi, T. (1999). The organization of verbs of knowing: Evidence for cultural commonality and variation in theory of mind. *Memory and Cognition, 27*, 813–825.

Simons, D. J., and Levin, D. T. (1998). Failure to detect changes to people in a real-world interaction. *Psychonomic Bulletin and Review, 5*, 644–649.

Wells, G. A., Small, M., Penrod, S., Malpass, R. S., Fulero, S. M., and Brimacombe, C. A. E. (1998). Eyewitness identification procedures: Recommendations for lineups and photospreads. *Law and Human Behavior, 22*, 1–39.

Xu, F., and Carey, S. (1996). Infants' metaphysics: The case of numerical identity. *Cognitive Psychology, 30*, 111–153.

Chapter 1

Development of Knowledge about Vision

John H. Flavell

A developmental psychologist shows a 5-year-old girl a candy box with a picture of candy on it and asks her what is in it. "Candy," the girl replies. She then gets to look inside the box and, to her surprise, sees that it actually contains, not candy, but a little doll. She is then asked what another child who had not yet opened the box would think was in it. "Candy!" says the child, amused at the deception. The experimenter then presents a 3-year-old boy with this same false-belief task. His answer to the first question is the expected "Candy," but his response to the second is a confident and unamused "Doll." Even more incredible, the boy also maintains that he himself had first thought that the candy box would contain a doll. Unlike the 5-year-old, the 3-year-old shows no evidence of understanding that either he or other people could hold a belief that is false.

Results such as this are found in currently flourishing research on the development of our knowledge and beliefs about the mental world—our folk psychology or naive theory of mind. To a greater extent than earlier metacognitive and social-cognitive approaches to the same domain, the theory of mind approach probes children's conceptions of the most fundamental components of the mind, such as beliefs and desires. In less than twenty years, this fast-growing area of research has spawned hundreds of articles and scores of books and monographs. Indeed, the spate of papers and posters on this topic at recent meetings of the Society for Research in Child Development reminded older participants of the way Piagetian research dominated the program in years past. To illustrate, a recent meta-analysis of false-belief studies alone—just one topic in this area—included 178 studies (Wellman, Cross, and Watson, 2001). Developmental findings in this area have also become of interest to philosophers of mind, who believe that these findings may help clarify philosophical disputes about the nature of folk psychology. (For reviews of work on this topic, see, for example, Baron-Cohen, Tager-Flusberg, and Cohen, 2000; Bartsch and Wellman, 1995; Flavell and Miller, 1998; Hughes, 2001; Mitchell and Riggs, 2000; Moore, 1996; and Wellman and Gelman, 1998.)

Why this intense research interest in the development of knowledge about the mental world? Numerous motives, ranging from self-preservation to simple curiosity, impel people the world over to try to make sense of themselves and other people, and doing that requires a folk psychology. Human social and cognitive life bereft of knowledge or beliefs about the mind seems virtually unimaginable, and the development of something that important and ubiquitous is surely worth learning about. In her lectures on this topic, Alison Gopnik likes to make this point in the following way. Imagine what it would be like for you to give a lecture to an audience if you had no conception of mental states. The audience might appear to you as bags of meat with two small holes at the top. You would see these bags and the shiny things in their holes shift around unpredictably in a way that perplexed and terrified you, although of course you would not realize that you were perplexed and terrified. Gopnik's scenario may not be as imaginary as it seems. Autistic individuals, known to be deficient in knowledge about the mind, sometimes act as if they viewed other people as unpredictable and scary.

Several types of theories have been offered as explanations for the development of children's mentalistic understanding. One is the so-called theory theory (Gopnik and Meltzoff, 1997; Gopnik and Wellman, 1994; Perner, 1991; Wellman and Gelman, 1998). Theory theorists argue that our knowledge about the mind constitutes not a formal scientific theory but an informal, everyday "framework" or "foundational" theory. An important insight of this approach is that we acquire knowledge or beliefs, not just about each type of mental state considered in isolation, but also about how each one relates to other mental states, to sensory inputs, and to observable behaviors. This insight is particularly compelling in the case of knowledge about vision. On the one hand, there are some things we could learn about vision construed narrowly—about what might loosely be called "visual sensing" or "basic seeing." On the other hand, there are some very important things we could learn about what can happen in people's minds and behaviors once the visual stimulus has been detected, that is, about the myriad possible connections between basic seeing and other mental and behavioral phenomena. This chapter summarizes much of what infants and children have been found to learn in this area, both about basic seeing and about its mental and behavioral correlates.

Development during Infancy

There is research evidence that children have acquired some basic knowledge about vision by the age of 18–24 months. Most of this evidence concerns their developing understanding of the referential nature or "aboutness" of vision. That is, as they grow older, infants become increasingly aware that another person's gaze at an object is an action by that person directed at that object. In addition, they discover some of the implications of another person's gaze, for example, that the person's talk, expressed emotions, and other behaviors when interacting with them are likely to relate to the object of the person's gaze. There is also reason to think that by the end of infancy children are becoming increasingly aware that things happen inside people when they see: they receive information about the world and have visual and other subjective experiences. (For reviews of research on infants' knowledge about vision, see Butler, Caron, and Brooks, 2000; Carpenter, Nagell, and Tomasello, 1998; Corkum and Moore, 1998; Flavell and Miller, 1998; Moore and Corkum, 1994; Winer, 1991; and Woodward, 2003, in press.)

Looking as a Relation between Looker and Object

To have any chance of understanding the meaning of other people's visual acts, infants must obviously first pay attention to the people's eyes and then be able to follow the direction of their gaze. Early in the first year, babies prefer to look at eyes over other facial features (Maurer, 1985). They also show sensitivity to changes in gaze direction and may sometimes look in the general direction another person looks (Hood, Willen, and Driver, 1998). This critical ability—to follow the other person's gaze successfully—improves considerably between 6 and 18 months of age.

Can we conclude from infants' gaze following that they are aware that the gazer is related to—or at least looking at—the object? Although this seems reasonable, Moore and Corkum (1994) have cogently argued that we cannot draw such a conclusion. They argue that infants may have simply learned from experience that, when they follow a person's gaze, they will see something interesting. Their representation of the event may not include the person or the person-object relation at all—only the object (see also Butterworth and Jarrett, 1991). As Woodward (in press) puts it, in such a construal, the other person's gaze merely "spotlights" the looked-at object. Although Corkum and Moore (1998, p. 38) accept that understanding of vision as person-object connectedness is in place by the end of infancy or somewhat earlier, they doubt that younger infants grasp the referential nature of looking, despite some ability to follow gazes.

Two recent investigations provide some support for Corkum and Moore's claim. Butler, Caron, and Brooks, 2000, studied the gaze-following behavior of 14- and 18-month-olds under three conditions. In each condition, infants faced an experimenter who would conspicuously turn head and eyes to look in the direction of stationary targets placed a few feet away, one on the right and one on the left. In the no-screen condition, there were no visual obstacles to prevent the experimenter from seeing the targets. In the screen condition, opaque screens were interposed between the experimenter and the two targets such that, whereas the infant subjects could still see the targets, the experimenter clearly could not. In the window condition, each screen contained a large transparent window that allowed the experimenter full visual access to the targets, as in the no-screen condition. The window was at an angle that allowed the infants to see through it to the back wall; in addition, the experimenter waved at the infants through it to demonstrate its transparency.

The authors reasoned that infants who do not understand the referential nature of looking and its line of sight requirements would turn equally in all three conditions; if the experimenter looks, they look. In contrast, infants who better understand the link between looker and object would look toward the targets maximally when the experimenter would be able to see them (no-screen and window conditions) and minimally when not. Eighteen-month-olds showed the latter response pattern: They turned much more in both the no-screen and the window condition than in the screen condition. In contrast, 14-month-olds showed a mixed pattern. On the one hand, they turned less in the screen condition than in the no-screen condition. On the other hand, they turned at well above chance levels in the screen condition. More strikingly, they turned less often in the window condition than in the screen condition. In addition, whereas, among the 18-month-olds, 7 of 20 leaned forward to gaze at the inside of the screen in the screen condition, presumably to see what the experimenter might be finding to look at there, among the 14-month-olds, only 1 of 22 did. Brooks and Meltzoff (2003) showed that, during the second year of life, infants are likelier to follow an adult's head turn to look at a target if the adult's eyes are open or uncovered rather than closed or covered with a blindfold. Woodward (2003 and in press) also found that infants follow eye gaze before they understand that gaze expresses a relation between gazer and target object, although Woodward's method suggests an earlier age of transition than that indicated in Butler, Caron, and Brooks, 2000. Infants 7, 9, and 12 months of age were tested in a habituation paradigm in which they watched an experimenter look at one of two toys on a table. On each trial an experimenter made eye contact with the infant, said, "Hi," and then, "Look," as the experimenter turned to stare at one of the toys, and then stopped staring at it as soon as the infant looked away for 2 seconds. Infants saw the same event on subsequent trials until habituation. Then the positions of the two toys were reversed and two new kinds of test events were presented. On new toy trials, the experimenter continued to turn to the same side as during habituation, and thus looked at a new toy. On new side trials, the experimenter turned to the opposite side, thereby looking at the same toy as during the habituation trials. Woodward (in press) reasoned that if infants are representing the relation between the experimenter and the object the experimenter is looking at, then they should look longer on new toy trials, which present a new looker-object relation. If they attend only to a change in the experimenter's physical movements, then they might look longer when the experimenter turns to a different side (new side trials).

Woodward (2003, in press) found that infants of all three ages usually followed the experimenter's gaze to the looked-at object. However, the 7- and 9-month-olds looked equally on new toy and new side test trials, and also did not show a reliable increase in looking from habituation to test trials on either type of trial. "It was as if 7- and 9-month-olds identified the visible objects (the bear, the ball, and the actor) as being the same as during habituation, without considering the relations between them" (Woodward, 2003, pp. 303–304). In contrast, the 12-month-olds looked reliably longer on the new toy trials than on the new side trials and also recovered from habituation when presented with the new toy trials but not the new side ones.

How do infants learn that looking is a relation between looker and object? Woodward (2003) suggests two possibilities, both of which may be true. One possibility, elaborated in detail by Moore and Corkum (1994), is that repeated experience of joint attention on objects with adults serves as a vital crucible. According to this account, infants begin by associating their own visual experience of an object in these interactions with the adult's head and eye orientation toward the same object. In this way, they gradually come to realize that when they and other people gaze at objects, they are related to these objects via an inner experience of seeing them. The second possibility, proposed by Woodward herself (2003), is that infants gradually notice behavioral regularities associated with gaze. For example, having once learned that grasping involves a relation between people and objects, and noticing that people usually look at what they grasp, infants could eventually infer that looking also involves such a relation. Presumably, noticing the regular co-occurrence of people's looking with their touching, pointing, and object labeling could similarly contribute to this insight.

Finally, infants also show their burgeoning understanding of the referential nature of people's gaze, not merely by following it, but also by directing and checking it:

> Franco and Butterworth (1989); Butterworth, (1991) found that at around 12 to 16 months children not only point but also check the gaze of the adult whose attention they are trying to direct. They do that in two different ways. Before pointing, they check whether the adult is looking at them; and as they point, they check whether the adult is looking at the indicated object. The fact that infants do not just try to manipulate the other's gaze but also check on it indicate that they are aware of its importance. (Perner, 1991, p. 129)

(See also Carpenter, Nagell, and Tomasello, 1998; Moore and D'Entremont, 2001; for a different approach to the study of infant gaze following and attribution of intentionality, see Johnson, 2000; Johnson, Slaughter, and Carey, 1998.)

Implications of Looking

One important implication of looking that children discover by the end of infancy is that where people look is a clue to what object they are labeling. That is, babies learn the names for things by noting what object adults appear to be attending to when they say the label. Some clever studies of this kind of aboutness reading have been done during the past decade (see Baldwin and Moses, 1994; Moore, Angelopoulos, and Bennett, 1999; Tomasello, 1995; Woodward and Markman, 1998). Baldwin (1991, 1993; Baldwin and Moses, 1994) showed that infants 19–20 months of age sense that the verbal label an adult utters refers to the object the adult shows clear signs of visually attending to at that moment. These infants recognize that it does not refer to other perceptually salient objects the adult is not focused on: for example, an object that they, rather than the adult, are currently looking at, or an object that the adult calls to their attention but in such a way as to not appear to be labeling it. In short, infants of this age seem to recognize that it is an adult's visual focus rather than their own that gives clues as to the adult's referential intent. Moore, Angelopoulos, and Bennett (1999) confirmed these results and also showed that this referential understanding is more robust in 24-month-olds than in 18-month-olds.

These word-learning studies show that infants develop the ability to learn what an object is *called* by reading an adult's visual focus when the adult labels it. There is also evidence that they develop the ability to learn what an object is *like* by reading an adult's visual focus when the adult is expressing a positive or negative emotional reaction to it. That is, they can recognize that an adult's emotional display refers to a particular object just as they can recognize that an adult's spoken label refers to a particular object. Seeking or using information about objects' positive or negative qualities conveyed by adults' perceptible emotional reactions to these objects has been called "social referencing"; the developmental literature on social referencing has recently been reviewed by Moses and colleagues (2001), Mumme and Fernald (2001), and Repacholi (1998). Parents often present young children with this kind of evaluative information, as when they try to interest them in a new toy by acting as if it were the greatest thing ever ("Wow, look at *this*!" "See what *this* does!" etc.).

One question that has arisen in the social referencing literature is whether babies actually realize that an adult's expressions of emotion are about the object. An alternative possibility is that these expressions just alter the babies' mood, which in turn alters the babies' reactions to all objects, for example, dampening them when the mood thus induced is negative. However, the evidence now strongly suggest that, although such mood modification effects also can occur, by 12 months or so, infants do have some understanding that an adult's behavior is about the specific object the adult is looking at when expressing the positive or negative affect (Moses et al., 2001; Mumme and Fernald, 2003; Repacholi, 1998). For example, Moses and colleagues (2001) showed that, on hearing a female experimenter's emotional outburst of pleasure ("Nice!") or disgust ("Yecch!"), 12-month-olds immediately checked her face, followed her gaze to the object she was emoting about, and acted appropriately—for example, spending less time with and responding less positively to objects that she had "yecched." Repacholi (1998) has also presented impressive evidence for object-specific social referencing in 14-month-olds.

The research on social referencing shows that infants can recognize the implications for their behavior of other people's visual and emotional regard. Four experiments by Phillips, Wellman, and Spelke (2002) give evidence that infants can also recognize the implications of these actions for an adult's own behavior. In one of their experiments, 8- and 12-month-olds first saw an adult look at one (A) of two almost identical stuffed animals (A and B) with facial and vocal expression of interest and delight. Then a screen was closed briefly, and when it reopened, the infants saw the adult holding A. After habituating to this sequence, the infants were then shown two types of test trials in alternation. As in the habituation trials, one type of test trial was consistent with the principle that people will probably approach what they act as if they like. On these consistent trials, the adult first acted positively toward the second animal, B, and after the screen closed and reopened, was shown holding B, in accord with the principle. On the other, inconsistent trials, the adult began by acting positively toward A, but then grasped B instead, in violation of the principle. The 12-month-olds looked longer at the inconsistent event than at the consistent one, as if recognizing that looking at things with positive regard predicts approaching them. In contrast, the 8-month-olds looked equally at the two types of events. Wellman, Phillips, and Rodriguez (2000) found evidence for a more advanced understanding in 2½-year-olds: if an adult looks with positive affect at an object the child cannot see, that object is likely to be one the child regards as desirable rather than undesirable, whereas the opposite is true if the adult's affect is negative. Montgomery, Bach, and Moran (1998) found that 6-year-olds, but not 4-year-olds, showed a yet more advanced insight: that an object that is looked at for a long time is more likely to be a protagonist's goal than one that is only glanced at. Clearly, there are a number of developmental levels of social referencing.

Seeing as an Internal Psychological Event
A distinction within this category can be made between seeing as the receipt and use of information about the world and seeing as an action accompanied by a phenomenological experience. In the former, the emphasis is on the specific thing seen and the effects of seeing it on other mental states and behaviors. Seeing something results in obtaining information about it, and that information may then engender various beliefs, desires, intentions, and other mental and behavioral events. In the latter, the emphasis is on the act and subjective experience of seeing rather than on the specific object seen. There is at least suggestive evidence that some understanding of both the informational and the act-experiential aspects of seeing is present during late infancy or very early childhood.

Regarding the informational aspect, casual observation suggests that older infants, at least, often show their caretakers an interesting new object only once, even though their indulgent caretakers would probably be willing to reinforce additional showings with appropriate effusions of interest and approval. They may repeat other interchanges endlessly, to the point of adult tedium, but usually seem to feel the need to show things just once. Why? It seems possible that they somehow sense that the adult has received the new information on the first showing, and thereafter continues to "know it." They seem not merely to want the other person to look at or see the object—that would be as effectively accomplished on the nth showing as on the first—but in some sense to "know" what it is and that it is there. Such observations suggest that infants may at times be attributing to other people something inner and unobservable, even though we are presently at a loss to imagine what that attribution experience might be like for creatures so unknowledgeable and nonverbal.

O'Neill (1996) obtained experimental evidence consistent with this possibility. Young 2-year-olds had to ask a parent for help in retrieving a sticker dropped into one of two identical containers that were placed out of reach. With the child watching, the parent had either seen which container the sticker was dropped into or had not seen it because the parent's eyes were conspicuously closed. In their requests for help, the children gestured significantly more often when the parent had not seen which container held the sticker than when the parent had. As will be seen, there is more compelling evidence for the understanding that seeing leads to knowing in studies with preschool children. Nevertheless, casual observation and the findings in O'Neill, 1996, suggest that at least the rudiments are present by the close of infancy. Finally, the evidence presented in the previous section on the implications of looking is also suggestive. Older infants seem aware that people's looking is a clue to their referential and other intentions.

As to the act and experience of seeing, there is also evidence that may indicate some early understanding (Flavell and Miller, 1998; Winer, 1991). Many children correctly understand and use the words *look* and *see* by their second birthday (Bretherton and Beeghly, 1982). Older infants' mastery of Piagetian object permanence tasks shows that they understand that objects can be now visible, now not, all the while continuing to exist. Infants and young children sometimes deliberately manipulate their own and other people's visual experience, as when playing peekaboo games and when rapidly opening and closing their eyes just for the experience of it. The following interchange between the developmental psychologist Elizabeth Spelke and her then 25-month-old daughter Mae, who had just dropped a cereal spoon and was touching her belly, seems to reflect good awareness of the act and experience of seeing:

> *Liz*: Mae, do I have a belly?
> *Mae*: Yes.
> *Liz*: Can you see it?
> *Mae*: (looks at [Liz's clothed] stomach, then looks up) No. Can't see it.
> *Liz*: Do you have a bowl of cereal?
> *Mae*: Yes (looking at [Liz]—she does not look down).
> *Liz*: Can you see it?
> *Mae*: (giggles, doesn't look down) No can see it!
> *Liz*: You can't?
> *Mae*: (looking down) Yes. See it. (Spelke, personal communication)

There is other evidence as well. If asked to show a picture to an adult, a woman, say, who has covered her eyes with her hands, 18-month-olds will move the adult's hands or try to put the picture between the adult's hands and eyes. They tend to show pictures to another person in such a way that they can also continue to see them while the other person does, rather than turning them away from the self and facing them toward the other, as 24-month-olds tend to do (Lempers, Flavell, and Flavell, 1977). Accordingly, when asked to show a small picture glued to the inside bottom of an opaque cup, 18-month-olds tend to hold the cup low and tilt its opening back and forth so that both they and the other person can get alternating glimpses of it. Although not inclined to credit younger infants with knowledge that people's looking behaviors are accompanied by inner visual experiences, Perner (1991) regards the foregoing showing strategy as evidence that 18-month-olds probably do have this knowledge:

> But why do they show the picture in such a way that they themselves can see it at the same time? An interesting possibility is that they understand from their own experience when being shown something that showing must lead to an *inner experience* of seeing. Since they cannot have the other person's experience, the only way of ensuring that this critical part is not missing is to produce the experience in themselves. This, of course, can only be achieved by looking at the picture simultaneously with the other. (Perner, 1991, p. 140)

Other findings suggest that older infants have a rudimentary sense of self and some capacity to attribute emotional experiences to self and others (Flavell and Miller, 1998; Wellman, Phillips, and Rodriguez, 2000). They show evidence of a rudimentary sense of self, which would seem to be a prerequisite for attributing inner experiences. They sometimes appear to be trying to manipulate other people's emotional responses rather than, as in social referencing, just reading these responses for the information about reacted-to objects that they may provide. Even toddlers occasionally seem to try to change other people's feelings, or at least change their affective behavior. In the second year of life, they begin to comfort younger siblings in distress by patting, hugging, or kissing them, and may even bring a security blanket to an adult in pain (Zahn-Waxler et al., 1992). An awareness of self and of inner experiences may develop together: Bischof-Köhler (1991) found a high correlation in 16- to 24-month-olds between a test of early self-concept (mirror self-recognition) and empathic responses to a person in distress, even after partialing out chronological age. Although evidence that older infants have a sense of self and attribute emotional experiences to people obviously does not prove that they also attribute visual experiences, it does lend plausibility to the claim.

Some of the infant competencies discussed in this chapter have also been investigated in other primates, most notably chimpanzees. The evidence suggest that chimps are skilled at following the gaze of other chimps and humans. Whether or to what extent they make adaptive use of gaze information is currently the subject of controversy (Hare et al., 2000; Karin-D'Arcy and Povinelli, 2001; Theall and Povinelli, 1999), however, and even those who think they do (Hare et al., 2000) doubt that they conceive of seeing as an internal psychological event.

In focusing attention on the development of knowledge about vision during infancy, it is easy to forget the broader stream of social and theory-of-mind development of which it is a part. This stream can be characterized in a number of ways. According to Barrett, Richert, and Driesenga (2001), children begin by distinguishing between the movements of people and those of inanimate objects. As they learn that, unlike inanimate objects, people are self-propelled, they gradually learn that people are also purposive—not just self-propelled, but self-propelled toward goals. Later, children start to attribute internal, mental states to people, at first in a not fully representational way ("He feels hungry. He will act") and later representationally ("She thinks it is in the box, but it isn't"). Knowledge about vision informs and is informed by these larger developments, not only during, but also after infancy, and as we will now see.

Later Developments

Level-1 and Level-2 Understanding
Assuming that, at some quite early age, children begin to realize that people have inner visual experience or percepts, what do they know about these percepts? There is evidence for two roughly distinguishable developmental levels of early understanding about vision (Flavell, 1978, 1992; Flavell, Everett et al., 1981; Hughes and Donaldson, 1979; Masangkay et al., 1974). At the higher one, called "level 2," children clearly understand the idea of people having different perspectives or views of the same visual display. Level-2 children can represent the fact that, although both they and another person see the very same thing from different station points, the other person nonetheless sees it a bit differently, or has a somewhat different visual experience of it, than they do. For example, they realize that a cat they see right side up in a picture book will look upside down to someone who views the book wrong side up. At earlier-developing "level 1," children understand that the other person need not presently see something just because they do and vice versa. For example, they recognize that, whereas they see what is on their side of a vertically held card, another person, seated opposite, does not. However, they do not yet conceptualize and consciously represent the fact of perspective-derived differences between their and the other person's visual experience of something that *both* people currently see. Level-1 children know that others also see things and that they and others need not see the same things at any given moment. They may also be able to infer exactly what things others do and do not see, given adequate cues. Thus it is clear they are not profoundly and pervasively egocentric in the Piagetian sense: they definitely do have some knowledge about visual perception. Level-2 children also possess this same knowledge and ability, of course, but in addition are aware that the same things may look different to another viewing them from a different position. They may also be able to infer approximately how these things appear from that different position, again given adequate cues.

Flavell and colleagues have made direct tests of this hypothesized developmental sequence by comparing the same children's performance on level-1 and level-2 tasks, and have also explored the nature and development of various sorts of level-1 and level-2 knowledge and skills. The first tests were made by Masangkay and colleagues (1974), on whose tasks the child and the experimenter faced each other across a small table. To assess level-1 knowledge, a card with a picture of a cat on one side and a picture of a dog on the other was held vertically between the child and the experimenter, and the child was asked to indicate which animal the experimenter sees. Their 3-year-old participants had no difficulty whatever in looking at the cat, say, but nonegocentrically reporting that the experimenter sees the dog. To assess level-2 knowledge, a picture of a turtle was placed horizontally such that the turtle appeared upside down from one side of the table and right side up from the other. Although the 3-year-olds always correctly reported how the turtle appeared to them (thereby demonstrating they understood the meaning of "right side up" and "upside down"), only about a third of them consistently attributed the opposite orientation to the experimenter. In contrast, a group of 4-year-olds performed virtually without error on both tasks.

Further experiments by Flavell, Everett, and colleagues (1981) provided additional evidence that there is a real and robust difference between level-1 and level-2 knowledge. Furthermore, relevant experience appears not to readily induce level-2 thinking in level-1 children, even when that experience consists of literally supplying them with the correct answer to level-2 questions. (For a summary of other studies of level-2 knowledge, see Flavell, 1992.)

As to level-1 knowledge, the research evidence shows that children have acquired a surprisingly rich fund of it by 2½–3 years of age (Cox, 1980; Esterly, 1999; Flavell, 1978; Flavell, Everett et al., 1981; Flavell, Shipstead, and Croft, 1978, 1980; Gopnik, Slaughter, and Meltzoff, 1994; Hughes and Donaldson, 1979; Lempers, Flavell, and Flavell, 1977; McGuigan and Doherty, 1999). By the age of 2½–3 years, children act as if they know implicitly that the following four conditions must hold if another person is to see a visual target (Flavell, 1978; Lempers, Flavell, and Flavell, 1977): (1) at least one of the person's eyes must be open; (2) the person's eyes must be aimed in the general direction of the target; (3) there must be no vision-blocking object on the line of sight between person and target; (4) what the children see has no bearing on what the person sees; that is, the young child's knowledge about vision is fundamentally nonegocentric when dealing with level-1, "what is seen"–type problems.

Tacit knowledge of these four conditions permits children 2½–3 years of age to engender, prevent, and diagnose object seeing by another person. They can engender the other person's seeing of the target by pointing to it or verbally designating it, by getting the person, a man, say, to open his eyes and face toward the target, by moving or reorienting it so that it is in the person's line of sight, and by repositioning either the target or a visual occluder so that the occluder no longer blocks the person's view of the target. They can prevent the other person's seeing of the target by moving the target behind the occluder, or the occluder in front of the target, and by getting the person, a woman, say, to close her eyes or turn away from the target. Finally, they can diagnose or assess whether or not the person currently sees the target by noting whether or not the four seeing conditions obtain. Thus the research evidence indicates that children of this age have enough knowledge about vision to be nonegocentric showers (e.g., they will orient a picture so that the other person, but not they, can see it), nonegocentric hiders (e.g., they will place an object where they, but not the other person, can still see it), and nonegocentric percept assessors (e.g., as Flavell, Shipstead, and Croft, 1980, have shown, children 2½–3 years of age know that their bodies are still visible to a person when their own eyes, but not the person's, are closed).

Although, as we have seen, infants have some ability to follow another person's gaze, this ability improves considerably during the early preschool period (Doherty and Anderson, 1999). In addition, McGuigan and Doherty (1999) found that 2-year-olds' ability to judge where another person is looking from eye direction alone was significantly correlated with their ability to prevent the person from seeing an object by interposing a screen between the person and the object—both level-1 abilities.

Flavell and colleagues (1991) observed a developmental increase from 3 to 5 years of age in a more advanced type of level-1 understanding: that an observer not only normally, but always and necessarily, sees targets via straight-line looking paths. For example, they found that 3-year-olds showed no understanding that another person cannot see objects through C-shaped or J-shaped looking tubes, even right after they themselves had the experience of not being able to see through tubes of lesser curvature than those. Examining more exotic forms of level 1–related cognition, Winer and colleagues (see Winer and Cottrell, chapter 5, this volume) found a decrease with age in participants' belief in something akin to the extramission theory of visual perception held by Plato, Euclid, and other ancient thinkers: namely, that there are emissions from the eye during the act of vision. For example, many children and a number of adults responded affirmatively to the question: "When people look at something or someone, do you think that rays or energy or something else go out from their eyes?" Similarly, Cottrell, Winer, and Smith (1996) report that many adults as well as children believe that one can sometimes feel the stares of an unseen other person. (Is "My ears are burning" the auditory counterpart?) Finally, there is evidence that blind children show an understandable delay in their grasp of basic level-1 conditions of seeing (Bigelow, 1991; Warren, 1994).

There have also been additional studies of level-2 understanding. In Flavell, Flavell, and colleagues, 1981, children 4½, 5, and 5½ years of age were tested for their knowledge of three spatial perspective-taking rules: (1) any object will appear the same to the self and to another person if both view it from the same position; (2) a heterogeneous-sided object (in this study, a tangle of wire) will appear different to the two observers if they view it from different sides, and (3) a homogeneous-sided object (a cylinder) will appear the same to the two if they view it from different sides. The data suggested that knowledge of at least rules 1 and 2 undergoes development during this age period and that 5½-year-olds have a good grasp of all three rules. In Flavell, Flavell et al., 1980, children 3, 3½, and 4½ years of age were tested for a different form of level-2 knowledge about visual perception, namely, knowledge that one observer stationed closer to a small object will be able to see it better than a second observer stationed farther away on roughly the same line of sight, whereas the two observers will be able to see it equally well if stationed side by side at the same distance from it. The data suggested that this knowledge also undergoes considerable development during the preschool period, with many 4½-year-olds seemingly possessing it in the form of a general rule. Finally, Pillow and Flavell (1986) showed that 4-year-olds are more aware than 3-year-olds of how the apparent size and shape of an object changes with changes in its distance and orientation with respect to the observer (see also Granrud, chapter 3, this volume). This is further evidence for a developing attentiveness during the preschool years to the way things appear perceptually.

Attention

In the sense that they come to understand that people show by their gaze direction and other actions that they are psychologically directed toward various objects and events in the world, infants clearly could be said to possess at least a rudimentary understanding of attention. Indeed, some developmentalists are inclined to credit infants with a quite rich understanding of attention (e.g., Baron-Cohen, 1993). We have also just seen that children begin with a more connections-like, whether-perceived-or-not, level-1 conception of perception and subsequently go on to develop a more representation-centered, how-it-is-perceived, level-2 conception.

There is evidence that children also go on to acquire other important insights about attention (Fabricius and Schwanenflugel, 1994; Flavell, Green, and Flavell, 1995; Miller, 1985; Parault and Schwanenflugel, 2000; Pillow, 1988, 1989a, 1995). First, attention is selective. We do not see or hear everything that is in our field of vision or in earshot; perceptibility does not guarantee perception. Even the things we perceive we may not devote much attention to, and therefore may not comprehend, reflect on, or remember. Second, attention entails constructive processing of what has been attended to. It involves a level 2–like interpretation and elaboration of the sensory input, rather than just a level 1–like internal registering or copying of it; as a consequence, one person's cognitive representation of what has been perceived may differ from another person's. Third, attentional capacity is limited. If we try to pay full attention to one thing we will not normally be very aware of other things in the perceptual field—unless the other things are very attention capturing (e.g., visually salient or loud), in which case attention to the first thing will suffer correspondingly.

To illustrate some of these developmental acquisitions, let us consider the following sample studies. When Miller and Bigi (1977) asked children to select objects to surround the target in a visual search task in order to make the search for the target, a red triangle, harder, they found that younger children simply add a lot of objects, regardless of their color or shape. By age 8 or 9, however, children begin to realize, in addition, that surrounding the target with objects identical to the target in shape and color (other red triangles of various sizes) makes the target blend into its background and not be seen immediately even though it is "right in front of his eyes." In a related investigation, Fabricius and colleagues (1997) asked third graders, fifth graders, and adults, "Can somebody look at something, but not see it?" The modal answers and answer justifications at the three age levels were: no, with no justification given (third graders); yes, because of a vision or lighting problem (fifth graders); yes, because attention was elsewhere (adults).

Flavell, Green, and Flavell (1995) tested children 4, 6, and 8 years of age for their understanding that a person who is mentally focused on one thing will devote little or no simultaneous attention or thought to another, totally irrelevant thing. For example, a person busy trying to recognize the people in a group photograph will not at the same time pay much attention to the frame around the photograph. Whereas most of the 6- and 8-year-olds demonstrated an understanding that task-oriented thought and attention are selectively focused in this way, most of the 4-year-olds showed no such understanding. These results are consistent with evidence obtained by Miller and Bigi (1979) and Pillow (1989a) with regard to auditory attention (see also Montgomery, Bach, and Moran, 1998). Flavell, Green, and Flavell (1995) speculated that 4-year-olds may implicitly conceive of the mind as more like a lamp than a flashlight, that is, as a device that can radiate attention and thought in all directions at once rather than in only one direction at a time.

Finally, experiments by Fabricius, Schwanenflugel, and colleagues (see Parault and Schwanenflugel, 2000) have shown some intriguing further developments in children's understanding of attention and other mental phenomena after the age of 8. As examples, older children seem to acquire a clearer distinction between attention and comprehension, a more abstract, supramodal conception of selective attention, and a more process-oriented, constructivist conception of the mind (cf. Pillow, 1995).

Knowledge

Among studies testing young children's understanding of the importance of perceptual access in acquiring knowledge, some have found that even 3-year-olds tend to attribute knowledge of a box's contents to a person who looks inside the box rather than to one who just touches the box (Pillow, 1989b; Pratt and Bryant, 1990). Others, however, have found that young children have considerable difficulty in isolating perceptual access as a critical condition for knowledge (Perner and Ogden, 1988; Ruffman and Olson, 1989; Wimmer, Hogrefe, and Perner, 1988). For example, Lyon (1993) found that 3-year-olds tend to attribute knowledge of a box's contents to a doll that does not look inside the box but moves toward it, in preference to one that looks inside but moves away from it. In both this and another study by Lyon (1993), 3-year-olds tend to attribute knowledge on the basis of something like desire or engagement rather than perceptual access, whereas 4-year-olds tend to do so on the basis of perceptual access alone. Similarly, Montgomery and Miller (1997) found that, unlike 5-year-olds, 3-year-olds believe that listeners will not know information they have clearly heard if the speaker did not want them hear it (see also Koerber and Flavell, 1998). It seems, then, that children of this age will sometimes wrongly deny knowledge to a person with perceptual access as well as wrongly attribute knowledge to a person without access. Such results support Taylor's conclusion (1996, p. 296; see also Montgomery, 1992, p. 423) that "the bulk of the evidence suggest 3-year-olds often do not know much about the relation between perceiving and knowing."

There is also considerable development during the preschool period in children's understanding of the conditions that provide a person with knowledge (O'Neill and Chong, 2001). To illustrate, in Gopnik and Graf, 1988, 3-, 4-, and 5-year-olds learned about the contents of a drawer in three different ways: by seeing them, by being told about them, or by inferring them from a clue. Later they were asked how they knew about the drawer's contents. The oldest subjects had little difficulty identifying the specific source of their knowledge, but the youngest were quite poor at this task. Consistent with this evidence, Aksu-Koc (1988, chap. 8) found that, among Turkish children, 4-year-olds are more aware than 3-year-olds of verb endings in Turkish that tell the listener how the speaker knows about an event, namely, by actually witnessing it (one verb ending) versus being told about it or inferring it (a different verb ending). This also suggests a developing sensitivity during the preschool period to sources of knowledge. O'Neill and Chong (2001, p. 803) have summed up the research findings on this issue as follows: "3-year-olds are somewhat able to identify the source of their beliefs, but in many cases their performance is substantially poorer than that of 4- or 5-year-olds." Taylor, Esbenson, and Bennett, 1994, found that young preschoolers are also often unclear about when as well as how they acquired a piece of knowledge. For instance, they tend to say that they have known for a long time both familiar, long-known information and new information that the experimenter just taught them.

In addition to learning about access and sources, children also need to learn about aspectuality—what senses yield what type of knowledge. A number of investigations have documented substantial developmental changes during the preschool and early elementary school years in children's understanding of the modality-specific nature of knowledge (O'Neill, Astington, and Flavell, 1992; O'Neill and Chong, 2001; Perner and Ruffman, 1995; Pillow, 1993; Remmel, 1999; Robinson et al., 1997; Weinberger and Bushnell, 1994). For example, O'Neill and

Chong (2001) presented 3- and 4-year-olds with five scenarios, each requiring a different sensory action to be performed in order to identify an object's property: in the case of a visual property, the action of looking inside a paper bag to determine whether a ball inside was red or green. The experimenter modeled a sensory action (e.g., looking) and then the children did it. The children were then asked (1) to tell how they found out the ball was red or green, (2) to show how they found out, and (3) to indicate which body part a doll would need to use to find out. The results were striking. Even though the 3-year-olds were asked about their own knowledge and very recent experiences, and could respond nonverbally, they were only correct about half the time, performing considerably worse than the 4-year-olds. Although 4-year-olds are better than 3-year-olds at identifying the correct modality on such tasks, they frequently overestimate the knowledge that can be obtained from seeing (Robinson et al., 1997).

As children develop, they gradually come to construe the mind as a selective, representational, and interpretive device rather than as one that just copies the objects and events presented to the senses. This allows them to recognize that visual and other perceptual information needs to be adequate as well as merely present. Children's understanding of the modality-specific nature of perceptual input (aspectuality), just discussed, is an early step in this direction. They also come to appreciate other ways in which the input may fail to engender a clear and correct interpretation in the perceiver (Carpendale and Chandler, 1996; Flavell and Miller, 1998; Miller, 2000; Montgomery, 1992; Robinson et al., 1997). One way is that the input may not contain enough information to allow a correct interpretation or, in some cases, any interpretation at all. For example, preschoolers are apt to think that a naive other person can tell that a picture contains a giraffe even if only a small, nondescript part of the giraffe is visible to the person. In contrast, older children are more likely to realize that, although a naive other person does indeed see the giraffe (there is visual access), the person simply does not see enough of it to be able to identify it as a giraffe (Chandler and Helm, 1984; Taylor, 1988; but see Gopnik and Rosati, 2001, Perner and Davies, 1991, and Ruffman, Olson, and Astington, 1991, for evidence that older preschoolers can manage some tasks of this type). There is a similar age trend with respect to understanding something like the opposite: a person may sometimes be able to infer information to which the person does not have direct visual access (Sodian and Wimmer, 1987). In addition, research by Lagattuta and colleagues (Lagattuta and Wellman, 2001; Lagattuta, Wellman, and Flavell, 1997) shows that even preschoolers may recognize that seeing something that was previously associated with a sad event can trigger memories and feelings associated with that event—but only in a person who has had that sad experience.

Children also learn that visual information can be not just insufficient but downright misleading. Hundreds of studies have shown that older children have a more secure and articulate understanding than younger ones of false belief, deception, and appearance-reality discrepancies (see the references cited in the second paragraph of this chapter). Development in this area can be quite extended. For instance, Flavell, Green, and Flavell (1986) found that although 6- to 7-year-olds could easily manage the simple appearance-reality tasks that 3-year-olds fail (e.g., they could recognize that the experimenter's fake rock simultaneously looks like a rock and is really a sponge), their ability to reflect on and talk about visual appearances, realities, and appearance-reality relations remained very limited. In contrast, the appearance-reality knowledge of 11- to 12-year-olds and especially college students was richly structured and highly accessible. For instance, adult participants could identify and differentiate among realistic-looking nonfake objects, realistic-looking fake objects ("good fakes"), nonrealistic-looking fakes ("poor fakes"), and even fake-looking nonfakes. Doing this reflects the development of quite sophisticated knowledge about relations between visual input and cognitive response.

There is also a growing understanding of the cognitive effects of visual input that is inadequate by dint of being ambiguous rather than impoverished or misleading (Miller, 2000). Chandler and colleagues (see Carpendale and Chandler, 1996) found that not until they were 7 or 8 did children clearly understand that an ambiguous visual stimulus (a reversible figure) could be construed differently by different people (cf. Gopnik and Rosati, 2001). The same was true for lexical ambiguities (e.g., homophones) and ambiguous messages. A higher form of this understanding is needed to evaluate the evidence—often subtly ambiguous—for scientific and other knowledge claims. This kind of metacognition is useful when trying to judge how confident one should be that a given conclusion is warranted by a given complex body of evidence (Kuhn, 2001; Moshman, 1998).

Older children also discover that what gets known or believed depends on the perceiver as well as the quality of the available information. For example, they learn that people's preexisting biases or expectations may influence their interpretation of the perceptual evidence. In experiments by Pillow (1991) and Pillow and Weed (1995), child participants heard scenarios in which character A likes character C, but character B does not. C does something damaging, but with ambiguous intent—perhaps accidentally, perhaps on purpose. The participants' task was to predict A's and B's interpretation of C's action. Kindergarten and second-grade children were able to attribute the appropriate biased interpretations to A and B, whereas preschool children responded at chance. On the other hand, research by Ross and other social psychologists (e.g., Ross, Pronin, and Puccio, 2001; Ross and Ward, 1996) reminds us that the ability to attribute bias correctly both to others and, especially, to oneself is far from completely developed even in adults.

Eisbach (2001) tested 5-year-olds, 9-year-olds, and adults for their understanding that the same visual input can engender different trains of thought in different people, and even in the same person on different occasions. In one of her studies, two protagonists, A and B, saw the same depicted object (e.g., a strange-looking animal) and then had a succession of three thoughts, represented by empty thought bubbles. The participants were asked: "Do you think that A and B are having exactly the same thoughts, or do you think that some of their thoughts are different?" Most 5-year-olds thought they would be the same because both A and B saw the same object, whereas most 9-year-olds and adults thought they would be different because A and B were different people, had different past experiences, and so on (or, as one 9-year-old put it, "because their brains aren't the same, so they don't think exactly alike"). Similar age differences in judgments and explanations were found when the same protagonist viewed the same object on different occasions, each time experiencing a succession of three thoughts. Somewhat similarly, Winer (1989) found that third graders and sixth graders were more aware than kindergartners of perceptual adaptation effects, for example, that the sun will seem brighter to the same person coming out of a movie theater than coming out of a house.

Conclusion

It is obvious that there are many facts about vision that children and most adults do not acquire. Uncovering such facts is the task of the vision researcher. Moreover, some of the visual metacognition adults have acquired is inaccurate. For example, Levin, Scholl, and colleagues (see Scholl, Simons, and Levin, chapter 7, this volume) have shown that adults overestimate their ability to detect large between-view changes in scenes—a metacognitive shortcoming called "change blindness blindness." Recall also Winer and colleagues' data on extramission and unseen stares (see Winer and Cottrell, chapter 5, this volume; on adult shortcomings in other areas of metacognition, see also Diana and Reder, chapter 8; Keil, Rozenblit, and Mills, chapter 11; Rachlinski, chapter 12, all this volume; Gilovich and Savitsky, 1999; Ross, Pronin, and Puccio, 2001).

Nevertheless, this chapter documents a number of important truths about vision that children do acquire. One way to characterize development in this area is to say that children seem to acquire a succession of general rules plus a set of specific qualifications or restrictions on those rules. For example, they learn that people see things when their eyes are open (rule), but then need to learn that people do so only if their eyes are pointed in the right direction, if there is no intervening visual barrier, and if the things are not too small, too far away, too dimly lit, or too camouflaged (qualifications). Children learn that things look a certain way when they see them, but also that the things may present a different appearance to someone who sees them from a different vantage point. They learn that perceivers frequently acquire knowledge by looking at things, but also that for one reason or another perceiver A may not acquire knowledge of type B when looking at object C. They learn that seeing things triggers thoughts, but also that seeing them is apt to trigger different thoughts in different people. The usual case seems to be that, when they err, children err by overestimating the cognitive yield of a visual encounter. Thus they are apt to assume that, if one looks, one will automatically see all, and if one sees, one will automatically know all. This seems to be a sensible, adaptive way for development to proceed: first learn the proto-typical patterns, the ones that often or usually hold, and then tease out the exceptions. Cognitive and linguistic development often seems to proceed in this first-overshoot-then-correct fashion (cf. Jusczyk, 2002; Markman, 1992).

If one could further the development of visual metacognition beyond the usual, what dispositions or skills might one target? Here are my candidates:

1. Improve people's attentional strategies. Teach them when to skim and when to search thoroughly and reflect in depth on what they unearth.

2. Help them remember that appearances are often different from and better than the realities they conceal (think of advertising and packaging). A healthy skepticism can be very helpful in navigating through the world's visual enticements.

3. Encourage them, nevertheless, to cherish many visual appearances, in particular, to savor the beauty they see in art museums, theaters, and the world outside.

4. Make them aware of the important metacognitive shortcomings currently being identified by psychological research. Where feasible, also provide them with ways of reducing these shortcomings, or at least their negative effects. People not only need to develop metacognition; they also need to acquire accurate and useful knowledge about their metacognition.

References

Aksu-Koc, A. A. (1988). *The acquisition of aspects and modality.* Cambridge: Cambridge University Press.

Baldwin, D. A. (1991). Infants' contribution to the achievement of joint reference. *Child Development*, 62, 875–890.

Baldwin, D. A. (1993). Early referential understanding: Infants' ability to recognize referential acts for what they are. *Developmental Psychology*, 29, 832–843.

Baldwin, D. A., and Moses, L. J. (1994). Early understanding of referential intent and attentional focus: Evidence from language and emotion. In C. Lewis and P. Mitchell (Eds.), *Children's early understanding of mind: Origins and development* (pp. 133–156). Hillsdale, N.J.: Erlbaum.

Baron-Cohen, S. (1993). From attention-goal psychology to belief-desire psychology: The development of a theory of mind, and its dysfunction. In S. Baron-Cohen, H. Tager-Flusberg, and D. J. Cohen (Eds.), *Understanding other minds: Perspectives from autism* (pp. 59–82). Oxford: Oxford University Press.

Baron-Cohen, S., Tager-Flusberg, H., and Cohen, D. J., Eds. (2000). *Understanding other minds: Perspectives from autism.* 2d ed. Oxford: Oxford University Press.

Barrett, J. L., Rickert, R. A., and Driesenga, A. (2001). God's beliefs versus Mother's: The development of nonhuman agent concepts. *Child Development*, 72, 50–65.

Bartsch, K., and Wellman, H. M. (1995). *Children talk about the mind.* New York: Oxford University Press.

Bigelow, A. E. (1991). The effects of distance and intervening obstacles on visual inference in blind and sighted children. *International Journal of Behavioral Development*, 14, 273–283.

Bischof-Köhler, D. (1991). The development of empathy in infants. In M. E. Lamb and H. Keller (Eds.), *Infant development: Perspectives from German-speaking countries* (pp. 1–33). Hillsdale, N.J.: Erlbaum.

Bretherton, I., and Beeghly, M. (1982). Talking about inner states: The acquisition of an explicit theory of mind. *Developmental Psychology, 18*, 906–921.

Brooks, R., and Meltzoff, A. N. (2003). The importance of eyes: How infants' interpret adult looking behavior. *Developmental Psychology, 38*, 701–711.

Butler, S. C., Caron, A. J., and Brooks, R. (2000). Infant understanding of the referential nature of looking. *Journal of Cognition and Development, 1*, 359–377.

Butterworth, G. (1991). The ontogeny and phylogeny of joint visual attention. In A. Whiten (Ed.), *Natural theories of mind: Evolution, development and simulation of everyday mindreading* (pp. 223–232). Oxford: Blackwell.

Butterworth, G., and Jarrett, N. (1991). What minds have in common is space: Spatial mechanisms serving joint visual attention in infancy. *British Journal of Developmental Psychology, 9*, 55–72.

Carpendale, J. I., and Chandler, M. J. (1996). On the distinction between false belief understanding and subscribing to an interpretive theory of mind. *Child Development, 67*, 1686–1706.

Carpenter, M., Nagell, K., and Tomasello, M. (1998). Social cognition, joint attention, and communicative competence from 9 to 15 months of age. *Monograph of the Society for Research in Child Development, 63* (4, serial no. 255).

Chandler, M. J., and Helm, D. (1984). Developmental changes in the contributions of shared experience to social role-taking competence. *International Journal of Behavioral Development, 7*, 145–156.

Corkum, V., and Moore, C. (1998). The origins of joint visual attention in infants. *Developmental Psychology, 34*, 28–38.

Cottrell, J. E., Winer, G. A., and Smith, M. C. (1996). Beliefs of children and adults about feeling stares of unseen others. *Developmental Psychology, 32*, 50–61.

Cox, M. V. (1980). Visual perspective-taking in children. In M. V. Cox (Ed.), *Are young children egocentric?* (pp. 61–79). New York: St. Martin's Press.

Doherty, M. J., and Anderson, J. R. (1999). A new look at gaze: Preschool children's understanding of gaze direction. *Cognitive Development, 14*, 549–571.

Eisbach, A. O. (2001). Children's developing knowledge about diversity in thought. Ph.D. diss., Stanford University, Stanford, Calif.

Esterly, J. B. (1999). Developmental changes in children's understanding of visual perception between twenty-four and thirty-six months. Poster presented at the biennial meeting of the Society for Research in Child Development, Albuquerque, April.

Fabricius, W., Schick, K., Prost, J., and Schwanenflugel, P. (1997). We don't see eye to eye: Development of a constructivist theory of mind. Poster presented at the biennial meeting of the Society for Research in Child Development, Washington, D.C., April.

Fabricius, W. V., and Schwanenflugel, P. J. (1994). The older child's theory of mind. In A. Demetriou and A. Efklides (Eds.), *Intelligence, mind, and reasoning: Structure and development* (pp. 111–132). Amsterdam: Elsevier.

Flavell, J. H. (1978). The development of knowledge about visual perception. In C. B. Keasey (Ed.), *Nebraska Symposium on Motivation, 25*, 43–76. Lincoln: University of Nebraska Press.

Flavell, J. H. (1992). Perspectives on perspective taking. In H. Beilin and P. Pufall (Eds.), *Piaget's theory: Prospects and possibilities* (pp. 107–139). Hillsdale, N.J.: Erlbaum.

Flavell, J. H., Everett, B. A., Croft, K., and Flavell, E. R. (1981). Young children's knowledge about visual perception: Further evidence for the Level 1–Level 2 distinction. *Developmental Psychology, 17*, 99–103.

Flavell, J. H., Flavell, E. R., Green, F. L., and Wilcox, S. A. (1980). Young children's knowledge about visual perception: Effect of observer's distance from target on perceptual clarity of target. *Developmental Psychology, 16*, 10–12.

Flavell, J. H., Flavell, E. R., Green, F. L., and Wilcox, S. A. (1981). The development of three spatial perspective-taking rules. *Child Development, 52*, 356–358.

Flavell, J. H., Green, F. L., and Flavell, E. R. (1986). Development of knowledge about the appearance-reality distinction. *Monographs of the Society for Research in Child Development*, *51* (1, serial no. 212).

Flavell, J. H., Green, F. L., and Flavell, E. R. (1995). The development of children's knowledge about attentional focus. *Developmental Psychology*, *31*, 706–712.

Flavell, J. H., Green, F. L., Herrera, C., and Flavell, E. R. (1991). Young children's knowledge about visual perception: Lines of sight are always straight. *British Journal of Developmental Psychology*, *9*, 73–88.

Flavell, J. H., and Miller, P. H. (1998). Social cognition. In D. Kuhn and R. S. Siegler (Eds.), *Handbook of child psychology*. Vol. 2: *Cognition, perception, and language*. 5th ed. (pp. 851–898). New York: Wiley.

Flavell, J. H., Shipstead, S. G., and Croft, K. (1978). Young children's knowledge about visual perception: Hiding objects from others. *Child Development*, *49*, 1208–1211.

Flavell, J. H., Shipstead, S. G., and Croft, K. (1980). What young children think you see when their eyes are closed. *Cognition*, *8*, 369–387.

Franco, F., and Butterworth, G. (1989). Is pointing an intrinsically social gesture? Paper presented at the Annual Conference of the Developmental Section of the British Psychological Society, University of Surrey. September.

Gilovich, T., and Savitsky, K. (1999). The spotlight effect and the illusion of transparency: Egocentric assessments of how we are seen by others. *Current Directions in Cognitive Science*, *8*, 165–168.

Gopnik, A., and Graf, P. (1988). Knowing how you know: Young children's ability to identify and remember the sources of their beliefs. *Child Development*, *59*, 1366–1371.

Gopnik, A., and Meltzoff, A. N. (1997). *Words, thoughts, and theories*. Cambridge, Mass.: MIT Press.

Gopnik, A., and Rosati, A. (2001). Duck or rabbit? Reversing ambiguous figures an understanding ambiguous representations. *Developmental Science*, *4*, 175–183.

Gopnik, A., Slaughter, V., and Meltzoff, A. (1994). Changing your views: How understanding visual perception can lead to a new theory of mind. In C. Lewis and P. Mitchell (Eds.), *Origins of an understanding of mind* (pp. 157–181). Hillsdale, N.J.: Erlbaum.

Gopnik, A., and Wellman, H. M. (1994). The "theory" theory. In L. A. Hirschfeld and S. A. Gelman (Eds.), *Mapping the mind: Domain specificity in cognition and culture* (pp. 257–293). Cambridge: Cambridge University Press.

Hare, B., Call, J., Agnetta, B., and Tomasello, M. (2000). Chimpanzees know what conspecifics do and do not see. *Animal Behaviour*, *59*, 771–785.

Hood, B. M., Willen, J. D., and Driver, J. (1998). Adult eyes trigger shifts of visual attention in human infants. *Psychological Science*, *9*, 131–134.

Hughes, C. (2001). From infancy to inferences: Current perspectives on intentionality. *Journal of Cognition and Development*, *2*, 221–240.

Hughes, M., and Donaldson, M. (1979). The use of hiding games for studying the coordination of perspectives. *Educational Review*, *31*, 133–140.

Johnson, S. C. (2000). The recognition of mentalistic agents in infancy. *Trends in Cognitive Sciences*, *4*, 22–28.

Johnson, S., Slaughter, V., and Carey, S. (1998). Whose gaze will infants follow? The elicitation of gaze-following in 12-month-olds. *Developmental Science*, *1*, 233–238.

Jusczyk, P. W. (2002). How infants adapt speech-processing capacities to native-language structure. *Current Directions in Psychological Science*, *11*, 15–18.

Karin-D'Arcy, M. R., and Povinelli, D. J. (2001). Do chimpanzees know what each other see? University of Louisiana at Lafayette, New Iberia.

Koerber, S., and Flavell, J. H. (1998). Children's understanding of sensory access as a necessary and sufficient condition for auditory perception. Stanford University, Stanford, Calif.

Kuhn, D. (2001). How do people know? *Psychological Science*, *12*, 1–8.

Lagattuta, K. H., and Wellman, H. M. (2001). Thinking about the past: Early knowledge about links between prior experience, thinking, and emotion. *Child Development, 72*, 82–102.

Lagattuta, K. H., Wellman, H. M., and Flavell, J. H. (1997). Preschoolers' understanding of the link between thinking and feeling: Cognitive cuing and emotional change. *Child Development, 68*, 1081–1104.

Lempers, J. D., Flavell, E. R., and Flavell, J. H. (1977). The development in very young children of tacit knowledge concerning visual perception. *Genetic Psychology Monographs, 95*, 3–53.

Lyon, T. D. (1993). Young children's understanding of desire and knowledge. Ph.D. diss., Stanford University, Stanford, Calif.

Markman, E. M. (1992). Constraints on word learning: Speculations about their nature, origin, and domain specificity. In M. R. Gunnar and M. P. Maratsos (Eds.), *Modularity and constraints in language and cognition: The Minnesota Symposium on Child Psychology* (pp. 59–101). Hillsdale, N.J.: Erlbaum.

Masangkay, Z. S., McCluskey, K. A., McIntyre, C. W., Sims-Knight, J., Vaughn, B. E., and Flavell, J. H. (1974). The early development of inferences about the visual percepts of others. *Child Development, 45*, 357–366.

Maurer, D. (1985). Infants' perception of facedness. In T. M. Field and N. A. Fox (Eds.), *Social perception in infants* (pp. 73–100). Norwood, N.J.: Ablex.

McGuigan, N., and Doherty, M. J. (1999). The relation between hiding skill and judgment of eye-direction in preschool children. University of Stirling, Scotland.

Miller, P. H. (1985). Children's reasoning about the causes of behavior. *Journal of Experimental Child Psychology, 39*, 343–362.

Miller, P. H., and Bigi, L. (1977). Children's understanding of how stimulus dimensions affect performance. *Child Development, 48*, 1712–1715.

Miller, P. H., and Bigi, L. (1979). Development of children's understanding of attention. *Merrill-Palmen Quarterly, 25*, 235–250.

Miller, S. A. (2000). Children's understanding of preexisting differences in knowledge and belief. *Developmental Review, 20*, 227–282.

Mitchell, P., and Riggs, K. J., Eds. (2000). *Children's reasoning and the mind.* Hove, England: Psychology Press.

Montgomery, D. E. (1992). Young children's theory of knowing: The development of a folk epistemology. *Developmental Review, 12*, 410–430.

Montgomery, D. E., and Miller, S. A. (1997). Young children's attributions of knowledge when speaker intent and listener access conflict. *British Journal of Developmental Psychology, 15*, 159–175.

Montgomery, D. E., Bach, L. M., and Moran, C. (1998). Children's use of looking behavior as a cue to detect another's goal. *Child Development, 69*, 692–705.

Moore, C. (1996). Theories of mind in infancy. *British Journal of Developmental Psychology, 14*, 19–40.

Moore, C., Angelopoulos, M., and Bennett, P. (1999). Word learning in the context of referential and salience cues. *Developmental Psychology, 35*, 60–68.

Moore, C., and Corkum, V. (1994). Social understanding at the end of the first year of life. *Developmental Review, 14*, 349–372.

Moore, C., and D'Entremont, B. (2001). Developmental changes in pointing as a function of attentional focus. *Journal of Cognition and Development, 2*, 109–129.

Moses, L. J., Baldwin, D. A., Rosicky, J. G., and Tidball, G. (2001). Evidence for referential understanding in the emotions domain at twelve and eighteen months. *Child Development, 72*, 718–735.

Moshman (1998). Cognitive development beyond childhood. In D. Kuhn and R. Siegler (Eds.), *Handbook of child psychology. Vol. 2: Cognition, perception, and language.* 5th ed. (pp. 947–978). New York: Wiley.

Mumme, D. L., and Fernald, A. (2003). The infant as onlooker: Learning from emotional reactions observed in a television scenario. *Child Development, 74*, 221–237.

O'Neill, D. K. (1996). Two-year-olds' sensitivity to a parent's knowledge state when making requests. *Child Development, 67*, 659–677.

O'Neill, D. K., Astington, J. W., and Flavell, J. H. (1992). Young children's understanding of the role that sensory experiences play in knowledge acquisition. *Child Development, 63*, 474–490.

O'Neill, D. K., and Chong, S. C. F. (2001). Preschool children's difficulty understanding the types of information obtained through the five senses. *Child Development, 72*, 803–815.

Parault, S. J., and Schwanenflugel, P. J. (2000). The development of conceptual categories of attention during the elementary school years. *Journal of Experimental Child Psychology, 75*, 245–262.

Perner, J. (1991). *Understanding the representational mind*. Cambridge, Mass.: MIT Press.

Perner, J., and Davies, G. (1991). Understanding the mind as an active information processor: Do young children have a "copy theory of mind"? *Cognition, 39*, 51–69.

Perner, J., and Ogden, J. (1988). Knowledge for hunger: Children's problem of representation in imputing mental states. *Cognition, 29*, 47–61.

Perner, J., and Ruffman, T. (1995). Episodic memory and autonoetic consciousness: Developmental evidence and a theory of amnesia. *Journal of Experimental Child Psychology, 59*, 516–548.

Phillips, A. T., Wellman, H. M., and Spelke, E. S. (2002). Infants' ability to connect gaze and emotional expression to intentional action. *Cognition, 85*, 53–78.

Pillow, B. H. (1988). Young children's understanding of attentional limits. *Child Development, 59*, 38–46.

Pillow, B. H. (1989a). The development of beliefs about selective attention. *Merrill-Palmer Quarterly, 35*, 421–443.

Pillow, B. H. (1989b). Early understanding of perception as a source of knowledge. *Journal of Experimental Child Psychology, 47*, 116–129.

Pillow, B. H. (1991). Children's understanding of biased social cognition. *Developmental Psychology, 27*, 539–551.

Pillow, B. H. (1993). Preschool children's understanding of the relationship between modality of perceptual access and knowledge of perceptual properties. *British Journal of Developmental Psychology, 11*, 371–389.

Pillow, B. H. (1995). Two trends in the development of conceptual perspective-taking: An elaboration of the passive-active hypothesis. *International Journal of Behavioral Development, 18*, 649–676.

Pillow, B. H., and Flavell, J. H. (1986). Young children's knowledge about visual perception: Projective size and shape. *Child Development, 57*, 125–135.

Pillow, B. H., and Weed, S. T. (1995). Children's understanding of biased interpretation: Generality and limitations. *British Journal of Developmental Psychology, 13*, 347–366.

Pratt, C., and Bryant, P. E. (1990). Young children understand that looking leads to knowing (so long as they are looking through a single barrel). *Child Development, 61*, 973–982.

Remmel, E. (1999). Source memory and source knowledge in preschool children Understanding of aspectuality develops around 3½. Poster presented at the biennial meeting of the Society for Research in Child Development, Albuquerque, April.

Repacholi, B. M. (1998). Infants' use of attentional cues to identify the referent of another person's emotional expression. *Developmental Psychology, 34*, 1017–1025.

Robinson, E. J., Thomas, G. V., Parton, A., and Nye, R. (1997). Children's overestimation of the knowledge to be gained from seeing. *British Journal of Developmental Psychology, 15*, 257–273.

Ross, L., Pronin, E., and Puccio, C. (2001). Understanding misunderstanding: Social psychological perspectives. In T. Gilovich, D. Griffin, and D. Kahneman (Eds.), *Heuristics of intuitive judgment: Extensions and applications*. New York: Cambridge University Press.

Ross, L., and Ward, A. (1996). Naïve realism in everyday life: Implications for social conflict and misunderstanding. In T. Brown, E. Reed, and E. Turiel (Eds.), *Values and knowledge* (pp. 103–135). Hillsdale, N.J.: Erlbaum.

Ruffman, T. K., and Olson, D. R. (1989). Children's ascription of knowledge to others. *Developmental Psychology, 25*, 601–606.

Ruffman, T. K., Olson, D. R., and Astington, J. W. (1991). Children's understanding of visual ambiguity. *British Journal of Developmental Psychology*, 9, 89–102.

Sodian, B., and Wimmer, H. (1987). Children's understanding of inference as a source of knowledge. *Child Development*, 58, 424–433.

Taylor, M. (1988). The development of children's ability to distinguish what they know from what they see. *Child Development*, 59, 703–718.

Taylor, M. (1996). A theory of mind perspective on social cognitive development. In R. Gelman and T. Au (Eds.), *Handbook of perception and cognition*. Vol. 13: *Perceptual and cognitive development* (pp. 282–329). New York: Academic Press.

Taylor, M., Esbensen, B. M., and Bennett, R. T. (1994). Children's understanding of knowledge acquisition: The tendency for children to report they have always known what they have just learned. *Child Development*, 65, 1581–1604.

Theall, L. A., and Povinelli, D. J. (1999). Do chimpanzees tailor their gestural signals to fit the attentional states of others? *Animal Cognition*, 2, 207–214.

Tomasello, M. (1995). Joint attention as social cognition. In C. Moore and P. Dunham (Eds.), *Joint attention: Its origins and role in development* (pp. 103–130). Hillsdale, N.J.: Erlbaum.

Warren, D. H. (1994). *Blindness and children: An individual differences approach*. Cambridge: Cambridge University Press.

Weinberger, N., and Bushnell, E. W. (1994). Young children's knowledge about their senses: Perceptions and misconceptions. *Child Study Journal*, 24, 209–235.

Wellman, H. M., Cross, D., and Watson, J. (2001). Meta-analysis of theory-of-mind development: The truth about false belief. *Child Development*, 72, 655–684.

Wellman, H. M., and Gelman, S. A. (1998). Knowledge acquisition in functional domains. In D. Kuhn and R. S. Siegler (Eds.), *Handbook of child psychology*. Vol 2: *Cognition, perception, and language*. 5th ed. (pp. 523–573). New York: Wiley.

Wellman, H. M., Phillips, A. T., and Rodriguez, T. (2000). Young children's understanding of perception, desire, and emotion. *Child Development*, 71, 895–912.

Wimmer, H., Hogrefe, A., and Perner, J. (1988). Children's understanding of informational access as a source of knowledge. *Child Development*, 59, 386–396.

Winer, G. A. (1989). Developmental trends in the understanding of perceptual adaptation. *Journal of Experimental Child Psychology*, 48, 293–314.

Winer, G. A. (1991). Children's understanding of perception and perceptual processes. In R. Vasta (Ed.), *Annals of child development*. Vol. 8 (pp. 177–213). London: Jessica Kingsley.

Woodward, A. L. (2003). Infants' developing understanding of the link between looker and object. *Developmental Science*, 6, 297–311.

Woodward, A. L. (in press). Infants' understanding of the actions involved in joint attention. In N. Eilan, C. Hoerl, T. McCormack, and J. Roessler (Eds.), *Joint attention: Communication and other minds*. Oxford: Oxford University Press.

Woodward, A. L., and Markman, E. M. (1998). Early word learning. In D. Kuhn and R. S. Siegler (Eds.), *Handbook of child psychology*. Vol 2: *Cognition, perception, and language*. 5th ed. (pp. 371–420). New York: Wiley.

Zahn-Waxler, C., Radke-Yarrow, M., Wagner, E., and Chapman, M. (1992). Development of concern for others. *Developmental Psychology*, 28, 126–136.

Chapter 2

Action Analysis and Change Blindness: Possible Links

Megan M. Saylor and Dare A. Baldwin

As we view others moving about the world transitioning from one thing to the next, we are faced with a dizzying display of activity—arms snake in and out, legs retract and extend, objects rise and fall. Adding to the muddle, such action scenarios typically proceed in a continuous stream without clear pauses delineating individual actions. Yet recent research on adults' and infants' analysis of dynamic action has revealed that observers of action do not perceive a chaotic jumble of motion (as might be expected given the complexity of the stimulus), but rather perceive a sensible, discrete series of actions (e.g., Baird, Baldwin, and Malle, 1999; Baldwin et al., 2001; Zacks, Tversky, and Iyer, 2001). This research highlights our ability to analyze human action, as reflected in a remarkable degree of agreement about how actions are segmented across a variety of event types, even in the face of complex, continuously flowing stimuli. In particular, human action tends to be segmented into units linked with inferences about actors' goals and intentions (e.g., Baird, Baldwin, and Malle, 1999; Zacks, Tversky, and Iyer, 2001).

Observers' skill at systematically detecting structure in human action seems to suggest acute attention to details about actors' motions and their effects on objects, even though these details are embedded within massive and continuous changes in the motion stream. However, this stands in sharp contrast to a striking finding from the visual cognition literature. In particular, observers of action often miss what, on the face of it, ought to be obvious changes inserted into the flow of action sequences. For example, in one dramatic display of such change blindness, a confederate approached participants on a college campus and then asked for directions. In the course of the conversation, a door was carried between the two speakers, and the confederate was surreptitiously replaced with another individual. Remarkably, half of the participants failed to notice the switch of the person to whom they had been speaking (Simons and Levin, 1998)! Importantly, this does not represent just an isolated finding—in other demonstrations, adults have also failed to notice changes to central actors inserted into short films (Levin and Simons, 1997; see Simons and Levin, 1997, for a review).

A recent surge of interest in the change blindness phenomenon has yielded considerable information about the types of stimuli most likely to elicit it. In particular, this body of work has clarified that attention mediates change blindness. For one, observers are faster to notice changes to items of central interest than to items of marginal interest. Furthermore, focusing attention on change locations attenuates change blindness rates (see Simons, 2000, for a review). Together, these findings point to a central role of attention in alleviating change blindness. Yet this account, on its own, is unsatisfying. It has little power to predict when, and to what degree, change blindness will occur in everyday processing of action. To do so requires knowing what factors drive the allocation of attention in observers' spontaneous action processing.

In the present chapter, we take seriously the possibility that discerning actors' goals and intentions is a major thrust of everyday action processing. If so, this effort will dictate what is and is not attended to, and hence should influence change blindness in systematic ways. Put another way, when processing is oriented toward interpreting goals and intentions, attention is likely to be allocated to components of action sequences most relevant to actors' intentions. In what follows, we detail current research on adults' and infants' action processing vis-à-vis intention detection; our aim is to generate predictions from this work regarding the allocation of attention during action processing, and hence the likely locus of change blindness effects.

We suspect that much of the action processing we are concerned with here is implicit, automatic, and outside our conscious awareness. That is, processing others' everyday goal-oriented actions seems to occur relatively automatically and with little conscious consideration, except when incongruencies or confusions arise (in which case, problem solving may be triggered at the conscious level). But, even though the elemental computations seem unavailable to conscious reflection, we suspect the *outputs* of our action processing system, namely, inferences about goals and intentions, are available—at least potentially. These inferences are central to our metacognitions about action and are at the heart of our theory of mind. Of great interest are the ways these metacognitions affect action processing, an issue that makes contact with a number of other chapters in volume (see Flavell, chapter 1, and Levin and Beck, chapter 6) and one we will take up toward the end of the chapter.

Before we begin, a quick caveat: In this chapter we make no attempt to account for all change blindness phenomena. We focus only on effects that might arise in the context of analysis of complex, continuous action sequences involving everyday human behavior (see Simons, 2000, for a review of proposed explanations of change blindness). The change blindness literature considers processing of a considerably broader range of stimuli including, for example, an analysis of change blindness across simple visual displays (e.g., Mack and Rock, 1998), across static complex visual scenes (e.g., Pringle, Kramer, and Irwin, chapter 8, this volume; Grimes, 1996; Rensink, O'Regan, and Clark, 1997), and across dynamic reality-based action scenarios (e.g., Levin and Simons, 1997; Simons and Levin, 1998), where the participants' analysis more closely resembles day-to-day action analysis and any associated change detection. By focusing on one crucially important processing context, we hope to provide a starting account of possible links between intention detection and change blindness.

The Central Role of Meaning

Simons and Levin (1997; see also Simons, 2000), recently offered an account of the causal underpinnings of change blindness that centers on the role of meaning in adults' interpretation of static scenes and dynamic action displays. They proposed that adults' change blindness results from their extraction of a "first impression" or gist of the meaning of a given scene or event. On this view, we, as observers, are inclined to assume that the gist of a scene or action, once extracted, tends to remain stable; on this assumption, further analysis is not strictly necessary. As a result, certain types of change that occur after the first pass at meaning analysis may not be detected because they do not radically alter the gist. Consistent with this proposal, the semantic value of changes inserted into static scenes has been found to predict change blindness. Thus participants are slower to detect changes that involve objects or scenery not central to the "meaning" of a display (e.g., Rensink, O'Regan, and Clark, 1997; Henderson, Weeks, and Hollingworth, 1999). In these studies, semantic value is determined either by evaluating observers' mention of features in a display during a short verbal description (Rensink, O'Regan, and Clark, 1997) or by manipulating which objects "belong together" in a display (Henderson, Weeks, and Hollingworth, 1999).

Our proposal—that observers are strongly oriented toward determining actors' goals and intentions—offers another a priori basis on which to predict the meaningful properties of a given action scenario in a given context. After reviewing recent findings on the ways meaningful properties are gleaned from dynamic human action, we will use these findings as a basis for predictions about change blindness and how it may undergo systematic changes with context, with knowledge acquisition, and during the course of human development.

Adults' Action Analysis

Social psychologists have long noted that observers of action readily identify distinct acts in others' everyday behavior, even though the motions themselves typically flow continuously without clear pauses to demarcate the beginning and end of individual acts (Asch, 1952; Heider, 1958; Newtson, 1973). For example, Newtson and colleagues (1973; Newtson, Enquist, and Bois, 1977) showed adults continuous everyday action sequences, such as motorcycle repair, and asked them to indicate meaningful junctures within the motion stream. They found a high degree of consistency across adults in their identification of natural "break points" within the continuous action sequence. Baird et al. (1999) found that such break points coincide with observers' analysis of the actors' goals and intentions, and provided additional evidence that adults spontaneously segment the flow of motion at such break points in the course of processing. They showed adults continuous, everyday action sequences such as a female actor cleaning her kitchen (washing a dish, hanging a towel, putting ice cream in the freezer, and inserting a bowl into the dishwasher) and asked them to identify points at which goals and intentions were achieved. This first group of adult participants displayed remarkable consistency in the number of distinct intentional acts they noted, and the precise time at which individual acts were completed. Baird and colleagues then used these "end point" judgments to construct a modified video in which tones were overlaid either to coincide with the end point of an intentional act or to interrupt an intentional act midstream. A second group of adult participants viewed the video with end point and midpoint tones, and on a subsequent, tone-free viewing, indicated the time point within the action where they recalled tones having occurred on their previous viewing. The participants displayed substantially better recall for the placement of end point tones than midpoint tones, even though the tones were equivalent in duration, volume, and all other acoustic properties. A control study using the identical pattern of tones overlaid on a motion sequence devoid of human action properties (shifting patterns of colors) revealed no recall advantage for end point tones, indicating that the effect did not simply arise from memory for rhythmic characteristics within the tone sequences, but indeed reflected processing of a relation between tones and the action sequence being viewed. Together, these findings clarify that boundaries between intentional acts have some special status in adults' processing of continuous action. Moreover, the findings suggest that, in the course of action processing, adults extract units spanning the initiation to completion of intentions, and these segments structure their recall of action scenarios.

Other researchers have probed adults' organization of human action sequences. At issue is how adults relate distinct acts or events—once extracted—to one another in constructing and remembering complex action scenarios. In particular, Zacks et al. (2001) asked whether adults' processing of dynamic human action is hierarchically organized—with large action units (e.g., putting a sheet on a bed) subsuming smaller action units (e.g., putting the top end of the sheet on the bed, putting the bottom end on the bed, smoothing the sheet). Participants in Zacks et al., 2001, were asked to segment action sequences across a variety of tasks, including segmentation both as an action unfolded and after the action had been completed (i.e., from memory). In each of the tasks, participants' judgments about the location of action end points revealed alignment between end points of small action units and end points of large action units. In other words, participants appeared to be embedding small action units within large action units, thereby clarifying that their organization of dynamic human action can be characterized as hierarchical in structure (see also Newtson, 1973).

How, then, do adults segment dynamic human action into hierarchically organized action units in the absence of pauses demarcating individual actions? This is not yet fully clear. Baldwin and Baird (1999, 2001; Baird and Baldwin, 2001) speculate that adults recruit multiple sources of information to guide segmentation of action. One set of sources they class broadly as top-down world knowledge concerns the kinds of intentions that a given individual is likely to display in a given context. That is, on viewing someone cleaning a kitchen or making a bed, observers may use their existing knowledge of such activities and associated intentions to guide recognition of distinct acts (washing a dish, hanging a towel, spreading a sheet, tucking a sheet) within the action sequence. The hypothesis that knowledge-driven top-down processing assists segmentation of action is certainly plausible, given the documented role of top-down processing in other aspects of perception and cognition. On the other hand, Norris, McQueen, and Cutler (2000) have convincingly argued that top-down processes do *not* play a role in segmentation of speech. Whether they do so in the action domain is thus far from self-evident, and will be an interesting topic for future research.

Baldwin and Baird speculated that bottom-up processes involving low-level analysis of structured patterns within the motion stream likely also aid segmentation. The movements people engage in when pursuing everyday, object-oriented goals (e.g., cleaning a kitchen, photocopying papers, brushing teeth) seem to possess an inherent structure that coincides, at least probabilistically, with the initiation to completion of intentions (Baldwin and Baird, 1999; see also Newtson, Enquist, and Bois, 1977; Zacks and Tversky, 2001).

Such structure may take a variety of forms. For one, as people enact intentions on inanimate objects, a predictable configuration occurs in the physical and temporal characteristics of bodily motion. To act intentionally, we first locate relevant objects—typically entailing head turns as well as concomitant changes in gaze direction and trunk orientation—then move toward the objects specified by head/gaze/trunk orientation, and contact them. If observers are sensitive to such configural structure, this could assist them in segmenting dynamic action along intention boundaries.

Dynamic intentional action also seems to possess relevant statistical structure. Certain motions within the stream of behavior co-occur more frequently than others, often because they are causally linked in achieving a goal (e.g., in preparing food for cooking, the motion of slicing a vegetable is frequently preceded by the motion of grasping a knife, whereas slicing a vegetable is only infrequently preceded by grasping a towel). From the observer's point of view, then, a history of low rates of co-occurrence for two adjacent motions is a potential clue to segmentation, that is, low transitional probabilities predict boundaries between intentional acts.

At present, little is known about the structure of dynamic human action, and thus even these sketches of configural and statistical structure are highly speculative. Moreover, evidence that sensitivity to such structure assists adults in segmenting dynamic intentional action has been slim: one seminal study (Avrahami and Kareev, 1994) demonstrates that adults can learn to identify arbitrary sequences of action as units based solely on patterns of co-occurrence in their prior experience. However, research under way in collaboration with a number of colleagues has begun to directly confirm that adults readily use statistical and configural regularities to segment continuous, everyday intentional action.

Infants' Action Processing
The research just considered indicates that among other things, adults' processing of continuous, intentional action involves segmenting behavior into units that demarcate action along intention boundaries. An intriguing question arises concerning the emergence of such segmentation skill. In particular, when and how do infants make a start at identifying distinct acts within the continuous flow of dynamic intentional action?

The fact that infants developing normally can discern some basic information about others' intentions as early as the second year (see Baldwin and Baird, 2001; Tomasello, 1999, for reviews) implies that they can already segment at least some kinds of dynamic actions along intention boundaries. To date, however, little research has examined how children acquire skills for identifying distinct intentional acts within human action. Most infancy research has presented infants with "presegmented" action. For example, a few groundbreaking studies (Sharon and Wynn, 1998; Wynn, 1995, 1996) investigated infants' ability to individuate actions within a continuous stream, but with simplified, puppet-enacted motion such as jumping and head wagging, not with naturalistic, intentional action. An important starting point for current research, then, is to develop techniques for investigating infants' skills for analyzing and organizing everyday, dynamic action.

One way to test for infants' action segmentation skills is to evaluate whether they treat intention-relevant units of action as cohesive bodies. If they do, then disruptions to such units should strike them as unexpected. Baldwin et al. (2001) investigated this possibility by presenting 10- to 11-month-old infants with two digitized videos of continuous intentional action in a variant of the habituation-dishabituation paradigm. In one video, a woman notices a towel that has fallen on the floor, turns to pick it up, grasps it, and hangs it on a towel rack. In the other video, a woman notices an ice cream container that has been left on a counter, approaches the counter, grabs the container, moves to a freezer and grasps and opens the freezer door.

During the familiarization phase, infants viewed the videos repeatedly so that they were able to process and possibly segment the action sequence. Following familiarization, infants were presented with two test videos in which 1.5 sec still-frame pauses had been inserted into the flow of action. In one test video, the pause occurred after the woman had completed her intention (e.g., after she had grasped the towel) but before she hung the towel on the rack. These completing pauses preserved the structure of the intention unit (see figure 2.1). In a second test video, the pause was inserted before the woman had completed her intention (e.g., before she had grasped the towel). These interrupting pauses disrupted the structure of the intention unit (see figure 2.2). Baldwin and colleagues reasoned that infants

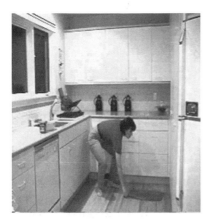

Figure 2.1
Completing still frame.

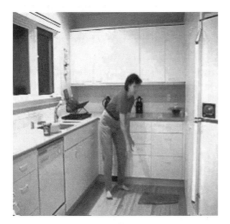

Figure 2.2
Interrupting still frame.

who had successfully segmented the continuous action scenario should be struck by the test videos in which pauses interrupted intention units.

As expected, infants' looking during the familiarization phase decreased across trials. When shown the test videos in which pauses coincided with intention boundaries, infants showed no recovery of interest; however, the test videos in which pauses interrupted intention units, struck infants as noteworthy. They looked longer at such interrupting test videos relative to both their last familiarization trial and to the completing test videos.

In other words, infants' attention was drawn to those videos in which relevant units of action—units with boundaries coinciding with the initiation and completion of intentional action—were disrupted. A control study clarified that the infants' longer looking at the interrupting test videos was not the result of a simple starting preference for the still-frame pauses accompanying such videos. That is, when infants watched the test videos without having had the opportunity for prior processing, they displayed equal interest in the interrupting and completing test videos (see figure 2.3).

Taken together, the findings from these two studies suggest that infants spontaneously identify "intention-relevant" units within continuously flowing intentional action. The boundaries of these units coincide with the initiation/completion of intentions, yet infants may or may not actually appreciate, on a conceptual level, the intentions that give rise to the units. That is, infants may extract intention-relevant units primarily through sensitivity to the patterned regularities they exhibit.

These studies highlight a strength of infants' action segmentation skills. In particular, even when they had not seen the actor or particular kitchen before, infants succeeded at identifying relevant segments within the action sequences. This

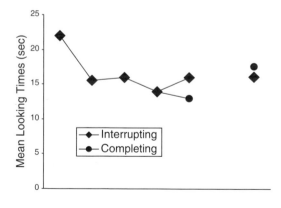

Figure 2.3
Infants' looking to familiarization and test videos.

finding points to the possibility that infants can extend segmentation skills to relatively unfamiliar action sequences. In other words, infants' segmentation skills may be robust enough to operate successfully in the absence of familiarity with the particulars of a given action sequence. However, these first studies involved repeated viewings of only two action scenarios within the same kitchen context (i.e., grasping a towel, putting ice cream away). Although repetition was a necessary feature of the familiarization-recovery experimental design, the studies' findings nevertheless, left questions about the scope and robustness of infants' skills for segmenting action unresolved. While it is possible that infants need considerable exposure to a given action scenario before they can detect structural regularities within it, it is equally likely that their action analysis skills are robust enough to operate in the absence of extensive familiarization.

One potential method for examining infants' action segmentation without requiring lengthy familiarization is the intermodal matching paradigm (e.g., Kuhl and Meltzoff, 1984; Spelke, 1979; Spelke, Born, and Chu, 1983; Spelke and Owsley, 1979). Researchers have used this technique to investigate infants' ability to coordinate information across different sense modalities (e.g., sight and sound). In such studies, infants watch two simultaneous presentations of a visual stimulus (e.g., mom's face and dad's face) and listen to a single sound stimulus that matches one of the visual displays but not the other (e.g., mom's voice). From very early in their first year, infants can coordinate information across different senses with longer looking to matching than nonmatching displays for a variety of stimuli including, for example, sound-to-mouth movement correspondences (Kuhl and Meltzoff, 1984) and sound-to-motion correspondences (Spelke 1979; Spelke, Born, and Chu, 1983).

Existing studies concerning infants' ability to detect sound-to-motion correspondences are particularly relevant for the present research. The abilities infants have displayed in some of these studies hint at skills for segmenting certain kinds of continuous motion displays. In particular, early studies by Spelke and colleagues (1979; Spelke, Born, and Chu, 1983) suggest that infants segment certain kinds of nonhuman motion, with trajectory changes signaling segment boundaries. Infants watched simultaneous videos of two distinct objects (e.g., a toy kangaroo and donkey) bouncing up and down such that trajectory changes were asynchronous with one another. A centrally presented sound corresponded to a trajectory change in just one object's motion path (e.g., a tone occurred when the kangaroo contacted the ground). This was dubbed the "matching display." Infants at 4 months looked longer at the matching than the nonmatching displays, revealing their sensitivity to the synchrony between the sounds and trajectory changes within continuous motion. In Spelke, Born, and Chu, 1983, 4-month-old infants were found to be sensitive to trajectory changes (i.e., transitions between up and down action) regardless of whether the object made contact with a surface or not; hence, it appeared to be an abrupt change in motion trajectory, rather than contact, that underlay infants' intermodal matching skill.

These early intermodal matching studies provide clear evidence that infants are sensitive to trajectory changes in *non*human motion sequences, hinting that such trajectory changes may function as segment boundaries in a segmentation process. Conceivably, then, the intermodal matching technique might provide a window on infants' attention to segment boundaries in *human* motion, and it can be used to probe such sensitivity without requiring lengthy, repeated presentation of a given motion scenario to infants. If infants are indeed sensitive to boundaries between actions within dynamic, human action, then they should look longer at displays in which action boundaries are synchronous with centrally presented tones relative to displays in which action boundaries do not correspond with tones.

To investigate this prediction, we presented 9- to 11-month-old infants with two simultaneous live-action displays in which actors manipulated a series of objects in a relatively novel manner (Saylor et al., 2002). Centrally presented tones matched completion points of one of the actors' actions and occurred randomly with respect to completion points of other actors' actions. In all action scenarios, motion was continuous.

Each object set was organized so that there was a central object of focus and several smaller objects that were used in relation to the central object. For example, one object set included a small, wooden shelf onto which the actor placed several objects (i.e., tea bags, a tea box, and small books) after wiping it with a sponge. Infants watched action scenarios involving four object sets altogether: a small, wooden shelf paired with a set of miniature, transparent drawers and a stand for hanging coffee mugs paired with a set of jars.

During the experimental session, infants saw four trial blocks of action. Within each trial block, the action sequences were repeated three times. On the first presentation, each action sequence was displayed without accompanying tones, which enabled us to obtain a baseline estimate of infants' starting level of interest in each of the action displays being presented. The second and third presentations were test trials. During the test trials, ten tones were played that matched the completion points of one actors' actions but were randomly associated with completion points of the other action sequence. For example, for the shelves one tone was played when the actor had completed each of the following actions: wiping out to the end of the top shelf (with a sponge), wiping out to the end of the bottom shelf, placing the sponge on the surface of the table, putting a bag of tea in a box, putting a second tea bag in a box, closing the lid on the box, placing the box of tea on the shelf, placing one book on the shelf, placing another book on the shelf, and placing a third book on the shelf.

We found that infants looked longer at matching displays, indicating that they noted the correspondence between tones and completion points within the actors' continuous action sequences (see figure 2.4). Furthermore, infants' longer looking to the matching than nonmatching side could not be explained with recourse to a starting preference for the matching side; when no tones were present—during the baseline trials lacking accompanying tones—infants showed no preference for

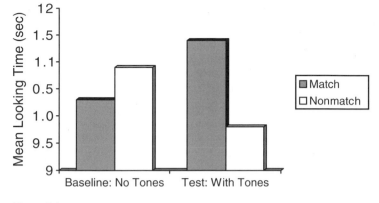

Figure 2.4
Infants' looking to matching versus nonmatching displays during salience and test trials.

either the matching or nonmatching action sequence. Finally, additional analyses revealed that the presence of tones induced a significant increase in infants' looking to the matching action relative to the silent, baseline viewing period. No such significant increase occurred for the nonmatching action when looking during the presence of tones was compared to looking during the baseline viewing period.

All in all, infants revealed a consistent pattern of preference for looking at the actions whose completion points matched the tones presented. Infants' ability to note correspondence between tones and completion points implies sensitivity to the very portions of the motion stream that demarcate boundaries between distinct intentional acts. These findings from the intermodal matching paradigm bolster the case for infants possessing skills for segmenting continuous intentional action, and provide new information about the robustness of infants' action processing. Infants watched four different, and relatively novel, action sequences. Moreover, they viewed two action sequences simultaneously, and saw each action sequence only once before their ability to detect completion points was probed. Infants' success at detecting correspondences between tones and completion points under these demanding conditions suggests that identifying boundaries between distinct acts is something they readily do for a variety of object-oriented actions.

Our findings to date clarify that infants as young as 10–11 months spontaneously segment dynamic human action, but how they do so is not yet clear. Infants lack much of the world knowledge that adults possess and hence would be unable to draw on detailed, specific knowledge of events to guide segmentation of continuous, intentional action. Moreover, at very early ages (i.e., before 9–12 months), infants may well lack a conceptual understanding of mental states such as intention (e.g., Barresi and Moore, 1996; Tomasello, 1999; but see Baron-Cohen, 1995; Premack, 1990), meaning that top-down approaches to appropriate segmentation of the behavior stream would not be available to them. Structure detection processes similar to those observed in adults by Baldwin and colleagues might be crucial for infants to begin segmenting dynamic human action appropriately along intention units.

This proposal—that low-level structure detection processes guide infants' discovery of relevant segments within the complex, dynamic flow of intentional action—has an analogue in the language development literature. Like human action, human speech is largely continuous, with few pauses between individual elements, such as words or clauses. However, identifying these elements within the continuous flow is crucial to processing speech. Researchers interested in the segmentation problem presented by language have found that infants as young as 7–8 months are capable of extracting structure from continuous speech based on both configural information coinciding with major clause boundaries (e.g., Hirsh-Pasek et al., 1987; Jusczyk et al., 1992; Jusczyk, 1997) and statistical information signaling word boundaries (e.g., Aslin, Saffran, and Newport, 1998; Saffran, Aslin, and Newport, 1996). These findings offer plausibility to our hypothesis that infants likewise capitalize on configural and statistical structure in the action domain to begin identifying distinct acts within the continuous flow of motion. Research under way with several colleagues directly investigates this possibility. If infants can indeed exploit structural regularities to identify relevant segments within continuous action, this will help to explain how they get started at achieving organized processing of the motion stream before they yet understand, at a conceptual level, the intentions being pursued on the actor's part.

Implications for Change Blindness
To this point, then, we have reviewed evidence indicating that both adults and infants spontaneously segment dynamic human action along intention boundaries and organize these units hierarchically. Segments—distinct acts within continuous motion—may be identified in part based on pattern recognition processes involving sensitivity to statistical and configural structure, and in part based on knowledge of the kinds of intentions given individuals are likely to undertake at given times in given contexts. Infants, lacking adults' enormous repertoire of world knowledge, are likely to rely more heavily on structure detection processes to guide segmentation, but presumably make use of their conceptual knowledge about intentions for segmentation purposes as it comes on line. Current evidence indicates that they do so at least as early as 9–12 months of age. A variety of predictions regarding change blindness, and possible developmental changes in change blindness, arise from these findings.

Intention Detection: Default? Automatic?   Intention-related processing of others' action should yield predictable effects concerning the loci of change blindness. Change blindness should be more likely to occur when goal-irrelevant changes are made to motion or context within an intentional action scenario. This prediction is consistent with the general finding that attentional focus predicts attenuation of change blindness (e.g., Pringle, Kramer, and Irwin, chapter 8, this volume; Rensink, O'Regan, and Clark, 1997; Scholl, 2000) because we expect attention will be preferentially directed toward goal-relevant aspects of intentional action. For example, an intention-laden interpretation of an actor approaching a mound of dirt with a shovel in hand might be that the actor intends to move the dirt with the aid of the shovel. In keeping with the analysis above, adults may be more likely to notice a change of the tool (e.g., into a rake) than a change of scenery (e.g., a tree changing locations). In other words, our reliance on intentional interpretations of human behavior may help us to detect changes relevant to such interpretations.

Of course, action scenarios, taken out of context, can be ambiguous with respect to what the actors' overarching intentions are. It should be possible to systematically influence the locus of change blindness by biasing viewers in advance toward one or another intentional interpretation. That is, goal-relevant aspects of motion and context will change depending on what intentions viewers are predisposed to attribute, and change blindness effects should change in concert.

Moreover, if we were to bias observers away from their default intention detection orientation toward some other mode of processing (e.g., asking people to report on the design features of the kitchen as opposed to reporting on the action), we might expect that the "standard" change blindness effects just described would be attenuated or entirely altered. A related question of real interest is the extent to which intention detection processing is actually under voluntary control. That is, at least certain aspects of intention-related processing may occur automatically, and if so, certain change blindness effects ought to be difficult to alter. Some evidence in fact exists regarding the automaticity of gaze direction detection (Driver et al., 1999; Langton and Bruce, 1999), which is a key component of intention-related processing of human action. The change blindness paradigm thus offers another methodology with which to examine such effects, and to further explore the extent to which intention detection is a relatively fixed default orientation in our approach to action processing.

A Window on Expertise and Development   If we are correct in suspecting that different intentional interpretations of dynamic action on the observer's part will determine the locus of change blindness, then we should expect the observer's knowledge to affect change blindness. One's depth of knowledge and level of understanding in a particular behavioral domain determines, in part, how richly structured one's intentional interpretation of a given action will be. For example, judges for Olympic-level gymnastic competitions possess representations of the intentional acts underlying gymnasts' athletic displays that are radically richer in structure than those of most ordinary observers.

Previous research on domain-specific expertise offers preliminary support for the proposal that different processing strategies might influence change blindness tendencies. In particular, expertise in a domain seems to change an individual's analysis of domain-relevant stimuli. For a domain of particular expertise adults display especially efficient processing and focused attention regarding domain-relevant features (e.g., Chase and Simon, 1973; Myles-Worsley, Johnston and Simons, 1988). Put another way, by using their domain-specific knowledge to guide them, experts may engage in more top-down processing of domain-relevant events than novices. For example, research into the effects of expertise on change blindness has revealed that experts in American football are faster to detect domain-relevant changes than novices, although they do not differ from novices on a change detection task involving scenes unrelated to football (Werner and Theis, 2000). Hence, there is starting evidence that expertise-based analysis strategies within domains influence change blindness tendencies.

To the extent that expertise influences change blindness, we should expect to see knowledge-related developmental differences in change blindness, as well. To illustrate, your and my interpretation of everyday acts such as supermarket checkout procedures will be significantly richer than that of a one-year-old child, in part because of our substantially greater knowledge of money, bar code technology, cash registers, and the like. This means we should expect to see significant developmental change in the locus of change blindness effects as children gain knowledge about action, and as their conceptual understanding of the intentions motivating action deepens. That is, adults ought to be more likely than young children to detect changes that have implications for an actor's central goal than changes that do not. Infants, in contrast, might show roughly equivalent levels of change blindness for goal-relevant and goal-irrelevant changes because they do not yet have the higher-level intentional interpretation to guide attention to goal-relevant aspects of a given scenario. In fact, this raises the counterintuitive possibility that infants' overall rates of change detection for intention-*irrelevant* changes may be higher than adults'. We are beginning to investigate these predicted developmental effects in collaboration with several others.

Another reason why change blindness in action processing should vary based on expertise is that lack of expertise should undercut our ability to direct processing toward information-rich "hot spots" within the motion stream. Put another way, processing that is less constrained may be associated with attention being more diffusely distributed across the action stimulus. Pringle, Kramer, and Irwin (chapter 8, this volume) found that breadth of attention predicts change blindness, with wider attentional breadth facilitating change detection. We might expect, then, that a novice would be more likely to detect changes at midpoints within the motion stream than would viewers who possess expertise in processing this form of action. That is, a novice in the realm of viewing gymnastics might well be better at detecting midpoint changes in Olympic gymnastic routines than would an official Olympics judge, although strikingly worse at interpreting the intentional content motivating the skater's motions. Infants, as "universal novices," might likewise distribute their attention more widely across the action stream and thus display an advantage in detecting midpoint changes relative to older children and adults with actions that are familiar, but conceptually challenging to process, such as supermarket checkout. If this pans out, it will then be possible to examine empirically the kinds of information and experience that promote enhanced action processing. That is, one could establish a novice pattern of processing, then manipulate the kind of input received concerning a given action, and subsequently detect learning by virtue of change blindness changes.

A Window on Structuring of Action   Research conducted by Zacks, Tversky, and Iyer (2001) also highlights the possibility that the gist extracted from action sequences might have implications for change blindness tendencies. Specifically, Zacks et al. (2001) found that adults vary their verbal descriptions of events depending on the hierarchical level of description they are instructed to provide. When asked to segment human action into coarse units (i.e., "the largest units that seem natural") adults' descriptions of events include specific information about objects and only general information about actions. In contrast, when they are asked to segment action into fine units (i.e., "the smallest units that seem natural"), adults supply more specific information about *actions* and more general information about objects. Zacks et al. (2001, p. 50; see also Newtson, 1973) interpreted these data as evidence that adults structure events hierarchically wherein "different objects are associated with different higher level functions or goals [and] different actions on the same object are associated with more refined functions or goals." Their findings yield a prediction regarding change blindness effects. In particular, if participants are told to focus on "large units of action," we should expect them to be faster to detect changes to the central object during a change detection task relative to when they are told to focus on small units. In contrast, if they are directed to "small units," we should expect adults to be faster to notice changes in a target action relative to when they are focused on large units. In sum, the particular hierarchical level at which action is processed might also have implications for the components of action toward which adults deploy their attention.

A Window on Segmentation of Dynamic Action   The evidence we discussed earlier regarding segmentation processes subserving adults' and infants' analysis of dynamic action also gives rise to some unique predictions regarding change blindness effects. Recall that Baird et al. (1999) found that adults are more accurate at recalling the location of tones placed at completion points within continuous intentional action than identical tones that interrupted intentional acts midstream, suggesting that completion points—boundaries between one intentional act and the next—have some special status in processing such action. Recall, as well, that 10- to 11-month-old infants spontaneously register completion points within continuous, intentional action (Baldwin et al., 2001; Saylor et al., 2002). These findings would seem to suggest that action processing targets the identification of completion points. It is likely, then, that completion points receive a disproportionate allotment of attentional resources relative to other portions of the motion stream. Given that change blindness appears to be attenuated when observers' attention is focused on change locations in a display (e.g., Scholl, 2000), one prediction is that observers might be more likely to detect changes inserted into completion points than comparable changes inserted into nontransition points of action sequences. Evidence reported by Newtson and Engquist (1976) is consistent with this idea, although it is important to note that these researchers interpreted their findings rather differently. They reported that adults are more likely to detect frames deleted from filmed intentional actions (e.g., motorcycle repair) when the deletions occur at "break points" (comparable to our notion of completion points) versus non-break points. However, one might question how general this result is. Frame deletions might generate this effect because of physical parameters associated with completion points, while other kinds of changes that alter physical parameters to the same degree at all points would not yield the effect. Research underway (Baldwin et al., in preparation) tests this issue via color changes rather than frame deletions. In pilot work, adults watched videos of everyday action (e.g., a woman peels a banana and eats it; a different woman packs clothing and shoes into a bag, zips it, and departs) into which color changes had been inserted into just one video frame. That is, the color shade of the hand in one particular frame was altered within a 30 frames/sec movie. Shade changes to the hand were either extreme and thus relatively easy to detect (e.g., the hand was made all pale yellow), or they were more subtle and hence more challanging to detect (e.g., the skin tone was slightly lightened). The frames including color changes occured either at points midstream within intentional acts or at points of completion dividing intentional acts (the completion point placements were derived from judgments of an independent group of adults asked simply to report on where goals and intentions were completed within the continuous flow of motion). When color changes were blatant, adults accurately detected them regardless of their position within the flow of intentional action, whereas when such changes were subtle, adults detected them significantly more often at completion points than at points midstream within intentional acts. These preliminary findings add to the Newtson and Engquist (1976) findings to confirm that processing resources are marshaled to identify boundaries between intentional acts in dynamic human action.

Completion points within intentional action may receive extra doses of attention for at least two, potentially compatible, reasons: (1) because they are central to the appropriate segmentation of the continuous flow; and (2) because of they may be especially information rich with respect to the content of actors' intentions. The seminal work of Newtson and Engquist (1976) provides some additional suggestive evidence that transition points are indeed information rich with respect to inferences about intentional content. When shown a series of still photographs depicting either only break points (at the transitions between intentional acts) or only non–break points (occurring in the midst of intentional acts) and asked to describe the overall action being carried out, adults were better able to divine the appropriate overall action when they viewed sequences of break point than non–break point stills. This finding hints that transitional phases within intentional action carry content-relevant information that is not available at points midstream in the execution of an intentional act. In other words, transitional information seems to be especially helpful in enabling observers to recognize what intention is being pursued. Interestingly, a direct analogue to this action recognition effect has been observed in object recognition. For example, Biederman (e.g., 1995) demonstrated that certain portions of an object's outline—the "junctures of concavity" that lie at boundaries between elemental "geon" units—are key to adults' ability to recognize objects. Deleting portions of objects' outlines at these junctures disrupts recognition to a greater degree than comparable deletions of nonjuncture portions. The emergence of parallel findings across object recognition and action recognition suggest that comparable mechanisms of higher-level interpretive processing are occurring in these cases. However, the Newtson and Engquist (1976) findings may not be informative about action processing in any kind of on-line, everyday sense, for the very reason that adults were not shown actual action, but instead saw only nondynamic depiction of several small slices of the original action stimulus. Whether these same effects would emerge if viewers were presented transitional versus nontransitional portions of action in full dynamic detail is an important question, one that is the focus of research under way.

Although it is unclear whether intention boundaries garner particular attention because they are important for segmentation, because they are information rich with respect to intentional content, or both, change blindness techniques offer a possible avenue for investigating this question. For example, certain actions seem to possess segmentable structure—like some kinds of modern dance—but at the same time seem to be largely devoid of any but the most global level of intentional content. On watching such actions, we can readily point to segments within the continuously flowing motion (e.g., the dancer hops, somersaults, sways back and forth sinuously, and the like). Yet we show little agreement about the intentional content of any of these individual acts and we tend to resist the request to interpret them. All that we tend to agree on is that the actor intends to dance. This asymmetry between what is segmentable and what is interpretable in terms of intentional content gives rise to unique predictions from the segmentation versus the intentional content accounts about the locus of change blindness effects. In the segmentation account, we should expect even for such content-sparse actions that change blindness will occur at higher rates for changes placed at segment boundaries—completion points—than for changes occurring midsegment. In the intentional account, change blindness differences for completion point versus midpoint changes should be reduced in content-sparse actions such as modern dance relative to content-rich everyday intentional actions such as kitchen cleanup.

Research using change blindness techniques with infants seems also to have the potential to address the debate as to whether completion points are privileged in processing because they are information rich, because they are crucial to segmentation, or both. As mentioned earlier, there are many action sequences infants cannot interpret in terms of higher-level intentional content: they cannot know what specific intention motivates the full action sequence simply because they do not know enough. Supermarket checkout actions, involving motions such as passing articles over a glass to be scanned to register their prices and pressing buttons on a cash register to complete a sale, again serve as an example. Infants cannot yet conceive of the intentions motivating these distinct acts, yet they may well be able to segment the flow of motion appropriately based on a sensitivity to structural information, inherent in the motion, that coincides with intention-relevant segments. If infants display greater change blindness for changes at completion points than at midpoints even for action sequences that place especially heavy demands on world knowledge they lack, this would support the segmentation account rather than the information-rich account.

Conclusion

We have proposed that both infants and adults process dynamic human action primarily to discern the goals and intentions motivating the actor's execution of that action. This proposal yields a range of predictions concerning the nature of the mechanisms subserving action processing and how attention will be allocated during such processing, which in turn leads to potential implications for change blindness. We suspect that action processing undergoes change—both in the course of normal human development and as a result of increasing expertise at any age with a specific type of action. Such expertise- and development-related changes in action processing seem likely to give rise to changes in change blindness. Techniques for probing change blindness—and the development of change blindness—thus may provide an altogether new window on basic processes subserving our processing of dynamic human action.

References

Asch, S. E. (1952). *Social psychology*. Englewood Cliffs, NJ: Prentice-Hall.

Aslin, R. N., Saffran, J. R., and Newport, E. L. (1998). Computation of conditional probability statistics by 8-month-old infants. *Psychological Science, 9*, 321–324.

Avrahami, J., and Kareev, Y. (1994). The emergence of events. *iCognition, 53*, 239–261.

Baird, J. A., and Baldwin, D. A. (2001). Making sense of human behavior: Action parsing and intentional inference. In B. F. Malle, L. J. Moses, and D. A. Baldwin (Eds.), *Intentions and intentionality: Foundations of social cognition* (pp. 193–206). Cambridge, MA: MIT Press.

Baird, J. A., Baldwin, D. A., and Malle, B. F. (1999). Adults' parsing of continuous action: The role of intention-based units. University of Oregon.

Baldwin, D. A., and Baird, J. A. (1999). Action analysis: A gateway to intentional inference. In P. Rochat (Ed.), *Early social cognition* (pp. 215–240). Hillsdale, NJ: Erlbaum.

Baldwin, D. A., and Baird, J. A. (2001). Discerning intentions in dynamic human action. *Trends in Cognitive Science, 5*, 171–178.

Baldwin, D. A., Baird, J. A., Saylor, M. M., and Clark, M. A. (2001). Infants detect structure in human action: A first step toward understanding others' intentions? *Child Development, 72*, 708–718.

Baldwin, D., Pederson, E., Craven, A., Andersson, A., and Walker, H. (In preparation). Adults display enhanced detection of changes at intention boundaries in dynamic human action. University of Oregon, Eugene, OR.

Baron-Cohen, S. (1995). *Mindblindness: An essay on autism and theory of mind*. Cambridge, MA: MIT Press.

Barresi, J., and Moore, C. (1996). Intentional relations and social understanding. *Behavioral and Brain Sciences, 19*, 107–154.

Biederman, I. (1995). Visual object recognition. In S. M. Kosslyn and D. N. Osherson, (Eds.), *Visual cognition: An invitation to cognitive science*. Vol. 2: *An invitation to cognitive science*. 2d ed. (pp. 121–165). Cambridge, MA: MIT Press.

Chase, W. G., and Simon, H. A. (1973). Perception in chess. *Cognitive Psychology, 4*, 55–81.

Driver, J., Davis, G., Ricciardelli, P., Kidd, P., Maxwell, E., and Baron-Cohen, S. (1999). Gaze perception triggers reflexive visuospatial orienting. *Visual Cognition, 6*, 509–540.

Grimes, J. (1996). One the failure to detect changes in scenes across saccades. In K. Akins (Ed.), *Perception: Vancouver studies in cognitive science*. Vol. 2 (pp. 89–110). New York: Oxford Press.

Heider, F. (1958). *The psychology of interpersonal relations*. New York: Wiley.

Henderson, J. M., Weeks, P. A., and Hollingworth, A. (1999). The effects of semantic consistency on eye movements during complex scene viewing. *Human Perception and Performance, 25*, 210–228.

Hirsh-Pasek, K., Kemler-Nelson, K. D., Jusczyk, P. W., Wright-Cassidy, K., Druss, B., and Kennedy, L. (1987). Clauses and perceptual units for young infants. *Cognition, 26*, 269–286.

Jusczyk, P. W. (1997). *The discovery of spoken language*. Cambridge, MA: MIT Press.

Jusczyk, P. W., Hirsh-Pasek, K., Kemler-Nelson, K. D., Kennedy, L., Woodward, A., and Piwoz, J. (1992). Perception of acoustic correlates of major phrasal units by young infants. *Cognitive Psychology, 24*, 252–293.

Kuhl, P. K., and Meltzoff, A. N. (1984). The intermodal representation of speech in infants. *Infant Behavior and Development, 7*, 361–381.

Langton, S. R. H., and Bruce, V. (1999). Reflexive visual orienting in response to the social attention of others. *Visual Cognition, 6*, 541–567.

Levin, D. T., and Simons, D. J. (1997). Failure to detect changes to attended objects in motion pictures. *Psychonomic Bulletin and Review, 4*, 501–506.

Mack, A., and Rock, I. (1998). *Inattentional blindness*. Cambridge, MA: MIT Press.

Myles-Worsley, M., Johnston, W. A., and Simons, M. A. (1988). The influence of expertise on X-ray image processing. *Journal of Experimental Psychology: Learning, Memory, and Cognition, 14*, 553–557.

Newtson, D. (1973). The dynamics of action and interaction. In L. B. Smith and E. Thelan (Eds.), *A dynamic systems approach to development: Applications* (pp. 241–264). Cambridge, MA: MIT Press.

Newtson, D., and Engquist, G. (1976). The perceptual organization of ongoing behavior. *Journal of Experimental Social Psychology, 12*, 436–450.

Newtson, D., Engquist, G., and Bois, J. (1977). The objective basis of behavior units. *Journal of Personality and Social Psychology, 35*, 847–862.

Norris, D., McQueen, J. M., and Cutler, A. (2000). Merging information in speech recognition: Feedback is never necessary. *Behavioral and Brain Sciences, 23*, 299–370.

Premack, D. (1990). The infant's theory of self-propelled objects. *Cognition, 36*, 1–16.

Rensink, R. A., O'Regan, J. K., and Clark, J. J. (1997). To see or not to see: The need for attention to perceive changes in scenes. *Psychological Science, 8*, 368–373.

Saffran, J. R., Aslin, R. N., and Newport, E. L. (1996). Statistical learning by 8-month-old infants. *Science, 274*, 1926–1928.

Saylor, M. M., Baird, J. A., Killingsworth, J., and Baldwin, D. A. (2002). Infants' on-line parsing of dynamic human action in an intermodal matching paradigm. University of Oregon.

Scholl, B. (2000). Attenuated change blindness for exogenously attended items in a flicker paradigm. *Visual Cognition, 7*, 377–396.

Sharon, T., and Wynn, K. (1998). Individuation of actions from continuous motion. *Psychological Science, 9*, 357–362.

Simons, D. J. (2000). Current approaches to change blindness. *Visual Cognition, 7*, 1–15.

Simons, D. J., and Levin, D. T. (1997). Change blindness. *Trends in Cognitive Sciences, 1*, 261–267.

Simons, D. J., and Levin, D. T. (1998). Failure to detect changes to people during real-world interactions. *Psychonomic Bulletin and Review, 5,* 644–649.

Spelke, E. S. (1979). Perceiving bimodally specified events in infancy. *Developmental Psychology, 15,* 626–636.

Spelke, E. S., Born, W. S., and Chu, F. (1983). Perception of moving, sounding objects by four-month-old infants. *Perception, 12,* 719–732.

Spelke, E. S., and Owsley, C. J. (1979). Intermodal exploration and knowledge in infancy. *Infant Behavior and Development, 2,* 13–27.

Tomasello, M. (1999). Having intentions, understanding intentions, and understanding communicative intentions. In P. Zelazo, J. Astington, and D. R. Olson (Eds.), *Developing theories of intention* (pp. 63–76). Mahwah, NJ: Erlbaum.

Werner, S., and Thies, B. (2000). Is "change blindness" attenuated by domain specific expertise? An expert-novice comparison of change detection in football images. *Visual Cognition, 7,* 163–173.

Wynn, K. (1995). Infants possess a system of numerical knowledge. *Current Directions in Psychological Science, 4,* 172–177.

Wynn, K. (1996). Infants' individuation and enumeration of actions. *Psychological Science, 7,* 164–169.

Zacks, J., and Tversky, B. (2001). Event structure in perception and conception. *Trends in Cognitive Sciences, 5,* 171–178.

Zacks, J., Tversky, B., and Iyer, G. (2001). Perceiving, remembering and communicating structure in events. *Journal of Experimental Psychology: General, 130,* 29–58.

Chapter 3

Young Children's Awareness of Their Own Lexical Ignorance: Relations to Word Mapping, Memory Processes, and Beliefs about Change Detection

William E. Merriman and John M. Marazita

The only good is knowledge and the only evil ignorance.

True knowledge exists in knowing that you know nothing. And in knowing that you know nothing, that makes you the wisest of all.

These well-known quotations of Socrates underscore the importance that the great philosopher placed on constant vigilance against ignorance. Modern cognitive psychologists have also emphasized the value of monitoring one's ignorance or lack of understanding when processing texts or messages (Flavell et al., 1981; Klin, Guzman, and Levine, 1997; Maki, 1998; Markman, 1981) or when attempting to master some body of knowledge (Nelson, 1996; Son and Metcalfe, 2000).

There have been few studies of preschool-age children's awareness of ignorance. In our investigations of the constraints that govern early word learning, we stumbled upon a link between preschoolers' awareness of ignorance and the consistency with which they chose a particular solution to a word reference problem: children who acknowledged their ignorance of novel words mapped them onto novel rather than familiar kinds more consistently than did other children (Merriman and Schuster, 1991). When asked, "Do you know what a zav is?" for example, those who said, "No," were more likely than the others to select a garlic press rather than a cup as the more likely referent of this term.

In this chapter, we will review recent work that has built upon this finding in various ways. We have obtained evidence for a more general construct, awareness of lexical ignorance, that not only encompasses the ability to identify a word as unknown, but also to identify something as having no known name. Age-related differences in these abilities have been documented, and a cognitive process that may underlie them has been explored. We have investigated preschoolers' estimation of their agemates' awareness of lexical ignorance, and have explored ways of promoting awareness. The results of follow-up studies of the tendency to map novel names onto novel kinds and to justify such mappings in terms of name knowledge have led us to hypothesize that those who possess more efficient basic memory processes are the first to become aware of their own lexical ignorance. Finally, the results of an empirical test of this last hypothesis not only provided support for it, but also revealed a possible link between such awareness and beliefs about change detection.

Developmental Trends in Two Types of Awareness

Children may be well served by the realization that they do not know the meaning of some word. It may save them from wasting effort trying to retrieve a meaning, and prompt them to request it or engage in contextual problem solving aimed at figuring it out. Also, such awareness might compel them to give more attention to the word, and any semantic information that might be introduced about it. These processes could also work in the opposite direction, from meaning to word. Youngsters may sense that they do not know the word to express some meaning or denote some referent, and such an insight may prevent them from conducting a vain search of memory for it. Such awareness might also prompt them to request the word, and increase the likelihood that the word and the link to its meaning or referent would be retained. We shall refer to the belief that some meaning lacks a word as "meaning-cued awareness" of lexical ignorance, and the belief that some word lacks a meaning as "word-cued awareness."

Word-Cued Awareness

When Smith and Tager-Flusberg (1982) asked preschoolers, "Is •• a word?" for each member in a list of familiar and novel (made-up) words, 4-year-olds answered correctly at a higher rate (.81) than 3-year-olds (.64). Chaney (1992) observed a comparable age difference in a similar task. Although results for familiar words were not separated from those for made-up ones in these two studies, most likely, the novel words gave the children more trouble than the familiar ones. Merriman and Bowman (1989, study 2) tested whether 2-, 2½- and 3-year-olds would say they knew familiar and unfamiliar words, then asked them to select exemplars for them. Even the oldest group rarely identified unfamiliar words as ones they did not know (.28), more often saying that they knew them (.48), although they did accept familiar words significantly more often than unfamiliar ones. The two groups of 2-year-olds rarely rejected either type of word, and did not accept familiar words significantly more often than unfamiliar ones. There was evidence of some awareness in the older 2-year-olds, however. Although nine produced identical patterns of response to familiar and unfamiliar labels, acceptances by the remaining seven exceeded rejections by a slightly greater margin for familiar than for unfamiliar labels ($p < .005$). The same pattern was evident in the 3-year-olds, but not in the younger 2-year-olds. These results are consistent with findings from transcript analyses of early spontaneous uses of the verb *know* (Bartsch and Wellman, 1995; Brown and Dunn, 1991; Furrow et al., 1992; Shatz, Wellman, and Silber, 1983). The first uses of this verb that clearly make reference to belief occur a few months before the third birthday, and such uses increase dramatically in the subsequent 18 months.

These trends have been corroborated. Marazita and Merriman (forthcoming) had 4-year-olds and 2½-year-olds listen to a story that contained familiar and novel (made-up) words, and after each sentence, say whether they knew one or two words in it. Merriman and Evey (in preparation) and Merriman and Brown (in preparation) administered this task to 4- and 3-year-olds. The 4-year-olds in these three studies virtually always accepted familiar words ($M = .92$), and tended not to accept novel ones (.24), whereas the 3-year-olds were nearly as accepting of familiar words (.83), but accepted about twice as many novel ones (.51). The 2½-year-olds tested by Marazita and Merriman, forthcoming, mostly accepted both types of words (.85 and .79, respectively; n.s.). As in Merriman and Bowman, 1989, study 2, most of these 2½-year-olds responded identically to the two types of words. Of those who did not, 8 accepted more familiar than unfamiliar words, whereas 4 children showed the opposite pattern. Although this finding was in the same direction as in the previous study, it was not significant. Thus 3-year-olds and older 2-year-olds may find it more difficult to identify a word as unknown when it has just occurred in a meaningful story than when it has not. Or perhaps the 2½-year-olds' repeated experience in Merriman and Bowman, 1989, study 2, of having to choose the novel word's referent after being asked whether they knew the word helped them to tune into their ignorance of it.

Meaning-Cued Awareness
Language transcripts indicate that some form of meaning-cued awareness may develop very early. One of the requests most frequently made by 1- and 2-year-olds is for something's name (i.e., "What dat?") (Brown, 1968; Smith, 1933). It is also among the most frequent requests that parents direct to their children (Brown, 1968). Presumably, toddlers ask for something's name when their own attempts to name it falter. What is not clear is whether they realize that they are doing this, that is, whether they believe that they do not know the name for something because they cannot generate a name for it. The same can be said about 2-year-olds' "invented" words (e.g., *darking* for the act of making something dark; Clark, 1982; 1993). It is not clear in these cases that the children believe they do not know the conventional forms that would convey the meanings they have in mind.

We have assessed youngsters' meaning-cued awareness. Marazita and Merriman (forthcoming) showed drawings of familiar and unfamiliar objects to 4- and 2½-year-olds, and asked them, "Do you know the name for this kind of thing?" Merriman and Evey (in preparation) and Merriman and Brown (in prepartion) administered this same task to 4- and 3-year-olds, and Marazita and Merriman (in preparation), to 4-year-olds. The oldest group's responses were similar to those for word-cued awareness: familiar objects were nearly always identified as having known names (.92), and unfamiliar objects were usually not

(.34). The younger children also nearly always claimed to know names for the familiar objects (.87 and .89 for the 3- and 2½-year-olds, respectively), but often also claimed this for the unfamiliar objects (.60 and .70, respectively). In even the youngest group, however, significantly more familiar than unfamiliar objects were identified as having known names.

Performance on the word- and object-cued tests was strongly linked in the 4- and 3-year-olds, suggesting that a common construct ties them together. For the four samples in this age range, correlation coefficients ranged from .55 to .72, and remained significant when receptive vocabulary size was partialed out, indicating that the underlying construct was not verbal ability, but something more specific. For the 2½-year-olds, the association may have been attenuated because of near-floor performance on the word-cued test, although the 8 of 32 children in this age group who identified more familiar than unfamiliar words as known also produced a significantly higher rate of correct responses on the object-cued test (.69) than the other children (.56). This relation also remained significant, by a one-tailed test, when receptive vocabulary size was partialed out.

For this chapter, we analyzed data from a published study of 4-year-olds' tendency to map novel verbs onto novel rather than familiar kinds of actions (Merriman, Marazita, and Jarvis, 1993, study 1). After the mapping test in this study, participants were asked, "What's she doing?" regarding each action presented in the test. For the actions they could not name, children varied considerably in whether they responded, "I don't know," which was considered a measure of meaning-cued awareness of lexical ignorance. This measure was significantly correlated not only with word-cued awareness (i.e., rate of responding, "No," when asked whether they knew various novel verbs) ($r = .60$), but also with the tendency to map novel verbs onto novel kinds ($r = .59$). Thus the unity of the awareness-of-lexical-ignorance construct in 4-year-olds is not limited to object reference, but also extends to action reference.

Explaining the Developmental Trends: Inference from a Global Impression of Novelty
Both the age-related increase in awareness and the increasing correlation between its two measures may be at least in part due to the acquisition of an additional means for judging lexical ignorance. Most 2- and 3-year-olds may only identify a lexical stimulus as unknown if they note their failure to generate its corresponding information. That is, they may need to notice that no specific semantic information for an unfamiliar word, or specific name for an unfamiliar referent or meaning, comes to mind. Although skill in detecting such mental nonoccurrences, or nonretrievals, ought to increase as experience with known and unknown stimuli accumulates, many preschoolers may be further assisted by a tendency to infer ignorance from a rapid, global impression of novelty that an unfamiliar stimulus evokes. There is considerable evidence that adults use such impressions to make a variety of quick decisions about their own knowledge (Jacoby, Woloshyn, and Kelley, 1989; Reder, 1987; Schwartz and Metcalfe, 1992).

In support of this proposal, Marazita and Merriman (forthcoming) found that the object-cued awareness of 4-year-olds, but not 2½-year-olds, was undermined by preexposure to unfamiliar kinds of objects. Only the older group was more likely to say that they knew the names for these objects when they had viewed them before the test than when they had not. If judgments had been based only on noting the nonretrieval of names, preexposure would not have undermined them. If anything, preexposure would have primed object encoding, making more resources available with which to note that the object's name could not be retrieved.

The claim that many 4-year-olds have some tendency to infer knowledge of an object's name from an immediate, global impression of the object's familiarity is consistent with evidence that this age group can make moderately accurate feeling-of-knowing judgments. Cultice, Somerville, and Wellman (1983) asked 4- and 5-year-olds to name photographs of persons. When the children could not name one, the children were asked to predict whether they could recognize the name "if I told you a lot of names." When given this very test, they recognized more of the names they predicted they would than of the ones they predicted they would not. Their predictions could not have been based on nonretrieval of these names: the children were only asked to make predictions for the names they had failed to recall. The predictions must have been based on a global feeling of familiarity that the photographs evoked, on whether information other than their names came to mind, or on both. We know of no studies of feeling-of-knowing judgments by children under 4.

Judgment of Another's Lexical Ignorance

This type of judgment has been explored in only one study, Merriman and Brown, in preparation, and only for word-cued awareness. When participants were asked to indicate whether "another kid who's [that child's age]" would know familiar and made-up words, both 3- and 4-year-olds tended to answer the same way as they did for themselves (rate of match = .91). There was a modest, but significant trend for the 3-year-olds to say more often that another child would know the made-up words than to claim this knowledge for themselves, whereas 4-year-olds would only occasionally respond this way and would also occasionally respond that another child would not know a familiar word that they themselves knew, a response that was very rare among the 3-year-olds.

The willingness to suppose that another child might know something that they themselves did not, or vice versa, is compatible with what Flavell and colleagues (Flavell, 1974; Masangkay et al., 1974) have dubbed "level-1" knowledge of visual perception. Most 2-year-olds possess level-1 knowledge, namely, the knowledge that, because seeing requires an unobstructed line of sight, another person may not see what one sees, and vice versa. They understand that only one of two people may know what is in a picture, for example, if the front of it is blocked for one of the viewers, and can represent a social situation as involving unshared ignorance.

The finding that 3-year-olds grant their agemates knowledge they admit to not possessing themselves is somewhat inconsistent, however, with their general tendency to view peers as less knowledgeable than themselves. For example, Gopnik and Astington (1988) allowed preschoolers to discover an object's deceptive identity (e.g., that what looked like a rock was really a sponge), then asked them what they first thought it was, as well as what someone else, who had not touched it, would think it was. They were more likely to judge that the other person would be fooled than to report that they themselves had been taken in.

Three-year-olds may be more likely to notice when another child has used an unfamiliar word than to notice when they themselves have used a word that another child does not understand. In the latter case, the listener may produce either no sign of comprehension failure or one the speaker fails to detect or interpret as such. The speaker may be preoccupied with the demands of speaking. In contrast, when they hear a child use an unfamiliar word, 3-year-olds' attention may be drawn to it as the cause of their failure to comprehend the child's message.

Experiences That May Promote Awareness

Merriman and Brown (in preparation) transformed the object-cued awareness test into a sorting task. Participants had to place objects into either a "know" bucket, which was marked with a picture of a self-satisfied child who was described as knowing names for things, or a "don't know" bucket, which had on it a picture of a puzzled child who did not know names for things. Corrective feedback was provided. Whereas 4-year-olds performed virtually perfectly on this task—better than they typically do when simply asked, "Do you know a name for this?"—3-year-olds did not perform substantially better than before.

It does not appear that 4-year-olds' better performance was due to the provision of corrective feedback. Nearly every child placed the first unfamiliar test object into the "don't know" bucket, compared to the two-thirds or so who have said they did not know the name for this object in our previous studies. So it must have been some other feature or features of the procedure that promoted object-cued awareness. It was probably the use of pictures to explain the difference between knowing and not knowing, although it could have been requiring participants to sort rather than to give yes-or-no responses. The latter explanation does not seem likely in light of the repeated demonstrations by Zelazo and colleagues (Jacques et al., 1999; Zelazo, Reznick, and Pinon, 1995) that young children find it more difficult to sort according to a rule than to make direct verbal judgments of how the rule applies.

Merriman and Evey (in preparation) found that more 3- and 4-year-olds showed word-cued awareness when they were first tested for their ability to repeat made-up words (e.g., "perplisteronk") than when they were not. The repetition test was developed by Baddeley, Gathercole, and colleagues (Baddeley, Papagno, and Vallar, 1988; Gathercole and Baddeley, 1990; Gathercole, 1995) as a measure of phonological short-term memory. Because instructions for this test identified the stimuli as "made-up words," it may have given the children a better idea both of what unfamiliar words sound like and of what kinds of cognitions they evoke— and, more important, fail to evoke.

Merriman and colleagues (1996) asked 24-month-olds whether they knew novel (unfamiliar) verbs before asking them to select an exemplar from a filmed pair of actions, one novel and the other familiar. In experiments 2–4, rates of denying knowledge of the verbs were very low, and similar to those reported for novel (unfamiliar) nouns, whereas, in experiment 1, the denial rate was significantly higher and was positively correlated with the rate of mapping novel verbs onto novel rather than familiar movements. A unique feature of experiment 1 was that, before the test, a film of six novel actions was presented three times. The intriguing possibility is that this experience promoted meaning-cued awareness of lexical ignorance, which in turn, promoted word-cued awareness. Viewing so many novel actions may have led some young 2-year-olds to realize that they did not know labels for these actions, which promoted the subsequent realization that they did not know meanings for the novel test verbs. The basis for this positive transfer may be that both novel actions and novel verbs fail to evoke a familiar, salient counterpart. The actions caused no verb to come to mind, and the verbs caused no actions to come to mind. The finding is also intriguing because it suggests that the capacity to comprehend the verb *know* in reference to mental states may be present near the second birthday, well before the age 2–9 to 3–0 suggested by analyses of child transcripts (Bartsch and Wellman, 1995; Brown and Dunn, 1991; Furrow et al., 1992; Shatz et al., 1983).

Relations to Novel Word Mapping

In Merriman et al., 1996, experiment 1, where young 2-year-olds displayed the highest levels of word-cued awareness, the more highly aware participants mapped novel verbs onto novel objects more consistently. Likewise, in Merriman and Bowman, 1989, study 2, the 2½- and 3-year-olds who admitted knowing more familiar than novel labels mapped the latter onto unfamiliar objects more often than did their agemates. Merriman and colleagues have also tested numerous samples of 4-year-olds on tests in which the children had, first, to say whether they know some novel word, then, to select its likely referent from a pair of novel (unfamiliar) and familiar kinds. Excluding a sample in which the rate of selecting novel kinds was at ceiling, and another in which the words were made to sound like the names of the familiar test objects, the average correlation between rates of denying knowledge of the novel words and mapping them onto novel kinds was .41, $p < .001$ (Marazita and Merriman, in preparation; Merriman and Bowman,

1989, study 1; Merriman and Schuster, 1991; Merriman, Marazita, and Jarvis 1993, three samples).

In Merriman and Bowman, 1989, study 4, after every trial in which a novel kind was selected as the likely referent of a test word, the experimenter asked, "How do you know this one is [, for example,] the zav?" Two types of answers were common: citing the familiar object's name (e.g., "Because this one [pointing to the familiar object] is a cup") and noting a property of the novel object (e.g., "Because it [pointing to the novel object] has balls inside"). Among the 4-year-olds, but not among the 2½-year-olds, those who showed greater awareness of word unfamiliarity offered the first type—familiar name justifications—more often than the other children.

Marazita and Merriman (forthcoming) also found that familiar name justifications were positively correlated with both word-cued and object-cued awareness in 4-year-olds, and that none of these measures was associated with general intelligence. Among 2½-year-olds, all who said they knew more familiar than novel (unfamiliar) words (6 of 6) offered at least one familiar name justification for novel word mapping, whereas only 7 of the 15 children who showed no word-cued awareness ever offered such a justification, Φ ($N = 22$) = .50, $p < .05$. In contrast to the 4-year-olds, the 2½-year-olds' object-cued awareness was not associated with familiar name justifications, and was as strongly related to general intelligence as to word-cued awareness. The reason a relation between word-cued awareness and justifications was obtained in Marazita and Merriman, forthcoming, but not in Merriman and Bowman, 1989, may be that a more valid measure of awareness was used: the latter study only asked participants whether they knew novel words, whereas the former asked them this about familiar words as well.

Why do children who know that they do not know novel words tend to map them onto novel kinds more consistently, and offer familiar name justifications for doing so? One reason may be that they tend to represent the mapping problem in terms of their own ignorance. They may encode the novel word as "one I don't know," the novel object as "one I don't know," and the familiar object as "one I know," then select the object that has the same description as the word. This metacognitive solution may reinforce an earlier developing solution that is simply based on avoiding label overlap (i.e., upholding the Mutual Exclusivity principle; see Markman and Wachtel, 1988; Merriman and Bowman, 1989).

Alternatively, the correlation may be explicable in terms of a third variable, efficient retrieval processes, which may independently promote awareness of lexical awareness and consistent label overlap avoidance. Karmiloff-Smith (1986) has argued that, because any particular metacognition will not develop until the cognition on which it is based has become overlearned, children may not take their failure to retrieve some piece of lexical information as a sign of ignorance until such retrieval processes have become overlearned. The more rapidly and reliably children retrieve the meanings of familiar words, the easier it should be for them to learn that not being able to retrieve a meaning for a word signifies ignorance of the word. Independent of these developments, efficient retrieval might promote avoidance of label overlap because such avoidance requires retrieving a familiar object's name and noting its mismatch with the novel word being mapped. If children fail either to retrieve the name or to compare it to the novel word in working memory, they will not realize there is any overlap to avoid. The next section presents, evidence for a link between awareness of lexical ignorance and retrieval efficiency.

Relations to Memory Processes

An intriguing correlational pattern led us to hypothesize that awareness of lexical ignorance might be related to the efficiency of basic memory processes. In many of our word mapping studies, half of the unfamiliar objects or actions, but none of the familiar ones, were presented for a few minutes before the test began. Our original motive for this preexposure manipulation was to examine whether youngsters would map novel words onto novel kinds (ones that they could not already name) or novel tokens (specific individuals that they had never encountered before) when these two types of novelty opposed each other.

In Merriman et al., 1993, study 1, as well as in a control condition of their study 2, 4-year-olds selected novel kinds less frequently on such opposition trials than on trials in which the choices differed only in kind novelty (i.e., in whether the choices had known names). On average, preexposure reduced the rate of selecting unfamiliar kinds from .85 to .70. However, in the "action context" condition of study 2, as well as in Marazita and Merriman, in preparation, 4-year-olds performed nearly identically on the two types of trials. Also, in Merriman and Schuster, 1991, preexposure reduced 4-year-olds' mapping rate from .90 to .77 when the familiar choice objects were typical-looking exemplars of their names, but did not alter it when the familiar objects were atypical-looking.

Our post hoc explanation was that preexposure had two opposing effects. It reduced preschoolers' tendency to select the unfamiliar kinds in the mapping test because it made these choices seem less novel. That is, it reduced the global impression of novelty that we believe only the more aware children consult. The countervailing effect was hypothesized to be repetition priming, that is, preexposure was presumed to reduce the difficulty of encoding these stimuli when they were encountered again in the mapping test. The two effects should have worked against each other in tests in which it was difficult to encode the choice stimuli and perform the other operations needed to reject the familiar choice (such as retrieving its name and noting the mismatch with the test word).

Consistent with this conjecture, the conditions in which preexposure did not undermine word mapping were those in which the difficulty of encoding the choices at test was greater. For example, encoding was presumably more difficult in the "action context" than in the control condition of Merriman et al., 1993, study

2. In the former condition, children had to pick out a novel noun's referent from a pair of simultaneous videotapes in which different objects were being addressed by the same action. For example, they were asked, "Show me the one of the man patting the jegger," regarding someone patting a spoon versus someone patting a garlic press. In the control condition, a pair of videotaped static objects was presented, and a simple object request was posed (e.g., "Show me the jegger").

Encoding difficulty was also presumably greater when the familiar choices were atypical- rather than typical-looking. The children would have needed to sustain attention longer to establish a visual representation of an atypical object and retrieve its name than to do so for a typical one. As noted, a negative preexposure effect was only found with typical-looking objects. Also, in Marazita and Merriman, in preparation, where no effect of preexposure was observed, all of the familiar choice objects were atypical-looking. In Merriman et al., 1993, study 2, where the effect was observed in static contexts, the objects were typical-looking.

What was the evidence linking awareness of lexical ignorance to the efficiency of retrieval processes? The correlation between word-cued awareness and consistency of mapping novel words onto unfamiliar objects was lower for preexposed than for non-preexposed unfamiliar objects *only when it was relatively easy to encode these objects*. As noted, the easy encoding conditions were also the ones in which preexposure reduced children's tendency to map novel labels onto unfamiliar objects.

This correlational pattern can be explained if the two hypothesized effects of preexposure (global novelty reduction and repetition priming) were actually greater in those children who were more aware of their own lexical ignorance. On the word mapping problems in which it was rather easy to encode the choice objects, only reduced novelty should have influenced performance. On these problems, those with greater awareness were more negatively affected by preexposure than those with lesser awareness. Hence the correlations were lower for preexposed than for non-preexposed trials. On mapping problems in which encoding was more difficult and the positive effect of repetition priming should have offset the effect of reduced novelty, the correlations were no different for preexposed than for non-preexposed trials because repetition priming was stronger among the children with higher levels of awareness.

Repetition priming occurs to the extent that children's encoding of an object at test benefits from activation of the representation they initially formed of the object during preexposure. That is, superior encoding and retrieval processes are responsible for superior repetition priming. Thus our claim that children who are more aware of their ignorance have superior repetition priming implies that they should also have superior encoding and retrieval processes.

If this conclusion is valid, then awareness of lexical ignorance ought to be positively correlated with recognition memory, which is considered an index of basic encoding and retrieval efficiency. In Marazita and Merriman, in preparation, which examined this link by using a short-term visual recognition test, also known as "successive perceptual matching" (Krueger and Chignell, 1985), 4-year-olds were told that they would see drawings of two objects one after the other, and instructed to say whether the pairs were the same or different. On each trial, the first picture appeared for 2.25 sec, the screen was dark for 2.75 sec, then the second picture appeared. "Different" pairs shared the same basic configuration of parts, but differed in the size, shading, or styling of a part or two. Both the word- and object-cued tests of awareness were associated with recognition ($r = .32$ and $.34$, respectively; both $p < .05$). Children who averaged above the median on the awareness tests answered correctly on recognition trials more often (.73) than the lower-scoring children did (.61). Receptive vocabulary size was also related to matching ($r = .28$; $p = .05$), but an awareness score based on the two tests combined remained significantly related to matching by a one-tailed test when receptive vocabulary size was partialed out.

Relations to Beliefs about Change Detection

In the recognition test just described, the high- and low-awareness children differed on "same" trials, where their rate correct averaged .89 and .65, respectively, but responded identically on "different" trials, where it averaged .58 for both groups. So not only were they more accurate overall, but the high-awareness preschoolers showed a bias to respond "same" on this test. This bias may be indicative of a belief that perceptual impressions of stimulus change are less reliable than perceptual impressions of stimulus constancy, at least in some circumstances. According to Krueger (see Krueger and Chignel, 1985; Krueger, Stadtlander, and Blum, 1992), because encoding processes are not perfect, mental representations of the first or second picture of a perceptual matching trial can be distorted. Errors can also occur in the process of comparing the two representations. Such "noisy" encoding and comparison processes are more likely to cause identical stimuli to appear different than to cause mismatching stimuli to appear identical. The latter mistake would only occur if both the first and second picture happened to be distorted by noise in the very same way. For this reason, adults trust their impressions of sameness, or constancy, more than their impressions of difference, or change. This disposition may contribute to adults' difficulty detecting change, or change blindness (Simons and Levin, 1998), in situations where they suspect that a change may have occurred, but are unsure.

Under some conditions, as when a pair of pictures is presented very rapidly, or the pictures are extremely complex, adults may decide that they have failed to encode all of the features of one or both of the pictures. In these cases, according to Krueger, Stadtlander, and Blum (1992), adults often attribute an impression that the pictures differ to having missed a feature in one, but detected it in the other, and so discount the impression of change. If time or memory does not permit a recheck of the perceived change, they tend to decide that the pictures match.

Preschool-age children who are the first to become aware of their own lexical ignorance may also tend to be the first to realize that their impressions of stimulus change can be wrong. Both this realization and the judgment of lexical ignorance presuppose an appreciation of representational inadequacy. In the case of lexical ignorance, representations are inadequate because they are incomplete (e.g., no meaning is stored with some word). In the case of illusory change, representations are inadequate because they do not match reality. In both cases, detection of the inadequacy requires noting how one's own representation of a stimulus falls short of some ideal representation.

To learn that one's perceptions of change are sometimes illusory may depend on having "false novelty" experiences, ones in which a stimulus initially appears to be novel, but is later discovered to be familiar. For example, preschoolers may not at first recognize a person, but after further processing, realize who it is. Or they may look for a toy where they left it, and decide it is not there (i.e., that the situation has changed), but then look again, and find it. Or someone else may point out their error. Such experiences may teach them to distrust their own impressions of change, or novelty, and cause them to recheck stimuli before deciding that they really are new or different. Preschoolers may not understand why their impressions of change can be false (e.g., noise in encoding or comparison, failure to detect a feature); our claim is only that some preschoolers have taken the first step of learning to recheck them. They can only learn this lesson if they contrast mismatching initial and subsequent representations of the same stimulus. Likewise, they can only learn what it means to not know something if they contrast their representations of unfamiliar things, which lack a certain type of information, with their representations of familiar things, which possess that information.

Gopnik and Astington (1988) and Wimmer and Hartl (1991) found that most 4-year-olds, but only a minority of 3-year-olds, were able to remember their initial representations of a deceptive situation. That is, after the deception was revealed, the 3-year-olds tended to insist that they initially held the true belief about the situation. Better performance has been elicited from 3-year-olds by rewording the questions (Lewis and Osborne, 1990) or by having them mail a card depicting their false belief right after forming it (Mitchell and Lacohee, 1991). Nevertheless, recall of one's own inaccurate representation of a situation increases over the preschool years. Being able to recall an inadequate representation is a prerequisite for comparing it with the adequate one, and learning a lesson about the potential inadequacy of representations.

Conclusions

Word- and object-cued awareness begin to emerge toward the last quarter of the third year, and increase substantially over the next two years. These types of awareness are strongly associated with each other, at least after the third birthday, even with statistical adjustments made for their relations to vocabulary size. Emergence of a tendency to infer one's own ignorance from a rapid, global impression of novelty may underlie the developmental increase in these types of awareness, as well as the increasing association between them. Preexposure was found to reduce object-cued awareness in older, but not in younger, preschoolers.

By and large, preschoolers project their own instances of name knowledge and ignorance onto children their own age, with 3-year-olds being more likely to grant knowledge to agemates that they do not claim for themselves than to do the opposite. This asymmetry may reflect the greater frequency of experiences in which another child is discovered to "know a word I don't know" than to "not know a word I know." Although no studies have directly examined ways of promoting awareness of lexical ignorance, the highest levels of awareness have been documented in studies where certain procedures may have boosted it. These procedures have included using pictures of knowing and puzzled children to teach the "know/not know" distinction, and presenting a series of unfamiliar words or kinds before testing awareness.

Those who show greater awareness of their lexical ignorance also tend to map novel words onto novel kinds more consistently, and to justify such mappings in terms of name knowledge. These associations may reflect individual differences in the application of a metacognitive solution to word mapping, in the efficiency of basic retrieval processes, on in both. The more rapidly and reliably that lexical information is retrieved, the easier it should be to learn that nonretrieval signifies ignorance. Indirect support for the retrieval efficiency hypothesis was found in the manner in which correlations between word-cued awareness and the consistency of mapping novel words onto novel kinds depended on whether the novel kinds had been preexposed. Direct support was obtained in a study documenting a positive association between awareness of lexical ignorance and visual recognition, an index of basic encoding and retrieval efficiency.

Awareness was also related to a "same" response bias in visual recognition judgments, suggesting that preschoolers who are more aware of their own ignorance may also be less willing to trust their own impressions of stimulus change in some circumstances. Krueger and colleagues have argued for the rationality of placing less trust in impressions of change than in impressions of constancy in the recognition task that we used. Development of a general appreciation for the potential inadequacy of representations may underlie the link between children's awareness of their own lexical ignorance and their distrust in perceptions of change.

Future Directions

Although very few young 2-year-olds show an awareness of their own lexical ignorance, it remains to be seen whether it can be evoked from larger numbers with simpler procedures or brief training. We also know nothing about continuity in this type of awareness from toddlerhood to adulthood. For example, are individual differences in preschoolers' awareness of their own ignorance predictive of later sensitivity to ambiguity, contradiction, or omission as sources of text comprehension difficulty (Markman, 1981) or of later resistance to false cues of knowing (Mitchell and Robinson, 1990) or remembering (Ackil and Zaragoza, 1998)?

The scope of preschoolers' knowledge of ignorance needs to be established. Lexical knowledge is an instance of knowledge of what, as opposed to how, where, when, whom, or why. We do not know whether awareness of lexical ignorance is part of a broader construct that includes other forms of what knowledge, such as what a sentence means, what one ate for breakfast, or even forms of how and other wh- type knowledge. It will also be important to examine links between awareness of one's own ignorance and understanding of the causes of other's ignorance. Would ignorance-aware children be more likely to understand that a person might not know something if they lacked perceptual access to it (Pillow, 1989; Pratt and Bryant, 1990)?

Our hypotheses regarding the roles of retrieval efficiency and rapid, global impressions of novelty need further empirical evaluation. Also, none of the current accounts of the development of theory of mind (see Wellman and Gelman, 1997) has addressed findings about children's awareness of their own lexical ignorance. Doing so may serve both to improve these accounts and to deepen our understanding of the development of awareness of ignorance.

Word- and meaning-cued awareness ought to promote vocabulary development. Preschoolers who know that they do not know some word or meaning ought to be more likely to learn them than those who lack this insight. Such awareness is associated with how consistently these children will map novel words onto unfamiliar rather than familiar kinds, but concurrent relations between measures of awareness and vocabulary size have been found to be rather modest. The power of measures of awareness to predict gains in vocabulary over time may prove to be stronger. We also need to find out how reliably preschoolers become aware of their own ignorance in situations where they typically encounter new words or meanings, and how they proceed whenever this awareness takes hold.

Finally, the link we have documented between awareness of lexical ignorance and a "same" bias in perceptual matching may serve to illustrate an insight that ties together diverse forms of metacognition. A general appreciation for representational inadequacy may encompass not only awareness of ignorance and distrust in perceived change, but also the various sensitivities to multiple representation that have been the focus of much theory-of-mind research (e.g., understanding of false belief, perspective taking, representational change, and the appearance-reality distinction). It may also include distrust in perceived sameness in certain circumstances, such as when comparing very complex pictures side by side, knowing they might differ in only a single feature (as in Vurpillot's 1968 classic apartment building comparison task). In these circumstances, preschoolers may have to resist a strong sense of the sameness of the pictures in order to complete an exhaustive comparison of their features. Future research should not only test the validity of awareness of representational inadequacy as a general construct, but also explore whether this construct predicts the acquisition of strategies that promote building complete, accurate representations of things. For example, preschoolers who appreciate representational inadequacy may be more likely than their agemates to ask what unfamiliar words mean or to search stimuli that they have perceived to be different for the source of this impression. Appreciation for representational inadequacy may prove to be not only a broad metacognitive construct, but also one central to explaining a variety of improvements in cognitive processing during childhood.

References

Ackil, J. K., and Zaragoza, M. S. (1998). Memorial consequences of forced confabulation: Age differences in susceptibility to false memories. *Developmental Psychology, 34,* 1358–1372.

Baddeley, A. D., Papagno, C., and Vallar, G. (1988). When long-term learning depends on short-term storage. *Journal of Memory and Language, 27,* 586–596.

Bartsch, K., and Wellman, H. M. (1995). *Children talk about the mind.* New York: Oxford University Press.

Brown, J. R., and Dunn, J. (1991). "You can cry, mum": The social and developmental implications of talk about internal states. *British Journal of Developmental Psychology, 9,* 237–256.

Brown, R. (1968). The development of Wh questions in child speech. *Journal of Verbal Learning and Verbal Behavior, 7,* 279–290.

Chaney, C. (1992). Language development, metalinguistic skills, and print awareness in 3-year-old children. *Applied Psycholinguistics, 13,* 485–514.

Clark, E. V. (1982). The young word-maker: A case study of innovation in the child's lexicon. In E. Wanner and L. R. Gleitman (Eds.), *Language acquisition: The state of the art.* Cambridge: Cambridge University Press.

Clark, E. V. (1993). *The lexicon in acquisition.* New York: Cambridge University Press.

Cultice, J. C., Somerville, S. C., and Wellman, H. M. (1983). Preschoolers' memory monitoring: Feeling-of-knowing judgments. *Child Development, 54,* 1480–1486.

Flavell, J. H. (1974). The development of inferences about others. In T. Mischel (Ed.), *Understanding other persons.* Oxford: Blackwell, Basil, and Mott.

Flavell, J. H., Speer, J. R., Green, F. L., and August, D. L. (1981). The development of comprehension monitoring and knowledge about communication. *Monographs of the Society for Research in Child Development, 46* (serial no. 192).

Furrow, D., Moore, C., Davidge, J., and Chiasson, (1992). Mental terms in mothers' and children's speech: Similarities and relationships. *Journal of Child Language, 19,* 617–631.

Gathercole, S. E. (1995). Is nonword repetition a test of phonological memory or long-term knowledge? It all depends on the nonwords. *Memory and Cognition, 23,* 83–94.

Gathercole, S. E., and Baddeley, A. D. (1990). The role of phonological memory in vocabulary acquisition: A study of young children learning arbitrary names for toys. *British Journal of Psychology, 81,* 439–454.

Gopnik, A., and Astington, J. W. (1988). Children's understanding of representational change, and its relation to the understanding of false belief and the appearance-reality distinction. *Child Development, 59,* 26–37.

Jacoby, L. L., Woloshyn, V., and Kelley, C. M. (1989). Becoming famous without being recognized: Unconscious influences of memory produced by dividing attention. *Journal of Experimental Psychology: General, 118,* 115–125.

Jacques, S., Zelazo, P. D., Kirkham, N. Z., and Semcesen, T. K. (1999). Rule selection versus rule execution: An error-detection approach. *Developmental Psychology, 35,* 770–780.

Karmiloff-Smith, A. (1986). From meta-processes to conscious access: Evidence from children's metalinguistic and repair data. *Cognition, 23,* 95–147.

Klin, C. M., Guzman, A. E., and Levine, W. H. (1997). Knowing that you don't know: Metamemory and discourse processing. *Journal of Experimental Psychology: Learning, Memory, and Cognition, 23,* 1378–1393.

Krueger, L. E., and Chignell, M. H. (1985). *Same-different* judgments under high speed stress: Missing-feature principle predominates in early processing. *Perception and Psychophysics, 38,* 188–193.

Krueger, L. E., Stadtlander, L. M., and Blum, A. J. (1992). Search for a singular word or nonword. *Journal of Experimental Psychology: Learning, Memory, and Cognition, 18,* 1331–1341.

Lewis, C., and Osborne, A. (1990). Three-year-olds' problems with false belief: Conceptual deficit or linguistic artifact? *Child Development, 61,* 1514–1519.

Maki, R. (1998). Prediction performance on text: Delayed versus immediate predictions and tests. *Memory and Cognition, 26,* 959–964.

Marazita, J. M., and Merriman, W. E. (Forthcoming). Young children's awareness of their own lexical ignorance.

Marazita, J. M., and Merriman, W. E. (In preparation). Relations among awareness of lexical ignorance, novel word mapping, and perceptual matching in early childhood. Ohio Dominican University and Kent State University.

Markman, E. M. (1981). Comprehension monitoring. In W. P. Dickson (Ed.), *Children's oral communication skills.* New York: Academic Press.

Markman, E. M., and Wachtel, G. F. (1988). Children's use of mutual exclusivity to constrain the meanings of words. *Cognitive Psychology, 20,* 121–157.

Masangkay, Z. S., McCluskey, K. A., McIntyre, C. W., Sims-Kinight, J., Vaughn, B., and Flavell, J. H. (1974). The early development of inferences about the visual percepts of others. *Child Development, 45,* 237–246.

Merriman, W. E., and Bowman, L. L. (1989). The mutual exclusivity bias in children's word learning. *Monographs of the Society for Research in Child Development, 54* (serial no. 220).

Merriman, W. E., and Brown, B. (In preparation). Preschoolers' judgments of their own and other children's lexical ignorance: Relations to a metacognitive strategy for word mapping. Kent State University.

Merriman, W. E., and Evey, J. A. (In preparation). Word- and object-cued awareness of lexical ignorance in early childhood: Discriminant relations to short-term verbal memory. Kent State University and Southern Indiana University.

Merriman, W. E., Evey-Burkey, J. A., Marazita, J. M., and Jarvis, L. H. (1996). Young two-year-olds' tendency to map novel verbs onto novel actions. *Journal of Experimental Child Psychology, 63,* 466–498.

Merriman, W. E., Marazita, J. M., and Jarvis, L. J. (1993). Four-year-olds' disambiguation of action and object word reference. *Journal of Experimental Child Psychology, 56,* 412–430.

Merriman, W. E., and Schuster, J. M. (1991). Young children's disambiguation of object name reference. *Child Development, 62,* 1288–1301.

Mitchell, P., and Lacohee, H. (1991). Children's early understanding of false belief. *Cognition, 39,* 107–127.

Mitchell, P., and Robinson, E. J. (1990). When do children overestimate their knowledge of unfamiliar targets? *Journal of Experimental Child Psychology, 50,* 81–101.

Nelson, T. O. (1996). Consciousness and metacognition. *American Psychologist, 51,* 102–116.

Pillow, B. (1989). Early understanding of perception as a source of knowledge. *Journal of Experimental Child Psychology, 47,* 116–129.

Pratt, C., and Bryant, P. (1990). Young children understand that looking leads to knowing (so long as they are looking into a single barrel). *Child Development, 61,* 973–982.

Reder, L. M. (1987). Strategy selection in question answering. *Cognitive Psychology, 19*, 90–137.

Schwartz, B. L., and Metcalfe, J. (1992). Cue familiarity but not target retrievability enhances feeling-of-knowing judgments. *Journal of Experimental Psychology: Learning, Memory, and Cognition, 18*, 1074–1083.

Shatz, M., Wellman, H. M., and Silber, S. (1983). The acquisition of mental verbs: A systematic investigation of first references to mental states. *Cognition, 14*, 301–321.

Simons, D. J., and Levin, D. T. (1998). Failure to detect changes to people in a real-world interaction. *Psychonomic Bulletin and Review, 5*, 644–649.

Smith, C. L., and Tager-Flusberg, H. (1982). Metalinguistic awareness and language development. *Journal of Experimental Child Psychology, 34*, 449–468.

Smith, M. E. (1933). Grammatical errors in the speech of preschool children. *Child Development, 4*, 183–190.

Son, L. K., and Metcalfe, J. (2000). Metacognitive and control strategies in study-time allocation. *Journal of Experimental Psychology: Learning, Memory, and Cognition, 26*, 204–221.

Vurpillot, E. (1968). The development of scanning strategies and their relation to visual differentiation. *Journal of Experimental Child Psychology, 6*, 632–650.

Wellman, H. M., and Gelman, S. A. (1997). Knowledge acquisition in foundational domains. In D. Kuhn and R. S. Siegler (Eds.), *Handbook of child psychology*. Vol. 2: *Cognition, perception, and language* (pp. 523–574). New York: Wiley.

Wimmer, H., and Hartl, M. (1991). Against the Cartesian view on mind: Young children's difficulty with own false beliefs. *British Journal of Developmental Psychology, 9*, 125–138.

Zelazo, P. D., Reznick, J. S., and Pinon, D. E. (1995). Response control and the execution of verbal rules. *Developmental Psychology, 31*, 508–517.

Chapter 4

Visual Metacognition and the Development of Size Constancy

Carl E. Granrud

In his 1860 book *A Treatise on Physiological Optics*, Hermann von Helmholtz described a memory from his childhood. While walking with his mother, he looked up and saw people high above in a chapel bell tower. Thinking that the people were dolls on a shelf, he asked his mother to reach up and take them down for him, which he believed she could do. Based on this memory, Helmholtz (1860) hypothesized that children misperceive the sizes of distant objects and that size constancy—accurate perception of objective size despite changes in distance and size of retinal image—is a learned ability that develops gradually during childhood.

Literature Review: Size Constancy in Children

Early in the twentieth century, researchers began empirical studies on the development of size perception in children, motivated primarily by the nature-nurture issue. Brunswik and his students in Vienna supported the nurture side of the debate, arguing that size constancy is a learned ability, whereas Koffka and his students in Berlin stood on the nature side of the debate, believing that size constancy is innate (Koffka, 1935). Each school reported research findings that appeared to support its side of the nature-nurture question. In Vienna, Beyrl (1926) found evidence that size constancy develops gradually, reaching adult levels of accuracy by about 11 years of age. In Berlin, Frank (1926) reported that accurate size constancy is present by 11 months, and that no changes in constancy occur between 11 months and 7 years of age.

Subsequent research has supported both Koffka's nativist view and the Helmholtz-Brunswik empiricist position. Studies with infants have found evidence of size constancy in 4-month-old (Day and McKenzie, 1981) and newborn infants (Slater, Mattock, and Brown, 1990), supporting the hypothesis that size constancy is an innate ability. On the other hand, many studies have confirmed Beryl's (1926) finding that size constancy performance improves significantly during childhood.

Although some degree of size constancy appears to be innate, the ability to estimate the sizes of distant objects improves substantially during childhood. In a typical size constancy experiment, the research participant views a standard object positioned at a distance between 1 and 1,000 m (this distance varies widely across different studies). The participant adjusts the size of a nearby variable object, or chooses from a set of comparison objects of varying size, to match the standard object's size. An accurate size match represents size constancy; an underestimation of size is referred to as "underconstancy" and an overestimation as "overconstancy." By about 10 years of age, children exhibit size constancy across a wide range of distances, and their size estimates do not differ significantly from those of adults (Beryl, 1926; Brislin and Leibowitz, 1970; Leibowitz, Pollard, and Dickson, 1967; Piaget, 1969). For children younger than 10 years of age, size-matching accuracy depends on viewing distance. When objects are viewed at distances of less than 3 m, children exhibit near-perfect size constancy by 4 years of age (Tronick and Hershenson, 1979). With distances between 3 and 15 m, young children typically exhibit underconstancy (Beryl, 1926; Piaget, 1969; Rapoport, 1967, 1969), although some studies have reported accurate size constancy by 5 years of age (Brislin and Leibowitz, 1970; Leibowitz, Pollard, and Dickson, 1967; Zeigler and Leibowitz, 1957). When viewing distance exceeds 15 m, young children exhibit considerable underconstancy (Brislin and Leibowitz, 1970; Leibowitz, Pollard, and Dickson, 1967; Zeigler and Leibowitz, 1957).

A Replication of Previous Findings

The goal of my recent research has been to investigate the causes of developmental changes in size constancy during childhood. When my students and I began to investigate the development of size constancy in children, our first step was to replicate a classic study by Zeigler and Leibowitz (1957). We wanted to establish the reliability of age-related changes in size constancy before attempting to investigate the causes of these changes. Two age groups were tested: 5-year-olds ($n = 20$) and college-aged adults ($n = 20$). Each participant viewed two standard objects, one at a time: a 51 cm tall rod at a distance of 30.5 m and a 5.1 cm tall rod at 3.05 m. The variable object was a rod positioned at a distance of 1.5 m whose height could be adjusted by an experimenter. Each participant was given four trials for each standard object: two ascending trials, in which the rod's height increased from a starting point of 0 cm, and two descending trials, in which the rod's height decreased from a starting point of 70 cm. The participant's task was to tell the experimenter when the variable object matched the standard object in height. The participant was then asked to direct the experimenter in making adjustments in the variable object's height to match the standard object as accurately as possible.

Figure 4.1 shows the results of this replication study. The dependent variable in the study was mean estimated size, averaged across four trials at each distance. We obtained results similar to those reported by Zeigler and Leibowitz 40 years earlier. The adults made accurate size estimates at both distances. The 5-year-olds

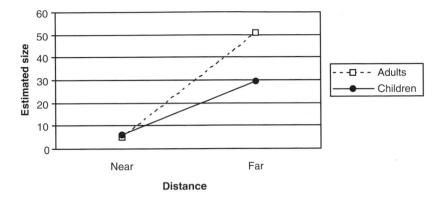

Figure 4.1
Mean estimated size (cm) of 5.1 cm rod at 3.05 m and 51 cm rod at 30.5 m by adults and 5-year-old children.

made accurate estimates at the near distance (3.05 m), but significantly underestimated size at the far distance (30.5 m).

After confirming the finding that young children underestimate the size of a distant object, we turned our attention to the question of what causes the change in size constancy performance that occurs between 5 years of age and adulthood. There seem to be two main possibilities. Improved size constancy could be caused by improvements in perceptual abilities. Alternatively, the development of size constancy could result from the development of cognitive abilities.

The Perceptual Learning and Cognitive Supplementation Hypotheses

Leibowitz (1974) proposed that developmental changes in size constancy result from improvements in perceptual abilities. His "perceptual learning" hypothesis is based on the relationship between perceived size and perceived distance. There is a large body of evidence indicating that the visual system achieves size constancy by registering information for an object's distance, then determining its physical size based on its distance and the size of its retinal image (e.g., Rock, 1983). In many situations, size constancy is achieved only if adequate depth information is available to support accurate distance perception (e.g., Holway and Boring, 1941; Harvey and Leibowitz, 1967). In addition, if depth cues such as accommodation, convergence, or binocular disparity are manipulated to change an object's perceived distance, perceived size also changes (e.g., Lawson, Gulick, and Park, 1972; Leibowitz and Moore, 1966; Leibowitz, Shinna, and Hennesy, 1972).

Leibowitz (1974) hypothesized that children underestimate distant objects' sizes due to inaccurate distance perception. He pointed out that, at near distances, depth cues such as accommodation, convergence, and binocular disparity provide precise information for distance, and that these cues support accurate size constancy when objects are nearby. But, as distance increases beyond a few meters, these cues no longer provide useful distance information, and pictorial depth cues, such as linear perspective and texture gradients, provide the main source of information for distance and size. Leibowitz proposed that children are less able than adults to perceive distance based on these depth cues. He hypothesized that children can achieve size constancy based on the oculomotor and binocular cues that are available at near distances, but that they cannot achieve size constancy based on pictorial depth cues when viewing distances are great. In support of this view, Leibowitz noted that young children's size estimates for distant objects are similar to those made by adults having poor depth cue information, as in the classic Holway and Boring (1941) study. According to Leibowitz's perceptual learning hypothesis, children gradually learn to use pictorial depth cues, and first achieve size constancy for distant objects at about 10 years of age. An important aspect of the perceptual learning hypothesis is the assertion that size constancy is a feature of perceptual experience. Adults' perception of a distant object's size is veridical, according to this view, whereas children's perception of size is inaccurate.

An alternative viewpoint is that developmental changes in size constancy result from cognitive development, and not from changes in perception. Building on ideas from several sources, including Rapoport, 1967, Tronick and Hershenson, 1979, and Wohlwill, 1963, Morreale and I (Granrud and Morreale, 2001) proposed what we call the "cognitive supplementation" hypothesis, according to which adults and children have the same perceptual experience. Perception of nearby objects' sizes is veridical, based on the rich depth cue information available. At greater distances, size perception is inaccurate for children and adults: both perceive distant objects as smaller than their actual sizes, due to poor depth cue information. However, according to this hypothesis, adults supplement their perceptual experience with deliberate cognitive strategies when making responses in size constancy tasks. For example, when they are asked to select a nearby comparison object that matches a distant standard object in size, they make accurate size judgments, or often overestimate size, by using strategies such as choosing a comparison object that is larger than the apparent size of the standard object. Young children, according to this hypothesis, respond based on perceptual experience without using cognitive strategies: they select a comparison object that matches the distant standard object's apparent size and, therefore, exhibit underconstancy. According to the cognitive supplementation hypothesis, the development of size constancy for distant objects results from development of the ability to engage in cognitive strategies that supplement perceptual experience.

Although researchers have conducted studies on size constancy in children since 1926, very little research has investigated the causes of developmental changes in size constancy performance, and neither the perceptual learning hypothesis nor the cognitive supplementation hypothesis has been firmly supported by empirical data. Our recent research has focused on testing the cognitive supplementation hypothesis.

Effects of Instructions in Size Constancy Tasks

Research investigating the effects of instructions provides evidence that adults' behavior in size constancy tasks is influenced by cognitive judgments. Leibowitz and Harvey (1969) have pointed out that instructions are the most effective independent variable in size constancy experiments. In response to varying instructions, adults exhibit size estimates ranging from substantial underconstancy to size constancy to overconstancy, without any changes in the target objects or viewing conditions. Because the information provided by varying instructions is verbal and conceptual and not visual in nature, it seems likely that the effects of varying instructions reflect cognitive judgments made by the observer, and not changes in how stimulus objects are perceived (Carlson, 1977).

With "objective size" instructions, participants are asked to match a standard object's physical size without regard to its apparent size; with "apparent size" instructions, they are asked to match a standard object's apparent size without regard to its physical size. Studies on the effects of instructions have used a variety of stimulus objects and distances, and they have reported varying results. When distant objects are viewed and apparent-size instructions are used, adult participants sometimes exhibit size constancy, but in most studies they show underconstancy. When objective-size instructions are used, adults typically exhibit size constancy or overconstancy. A consistent finding across many studies is that adults make larger size estimates with objective size instructions than with apparent size instructions (Carlson, 1960, 1962; Epstein, 1963; Gilinsky, 1955; Leibowitz and Harvey, 1967, 1969; Predebon, Wenderoth, and Curthoys, 1974).

It is difficult to know what adults experience as "perceived size" in size constancy experiments. As Leibowitz and Harvey (1969) point out, size constancy experiments measure size-matching behavior in adults; they do not measure perceived size directly. However, the following interpretation of the effects of instructions is plausible. When apparent-size instructions are used, adults' underconstancy responses may approximate perceived size. When objective size instructions are used, it is likely that adults begin with their perception of the standard object's size, then use a cognitive strategy, based on their knowledge about the effects of distance on apparent size, to make a size estimate. These size estimates are sometimes accurate but often fall in the range of overconstancy (e.g., Carlson, 1960, 1962; Gilinsky, 1955; Wohlwill, 1963). Cognitive strategies seem most clearly evidenced in cases of overconstancy. It is unlikely that distant objects are ever perceived as larger than their actual sizes. Therefore, when research participants exhibit overconstancy, they are probably making a cognitive judgment that overcompensates for the diminished perceived size of the distant standard object (Wohlwill, 1963).

The powerful effects that instructions have on size estimates indicate that adults' behavior in size constancy tasks is influenced by cognitive factors. Do young children exhibit underconstancy for distant objects because they lack the cognitive abilities, or knowledge about perception, necessary for supplementing their perceptual experience? Rapoport (1967) addressed this question by investigating the effects of instructions on children's performances in a size constancy task. She found that 10- to 20-year-olds exhibited significantly greater underconstancy with apparent-size instructions than with objective-size instructions when viewing a standard object at a distance of 9.14 m. In contrast, size estimates by 5-, 7-, and 9-year-olds did not differ between the two instruction conditions. These age groups showed underconstancy in both conditions when viewing a standard object at a distance of 7.32 m. Because instructions influenced the older group but not the younger group, Rapoport (1967) concluded that the change in size constancy performance from early childhood to adulthood results from the development of cognitive abilities and not from a change in perceptual abilities.

Although Rapoport's 1967 findings are consistent with the cognitive supplementation hypothesis, her results are open to plausible alternative explanations. First, as Rapoport (1969) herself would point out, it is possible that the younger children did not understand the difference between the two instruction sets. If this were the case, no difference in size matching performance would be expected in the two instruction conditions. Second, the distance of the standard object was confounded with age. Thus it is unclear what caused the difference in performance between the younger and older groups, a difference in size constancy abilities or the difference in viewing distance used with the younger and older groups. Given these threats to validity, Rapoport's 1967 study does not clearly demonstrate that young children are unaffected by varying instructions. Nor does it provide solid evidence for the cognitive supplementation hypothesis.

In her 1969 study, Rapoport asked 5-, 7- and 10-year-old children and adults to select the largest or smallest object from a set of five objects positioned at different distances up to 6.22 m, and to describe how they had done so. Adults, who on average exhibited accurate size constancy, frequently reported using explicit strategies, such as comparing the target objects to their supporting bases. The children, who on average exhibited underconstancy, typically did not report using cognitive strategies, but instead selected the objects based on how they "looked." These results are consistent with the hypothesis that adults use cognitive strategies to achieve size constancy, whereas children do not. However, the reports on strategy use were essentially anecdotal in nature. No systematic data on the participants' qualitative responses were presented in Rapoport, 1969. Although Rapoport's findings (1967, 1969) are suggestive, additional research testing the cognitive supplementation hypothesis is clearly warranted.

A Test of the Cognitive Supplementation Hypothesis

When my students and I began working on the topic of size constancy in children, we wanted to test the cognitive supplementation hypothesis, but had not yet developed a good method for doing so. We were conducting a study designed to replicate the findings of Shallo and Rock (1988) when an 8-year-old girl gave us an idea for how to investigate the role of cognitive factors in the development of size constancy. Children in the study viewed a standard object (a white circle, 61 cm in diameter) at a distance of 61 m. Their task was to identify which of nine nearby comparison objects matched the standard object in size. The girl stepped up to the viewing position, inspected the standard and comparison objects, then spontaneously began to describe her thoughts.

"When things are far away," she said, "they look smaller than they really are. That circle is pretty far away, so it looks really small. But I know that it's a lot bigger than it looks. It's probably the same size as the biggest one." She then chose the largest comparison object, 76.2 cm in diameter, as matching the 61 cm standard object, exhibiting 25% overconstancy. It seemed clear that this girl was making a distinction between what she perceived and what she knew. Moreover, she seemed to be using a deliberate cognitive strategy, based on knowledge about the relationship between distance and apparent size, to compensate for the diminished apparent size of the distant standard object. That same day, we outlined a study to test the cognitive supplementation hypothesis.

We hypothesized that children who, like the 8-year-old in our study, understood and could describe the effects of distance on apparent size would behave like adults in size constancy tasks. We predicted that these children, regardless of age, would engage in cognitive strategies to supplement their perceptual experience and, as a result, would exhibit accurate or near-accurate size constancy. We further predicted that children who did not yet understand the effects of distance on apparent size, or could not describe this relationship, would respond based on objects' perceived sizes and would exhibit significant underconstancy for distant objects.

To our knowledge, only one previous study, Pillow and Flavell, 1986, had investigated children's understanding of the relationship between distance and apparent size. In one of Pillow and Flavell's experiments, 3- and 4-year-old children were positioned in front of a window and asked whether an object would look big or little if it were moved "far away across the street" and big or little if it were moved "right up close to your eyes." Both age groups performed significantly better than chance, although the 4-year-old group performed significantly better than the 3-year-old group. The children were also asked whether the object would "really and truly be big (or little) or just look big (or little)." Both age groups performed better than chance on this question and the two groups did not differ significantly. These results, and other similar findings reported in Pillow and Flavell, 1986, suggest that, by 3 years of age, children have some understanding that objects' apparent sizes decrease as their distances increase. But acquisition of this understanding may be gradual as suggested by the age differences found in Pillow and Flavell, 1986.

Our study (Granrud and Morreale, 2001) tested the hypothesis that increases in knowledge about the relationship between distance and apparent and projective size, or increases in the ability to apply this knowledge in making size estimates, are responsible for the development of size constancy in childhood. We tested a sample of 79 children 5 to 10 years of age. The study had two parts. The first part was a size constancy task. The second was a "perceptual knowledge" test designed to assess children's understanding of the relationship between objects' distances and their apparent and projective sizes. Our central prediction was that score on the perceptual knowledge test would correlate with size constancy performance. High scorers were expected to show adultlike behavior, exhibiting size constancy or overconstancy when estimating distant objects' sizes, whereas low scorers were expected to exhibit underconstancy for distant objects. We further predicted that perceptual knowledge test score would predict size constancy performance better than would age.

The size constancy task consisted of two trials conducted outdoors on a large playing field. In each trial, the child viewed one circular standard object and nine nearby, circular comparison objects. The child's task was to point to the comparison object that matched the standard object in size. For one trial, referred to as the "near-distance condition," the standard object, a white circle 45 to 61 cm in diameter (the specific size was chosen randomly for each trial), was presented at a distance of 6.1 m. For the other trial, the "far-distance condition," the standard object was presented at 61 m. The dependent variable for the size constancy task was the percentage by which the participant underestimated or overestimated the standard object's size.

The perceptual knowledge test consisted of ten items. Each item was designed to assess children's understanding of the effects of distance on apparent and projective size and their abilities to explain these effects. Item 1 consisted of a follow-up question asked immediately after the child responded in the far-distance condition of the size constancy task. All the children were asked to explain why they selected the comparison object as a match for the standard object. The remainder of the perceptual knowledge test was administered on a separate day, after the size constancy task had been completed.

For items 2 and 3 of the perceptual knowledge test, children were asked to predict changes in apparent and projective size that would result from changes in object distance. In items 4 through 10, children were asked questions about photographs. For each of these items, they were asked two questions. In part A, they were asked a two-alternative question. In part B, they were asked to explain their response in part A. For example, in part A, while viewing a photograph of two equal-sized cars at different distances, the children were asked whether the two cars were the same size or different sizes in real life. In part B, the experimenter said: "You said that the two cars are the same size (or different sizes). Why do you think that?" Other photographs showed pairs of objects such as two people or two electrical poles at different distances that had very different image sizes in the photographs.

For each item, the children received one point for correctly answering the two-alternative question, saying, for example, that the cars were the same size. They received one additional point for describing the relationship between distance and apparent or projective size in their response in part B, saying, for example, that one car looked bigger because it was closer than the other car. The maximum possible score on the perceptual knowledge test was 20 points. The children's scores on the perceptual knowledge test ranged from 1 to 20 points.

We made three specific predictions based on the cognitive supplementation hypothesis. First, based on the hypothesis that cognitive strategies are used to achieve size constancy at far distances, but not at near distances, we predicted that perceptual knowledge test score would correlate with size constancy performance in the far-distance condition, but not in the near-distance condition. Second, because overconstancy seems to result from deliberate strategy use, we predicted that high-knowledge children would exhibit overconstancy more often than would low-knowledge children. Finally, we predicted that children who scored high in perceptual knowledge and who made accurate size constancy responses would frequently describe explicit strategies that they used to make their size estimates in the far-distance condition. In contrast, we expected children who scored low in perceptual knowledge to report that they responded based on the standard objects' apparent sizes.

The results confirmed our first prediction. Score on the perceptual knowledge test was positively correlated with size constancy performance in the far-distance condition ($r = .64$), indicating that children who scored high in perceptual knowledge made more accurate size estimates, on average, than children who scored low in perceptual knowledge. Consistent with previous research, age was also positively correlated with far-distance size constancy performance ($r = .39$), indicating that size estimation accuracy tended to increase with increasing age. As expected, age and perceptual knowledge score were also correlated ($r = .64$). Neither perceptual knowledge score nor age was significantly correlated with accuracy in the near-distance condition.

Our partial correlation analysis to determine whether age was related to far-distance performance independent of perceptual knowledge indicated that the correlation between age and size constancy performance was an artifact of the correlation between age and perceptual knowledge. With the effects of perceptual knowledge partialed out, age accounted for no variability in size constancy performance, whereas perceptual knowledge score was significantly correlated with size constancy performance when the effects of age were partialed out. This result is consistent with the hypothesis that the acquisition of knowledge about perception, or the ability to apply this knowledge in making cognitive judgments about size, is primarily responsible for the improvement in far-distance size constancy that occurs between 5 and 10 years of age.

In an additional analysis, the sample was divided into two groups based on perceptual knowledge test scores. Children who scored above the median were placed in the high-knowledge group; those who scored below the median, in the low-knowledge group. Figure 4.2 shows the two groups' mean percentage error values in the near- and far-distance conditions. Negative percentage error values indicate underconstancy, an error value of zero would indicate perfect size constancy, and a positive error value would indicate overconstancy. The high-knowledge group exhibited near-accurate size constancy in the far-distance condition: their group mean deviated from perfect constancy by less than 1%. In contrast, the low-knowledge group exhibited underconstancy in the far-distance condition, underestimating the standard objects' sizes by more than 20% on average.

It is interesting to note that distance had opposite effects on the two groups. The low-knowledge group exhibited greater underconstancy at the far distance than at the near distance. This suggests that the low-knowledge participants based their responses on the standard objects' apparent sizes: with increasing distance, progressively greater underconstancy would be expected for observers responding to apparent size. The high-knowledge group's size estimates were more accurate in the far-distance condition than in the near-distance condition. This result would not be expected if this group's far-distance size estimates were based on perception. If accurate size constancy were a feature of perceptual experience, size perception should be at least as accurate for nearby objects as for more-distant objects because depth cues such as accommodation, convergence, motion parallax, and binocular disparity provide more precise distance information for nearby objects than for distant objects. The most plausible explanation for this result is that children in the high-knowledge group supplemented their perceptual

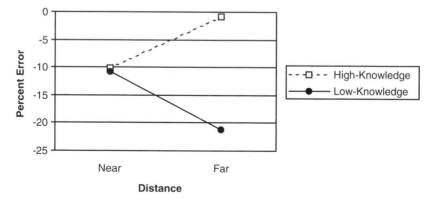

Figure 4.2
Mean percentage error in near- and far-distance conditions by high- and low-knowledge groups.

experience with cognitive strategies to make accurate size judgments in the far-distance condition. In the near-distance condition, they apparently responded to perceived size without engaging in cognitive supplementation.

A key result of the study, that the high- and low-knowledge groups' size estimates did not differ at the near distance, suggests that the two groups did not differ in perceptual abilities, attention, motivation, or task proficiency. If the high-knowledge group's more accurate size estimates at the far distance resulted from any of these variables, this group would be expected to exhibit more accurate size estimates at the near distance as well.

Our second main prediction was that, in the far-distance condition, the high-knowledge children would exhibit overconstancy significantly more often than would the low-knowledge children. This prediction was also confirmed by the results: 13 children in the high-knowledge group exhibited overconstancy in the far-distance condition, compared to 3 children in the low-knowledge group (a significant difference). When overconstancy occurs, it most likely reflects the use of deliberate strategies employed to compensate for the diminished apparent sizes of distant objects. The finding that overconstancy is associated with high perceptual knowledge suggests that the high-knowledge participants frequently used cognitive strategies to judge the distant objects' sizes.

To test our third prediction, we examined the children's responses to item 1 of the perceptual knowledge test, the follow-up question asking them to explain why they selected the comparison object as a match for the standard object in the far-distance condition. More than 50% of the children in the high-knowledge group reported using explicit cognitive strategies, compared to only 8% of the children in the low-knowledge group.

The following are examples of item 1 responses given by children in the high-knowledge group. A 10-year-old who made an accurate size match said: "As things get farther away, they look smaller, and since it looks about the same size as that one [pointing at a comparison object 43% smaller than the standard object], it would probably be a couple bigger: that one [points at the correct comparison object]." A 6-year-old who exhibited overconstancy said: "It looked small only because it was far away." Finally, a 10-year-old who made an accurate size match said: "I know if you go far it's gonna look smaller, so it will look like one of those [pointing at the three smallest comparison objects]; but I know it's really one of these bigger ones [points at the three largest comparison objects]." These descriptions seem to reveal deliberate strategies, based on knowledge about perception, that children in the high-knowledge group used in making their size estimates.

Children in the low-knowledge group typically reported that they did not know how they had gone about the task or that they responded based on how the objects "looked." For example, a 7-year-old girl said that she chose a comparison object 17% smaller than the standard object "because it looks the same size." A 5-year-old girl chose a comparison object 43% smaller than the standard object because, she said, "they're the same size." Finally, an 8-year-old who exhibited 14% underconstancy said, "I just looked at it for a few minutes, and it looked the same size."

Overall, the results provided strong support for the cognitive supplementation hypothesis. Children who scored high in perceptual knowledge exhibited near-accurate constancy in estimating the size of a distant object and frequently reported using strategies in making their size estimates, whereas low-scorers exhibited significant underconstancy and typically reported that they responded based on apparent size.

Effects of Instructions on Children's Size Constancy Performances

In our next study, we investigated the effects of instructions on children's performances in a size constancy task. Based on our first study, we hypothesized that high-knowledge children's performances would be affected by varying instructions, whereas low-knowledge children's performances would be unaffected by instructions. In this study, 60 children 5 to 11 years of age participated in the perceptual knowledge test and a size constancy task.

The size constancy task consisted of four trials. The standard object was positioned at 5 m for two trials (the near-distance condition) and 61 m for two trials (the far-distance condition). At each distance, apparent-size instructions were given for one trial and objective-size instructions were given for the other trial. With apparent-size instructions, the children were asked to select the comparison object that "looks the same size" as the standard object. With objective-size instructions, the children were asked to select the comparison object that "really is the same size" as the standard object. For each trial, the standard object was chosen randomly from three possible standard objects that were 45 to 61 cm in diameter.

In the far-distance condition, we expected high-knowledge children to exhibit near-accurate size constancy when given objective-size instructions and under-constancy when given apparent-size instructions. We also expected these children to report using explicit strategies for judging size when given objective-size instructions and to report responding based on how the standard object "looked" when given apparent-size instructions. We expected low-knowledge children to exhibit underconstancy, and to report that they responded to both types of instructions based on apparent size. In the near-distance condition, we expected that instructions would have no effect on size estimates and that perceptual knowledge score would not be related to size estimation accuracy.

As discussed earlier, Rapoport's 1967 study on the effects of apparent- and objective-size instructions on children's size estimates was vulnerable to an important threat to validity. It is possible that the 5- to 9-year-old children in the study did not understand the difference between the two types of instructions. To deal with this issue, our study included a pretest designed to assess children's understanding of apparent- and objective-size instructions. In the pretest, all children viewed two identical standard circles, 2.5 cm in diameter, and five comparison circles of varying sizes (all of the circles were viewed at a distance of approximately 35 cm). Four test trials were conducted. For two trials, a convex lens was placed over one standard circle, magnifying its image. The lens did not cover the other standard circle, and its apparent size remained unchanged. For the other two trials, a concave lens was placed over one standard circle, decreasing its image size.

Apparent-size instructions were given for one trial with each lens. On these trials, the children were asked to choose the comparison circle that "looks the same size" as the standard circle that was under the lens. A response was considered correct if the child chose a circle larger than 2.5 cm when the magnifying lens was used, and a circle smaller than 2.5 cm when the minimizing lens was used. Objective-size instructions were given for the other trial with each lens. On these trials, the children were asked to select the comparison circle that "really is the same size" as the standard circle under the lens. A response was considered correct if the child chose the 2.5 cm comparison circle. The instructions given in the pretest were identical to those used in the size constancy task. Children were included in the sample only if they answered correctly on all four trials of the pretest. The results from the pretest indicated that every child in the sample understood and could respond appropriately to apparent-size and objective-size instructions.

The sample was divided into two groups based on perceptual knowledge test scores. Children who scored above the median were placed in the high-knowledge group; those who scored below the median, in the low-knowledge group. Figure 4.3 shows mean percentage error values for the high-knowledge

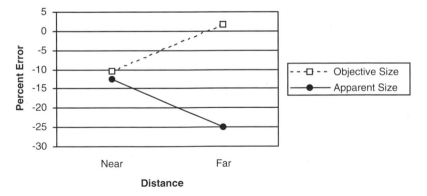

Figure 4.3
Mean percentage error for the high-knowledge group at the near and far distances with objective- and apparent-size instructions.

group with apparent- and objective-size instructions. In the far-distance condition, the high-knowledge group exhibited near-accurate size constancy in response to objective-size instructions and underconstancy in response to apparent-size instructions. In the near-distance condition, these children's size estimates were not affected by instructions. They exhibited significant underconstancy in response to both apparent- and objective-size instructions. Figure 4.4 shows mean percentage error values for the low-knowledge group. Instructions had no effect on this group. They exhibited significant underconstancy at both distances in response to both types of instructions. As predicted, there were no significant differences in size estimates between the high- and low-knowledge groups in the near-distance condition, which suggests that the two groups did not differ in perceptual abilities, attention, or motivation.

As in our first study, the children were asked to explain their size matches in the far-distance condition of the size constancy task. When objective-size instructions were given, 21 of the 30 children in the high-knowledge group described explicit strategies that they used in judging size. In the low-knowledge group, 25 out of 30 children reported that they responded based on apparent size. When apparent-size instructions were given, 29 out of 30 children in each group reported that they responded based on apparent size.

We also examined cases of overconstancy. As expected, overconstancy was exhibited predominantly by high-knowledge children responding to objective-size instructions. Because overconstancy most likely reflects the use of cognitive strategies, the finding that high perceptual knowledge scores are associated with overconstancy is consistent with the cognitive supplementation hypothesis.

The effects of instructions on children's size estimates and the children's self-reports also supported the cognitive supplementation hypothesis. When asked

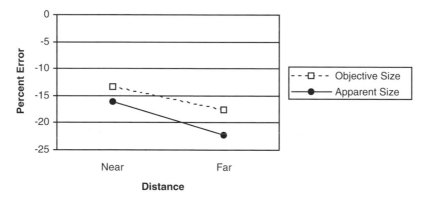

Figure 4.4
Mean percentage error for the low-knowledge group at the near and far distances with objective- and apparent-size instructions.

how big a distant object "looks," high- and low-knowledge children gave similar underconstancy responses, consistently reporting that they responded based on apparent size. These results suggest that children in both groups perceived the distant standard objects as smaller than their actual sizes. When children were asked how big a distant object "really is," low-knowledge children underestimated the object's size and reported that they responded based how the object looked. The pretest results indicate that these children understood and could respond appropriately to the two types of instructions, although they appeared to make no distinction between the distant standard objects' apparent and actual sizes. In contrast, children who scored high in perceptual knowledge generally made near-accurate size estimates in response to objective-size instructions, and they frequently reported using explicit strategies to infer the standard objects' actual sizes. These findings suggest that far-distance size constancy results from a cognitive judgment and is not a feature of perception.

Implications of the Perceptual Knowledge Test
Our findings suggest that age-related changes in far-distance size constancy between 5 and 10 years of age result from the development of cognitive, not perceptual, abilities. But what is the nature of this cognitive development? Does it involve the acquisition of knowledge about perception? Or is the ability to apply this knowledge in making size judgments the key factor in achieving size constancy?

The perceptual knowledge test results from both studies clearly indicate that knowledge about the relationship between distance and apparent and projective size is not an all-or-none achievement. For example, in item 2 of the knowledge test, children were asked whether an object moved far away would look big or small and whether an object moved close to their eyes would look big or small. They were then asked whether the object would "really and truly be small (or big)" or whether it would "just look small (or big)." Most 5-year-olds in each study answered the first part of this question correctly, and about half of the 5-year-olds answered both parts correctly. Thus most 5-year-olds could correctly predict apparent size changes that would result from distance changes, and many understood that the object's actual size would remain constant over changes in distance. These results are consistent with Pillow and Flavell's 1986 finding that children as young as three years of age performed significantly better than chance on a similar task. Thus most 5-year-old children have at least rudimentary knowledge about the relationship between distance and apparent size. Nevertheless, this age group exhibited substantial underconstancy in the far-distance conditions of both studies.

What accounts for the improvement in size constancy that occurs beyond 5 years of age? One possibility is that additional perceptual knowledge is needed before size constancy can be achieved. Alternatively, an inability to apply their knowledge in the use of explicit cognitive strategies may be the deficit that leads to underconstancy in 5-year-old children. Some items on the perceptual knowledge test asked a two-alternative question (e.g., "Are the two cars the same size or different sizes?"). Other items required a verbal explanation. In both studies, the items that required a verbal explanation were the best predictors of size constancy performance. Children who could describe the relationship between distance and apparent or projective size typically scored high in perceptual knowledge, exhibited size constancy in the far-distance condition, and were influenced by instructions. Children who were able to give correct answers to the two-alternative questions (e.g., "The two cars are the same size"), but were unable to describe why they gave their answers, typically fell into the low-knowledge group, showed underconstancy, and were not influenced by instructions. Thus knowing about the systematic relationship between apparent size and distance may not be sufficient for achieving size constancy. Advanced verbal abilities may be necessary to consciously formulate and apply strategies in making size estimates in real-world situations.

Revisiting the Perceptual Learning Hypothesis

Although our studies were not designed to test the perceptual learning hypothesis, it is interesting to note that this hypothesis cannot account for their results. For example, the perceptual learning hypothesis cannot explain the high-knowledge children's more accurate size estimates at the far distance than at the near distance. Based on this hypothesis, we would predict that size-matching accuracy in the near-distance condition should be as good as or better than accuracy in the far-distance condition because better depth cue information is available when objects are near. The finding that high-knowledge children made more accurate size estimates in the far-distance condition than in the near-distance condition cannot be explained in terms of depth cue sensitivity or developmental improvements in perceptual abilities.

Another result that conflicts with the perceptual learning hypothesis is the finding that explicit strategy use was associated with size constancy. In both studies, the majority of children who exhibited accurate size constancy described an explicit strategy that they used in making size judgments. If the development of size constancy resulted from increased sensitivity to depth cues, and not from the development of cognitive abilities, accurate size constancy should be achieved based on objects' appearances without any cognitive strategizing. Finally, the perceptual learning hypothesis cannot explain the phenomenon of overconstancy, which often occurs in studies of size constancy (e.g., Carlson, 1960, 1962; Gilinsky, 1955; Piaget, 1969; Wohlwill, 1963) and was exhibited by 20% of the participants in our first study and 32% of the participants in our second study.

Directions for Future Research

Our studies raised several interesting questions that we plan to pursue in future research. First, does the acquisition of knowledge about perception cause the development of size constancy in childhood? Second, what accounts for individual differences in perceptual knowledge within age groups? Finally, how do children, or adults for that matter, know when to use cognitive strategies to supplement perception and when to rely on perception alone?

Because of the correlational nature of our studies, it is important to note that the results do not demonstrate conclusively that either the acquisition of perceptual knowledge or development of the ability to verbally express this knowledge causes the development of size constancy. It is possible that a third, as yet unmeasured, variable, one correlated with performance on the perceptual knowledge test, causes the development of size constancy. More conclusive evidence that the development of size constancy results from the acquisition of perceptual knowledge could be obtained from a study that experimentally manipulated knowledge. Children who scored low on the perceptual knowledge test could be randomly assigned to two groups: a treatment group that received explicit training about the relationship between objects' distances and their apparent and projective sizes and a control group that received no training. If, after training, the treatment group showed more accurate size constancy than the control group, it would provide evidence that perceptual knowledge plays a causal role in the development of size constancy. We are currently planning this type of training study.

Another interesting question raised by our studies concerns individual differences in perceptual knowledge. Perceptual knowledge scores varied considerably within age groups, and differences in these scores were related to size constancy performance. For example, 6-year-old children who scored high in perceptual knowledge made more accurate far-distance size estimates than 8-year-olds who scored low in perceptual knowledge. What accounts for individual differences in perceptual knowledge and in different rates of acquisition of this knowledge? Specific experiences may play a role in the acquisition of perceptual knowledge. If so, we may be able to identify key experiences necessary for acquiring this knowledge in the training study described above. Another possibility is that the acquisition of perceptual knowledge is mediated by general cognitive abilities, such as those measured in IQ tests. The ability to apply this knowledge in size constancy tasks may also be influenced by IQ or verbal ability. We plan to pursue this issue by investigating the relationship between IQ, verbal ability, perceptual knowledge, and size constancy in a future study.

A third interesting issue involves how observers know when to engage in cognitive supplementation and when to rely on perception alone. The high-knowledge children in our studies used cognitive strategies at the far distance but seemed to respond to apparent size at the near distance. When we tested adults with viewing distances of 5 and 61 m, their behavior was similar to that of high-knowledge children. With objective-size instructions, adults made near-accurate size estimates at 61 m and exhibited significant underconstancy at 5 m. Adults and high-knowledge children seem to be sensitive to the quality of visual information available at near and far distances, and they know that cognitive supplementation is necessary at far distances. But, their metacognitive awareness is imperfect. Adults and high-knowledge children in our studies consistently underestimate size at distances of 5 to 6 m. They seem to assume that perceived size is veridical at these distances, and they do not appear to engage in cognitive strategies to supplement perception, as they do at greater distances. How children learn that cognitive supplementation is necessary to achieve size constancy for distant objects and what are the limitations in children's and adults' awareness of when perceived size is and is not veridical are issues we plan to pursue in future research.

Conclusions

A key question for theories of size constancy is whether size constancy is a feature of perception or the result of a cognitive judgment. A key question for developmental theories is whether age-related changes in size constancy result from improved perceptual abilities or from improved cognitive abilities. The results of our research, and findings from previous studies, suggest that different processes are used to achieve size constancy at near and far distances.

When objects are nearby, size constancy is probably a feature of perceptual experience. At viewing distances up to about 3 m, objects' physical sizes are perceived as approximately constant despite changes in distance and retinal image size, and size constancy appears to be achieved without cognitive supplementation of perception. In Tronick and Hershenson, 1979, children as young as 4 years of age exhibited near-perfect size constancy for objects at distances less than 3 m. Moreover, Tronick and Hershenson found size constancy in children who, in a separate part of the study, did not appear to understand that objects could have different objective and apparent sizes. This finding suggested that size constancy for near objects must be a feature of these children's perceptual experiences. If a child cannot distinguish between perceived size and objective size, it follows that the child's size estimates must be based on perceived size and not on a cognitive inference about objective size. Studies using near viewing distances have also found evidence of size constancy in 4-month-old (Day and McKenzie, 1981) and newborn infants (Slater, Mattock, and Brown, 1990). Size constancy at near distances, therefore, appears to be an innate perceptual ability.

At near distances, depth cues such as accommodation, convergence, binocular disparity, and motion parallax provide precise information for objects' distances, and this rich distance information seems to allow observers to achieve veridical size perception without the need for cognitive supplementation. In contrast, when viewing distances exceed about 3 m, size constancy cannot be achieved based on the oculomotor cues of accommodation and convergence (Harvey and Leibowitz, 1967; Leibowitz and Moore, 1966; Leibowitz, Shinna, and Hennesy, 1972) and distance perception based on motion parallax and binocular disparity becomes less precise (e.g., Ono and Comerford, 1977; Ono, Rivest, and Ono, 1986). When objects are far away, information for their absolute distances and sizes may be present in the pattern of light that reaches the eyes (Gibson, 1950), although, in most cases, the average human observer probably cannot use this information to achieve perfect size constancy. When viewing distances exceed a few meters, accurate size constancy most likely results from a cognitive judgment and not from direct perceptual experience.

In closing, let us return to the young Hermann von Helmholtz looking up at people in the bell tower. Why did he misjudge the scene that he was seeing? Why did he think that the people were dolls? The findings from numerous studies suggest that Helmholtz's experience may not have been unusual. Young children significantly underestimate the sizes of distant objects. But why did Helmholtz's mother not make the same mistake? Was her perception veridical? We would argue that Helmholtz and his mother both perceived the people as much smaller than their actual sizes. The difference between mother and child was in what they knew, not in what they saw. Our research suggests that young children underestimate distant objects' sizes because they do not supplement their perceptual experiences with cognitive strategies. Adults and older children, on the other hand, know that distant objects appear smaller than their actual sizes, and they use cognitive strategies to compensate for the diminished apparent sizes of distant objects. Based on our research thus far, it appears that the development of far-distance size constancy results from improvements in cognition, and not from changes in perception.

Acknowledgments

I gratefully acknowledge Melissa Granrud for her collaboration on both of the studies presented in this chapter, April Arnall for her help in conducting the study on the effects of instructions, and Daniel Levin for his helpful comments on the chapter.

References

Beyrl, F. (1926). Über die Grossenauffassung bei Kindern. *Zeitschrift für Psychologie, 100*, 344–371.

Brislin, R. W., and Leibowitz, H. W. (1970). The effect of separation between test and comparison on size constancy at various age-levels. *American Journal of Psychology, 83*, 372–376.

Carlson, V. R. (1960). Overestimation in size-constancy judgments. *American Journal of Psychology, 73*, 199–213.

Carlson, V. R. (1962). Size constancy judgments and perceptual compromise. *Journal of Experimental Psychology, 63*, 68–73.

Carlson, V. R. (1977). Instructions and perceptual constancy judgments. In W. Epstein (Ed.), *Stability and constancy in visual perception: Mechanisms and processes*. New York: Wiley.

Day, R. H., and McKenzie, B. E. (1981). Infant perception of the invariant size of approaching and receding objects. *Developmental Psychology, 17*, 670–677.

Epstein, W. (1963). Attitudes of judgment and the size-distance invariance hypothesis. *Journal of Experimental Psychology, 66*, 78–83.

Frank, H. (1926). Untersuchung über Sehgrossenkonstanz bei Kindern. *Psychologische Forschung, 7*, 137–145.

Gibson, J. J. (1950). *The perception of the visual world*. Boston: Houghton-Mifflin.

Gilinsky, A. S. (1955). The effect of attitude upon the perception of size. *American Journal of Psychology, 68*, 173–192.

Granrud, C. E., and Morreale, M. A. (2001). The role of perceptual knowledge in the development of size constancy. Poster presented at the meetings of the Society for Research in Child Development, Minneapolis, April.

Harvey, L. O. Jr., and Leibowitz, H. W. (1967). Effects of exposure duration, cue reduction, and temporary monocularity on size matching at short distances. *Journal of the Optical Society of America, 57*, 249–253.

Helmholtz, H. von. (1860). *A treatise on physiological optics*. Edited and translated by J. P. C. Southall. Reprint, New York: Dover, 1962.

Holway, A. H., and Boring, E. G. (1941). Determinants of apparent visual size with distance variant. *American Journal of Psychology, 54*, 21–37.

Koffka, K. (1935). *Principles of gestalt psychology*. New York: Harcourt Brace.

Lawson, R. B., Gulick, W. L., and Park, M. (1972). Stereoscopic size-distance relationships from line-drawn and dot-matrix stereograms. *Journal of Experimental Psychology, 92*, 69–74.

Leibowitz, H. W. (1974). Multiple mechanisms of size perception and size constancy. *Hiroshima Forum for Psychology, 1*, 47–53.

Leibowitz, H. W., and Harvey, L. O., Jr. (1967). Size matching as a function of instructions in a naturalistic environment. *Journal of Experimental Psychology, 74*, 378–382.

Leibowitz, H. W., and Harvey, L. O., Jr. (1969). Effect of instructions, environment, and type of test object on matched size. *Journal of Experimental Psychology, 81*, 36–43.

Leibowitz, H. W., and Moore, D. (1966). The role of changes in accommodation and convergence in perception of size. *Journal of the Optical Society of America, 56*, 1120–1123.

Leibowitz, H. W., Pollard, S. W., and Dickson, D. (1967). Monocular and binocular size matching as a function of distance at various age levels. *American Journal of Psychology, 80*, 263–269.

Leibowitz, H. W., Shinna, K., and Hennesy, R. (1972). Oculomotor adjustments and size constancy. *Perception and Psychophysics, 12*, 497–500.

Ono, H., and Comerford, J. (1977). Stereoscopic depth constancy. In W. Epstein (Ed.), *Stability and constancy in visual perception: Mechanisms and processes*. New York: Wiley.

Ono, M. E., Rivest, J., and Ono, H. (1986). Depth perception as a function of motion parallax and absolute distance information. *Journal of Experimental Psychology: Human Perception and Performance, 12*, 331–337.

Piaget, J. (1969). *The mechanisms of perception*. Translated by G. N. Seagrim. New York: Basic Books.

Pillow, B. H., and Flavell, J. H. (1986). Young children's knowledge about visual perception: Projective size and shape. *Child Development, 57*, 125–135.

Predebon, G. M., Wenderoth, P. M., and Curthoys, I. A. (1974). The effects of instructions and distance on judgments of off-size familiar objects under natural viewing conditions. *American Journal of Psychology, 87*, 425–439.

Rapoport, J. L. (1967). Attitude and size judgment in school age children. *Child Development, 38*, 1188–1192.

Rapoport, J. L. (1969). Size-constancy in children measured by a functional size-discrimination task. *Journal of Experimental Child Psychology, 7*, 366–373.

Rock, I. (1983). *The logic of perception*. Cambridge, MA: MIT Press.

Shallo, J., and Rock, I. (1988). Size constancy in children: A new interpretation. *Perception, 17,* 803–813.

Slater, A., Mattock, A., and Brown, E. (1990). Size constancy at birth: Newborn infants responses to retinal and real size. *Journal of Experimental Child Psychology, 49,* 314–322.

Tronick, E., and Hershenson, M. (1979). Size-distance perception in preschool children. *Journal of Experimental Child Psychology, 27,* 166–184.

Wohlwill, J. F. (1963). The development of "overconstancy" in space perception. In L. P. Lipsitt and C. C. Spiker (Eds.), *Advances in child development and behavior.* New York: Academic Press.

Zeigler, H. P., and Leibowitz, H. W. (1957). Apparent visual size as a function of distance for children and adults. *American Journal of Psychology, 70,* 106–109.

Chapter 5

The Odd Belief That Rays Exit the Eye during Vision

Gerald A. Winer and Jane E. Cottrell

More than a decade ago, one of us (Winer, 1991) noticed a statement by Piaget (1929) that children believe that, when they see, there are emissions from their eyes (he was commenting on a child's observation that the looks from two people "mix"). Piaget likened this belief to that of the ancient Greek philosopher Empedocles, who espoused what has come to be known as the "extramission theory of perception."

The fact that modern-day children, like ancient philosophers, could hold beliefs in visual extramission was surprising. If we assume that there might be a trend away from extramission beliefs with development, Piaget's observation represented a possible case of a parallel between the change in the history of scientific thought about vision and the course of thinking in ontogenesis, an idea that has fascinated psychologists (see Strauss, 1988).

The first step in our inquiry was to confirm that the ancients indeed believed in extramission. Here we made two discoveries that were surprising to us— albeit well known to historians of science. First, many ancient philosophers held extramission beliefs in one form or another. For example, Plato believed that a fiery essence emanated from the eye and merged with the object of regard before it returned to the eye. Euclid held an extramission notion also, as did other well-known philosophers such as al-Kindi (see Gross, 1999; Lindberg, 1976, 1992; Meyering, 1989) and Augustine (see Summers, 1987). This is not to say that all ancient or medieval philosophers believed in extramission. Aristotle, for example, believed in intromissions, as did Alhazan (see Lindberg, 1976).

Our second discovery was that extramission beliefs persisted until relatively late in the history of science. Even though the idea of visual intromission became relatively dominant by the early thirteenth century, chiefly through the work of Roger Bacon, Bacon continued to attribute some role to extramissions (Lindberg, 1992). Moreover, Leon Battista Alberti, who lived from 1404 to 1472, stated in his book on art, (Alberti, 1950) that rays both enter and leave the eye, and Leonardo da Vinci made extramissionist statements in his notebooks of 1490, although he would make only intromissionist statements two years later (Ackerman, 1978, pp. 126–128). Indeed, not until the early seventeenth century, possibly as a result of Johannes Kepler's theory of the retinal image (see Lindberg, 1976) was the extramission theory of perception finally put to rest in scientific circles.

Our next step was to confirm Piaget's finding of extramission beliefs in children. Piaget himself claimed to have found strong evidence of this belief in an unpublished report (see Piaget, 1974). Other investigators had also found evidence of what appeared to be extramission beliefs, but they did not seem to emphasize their importance and sometimes even claimed that they were not particularly meaningful. For example, Guesne (1985) expressly dismissed evidence of what appeared to be extramission beliefs as beliefs in the emission of rays and warned people not to attribute too much importance to them.

The first major foray into this field in our laboratory was Jane Cottrell's dissertation (1992; see also Cottrell and Winer, 1994). Cottrell asked a number of purely verbal questions about whether anything such as rays, mind waves, or energy went into or out of the eye, or both, during the act of vision. She also included pictorial item that showed three profiles of a face, with arrows pointing toward, away from, and both toward and away from the eye, respectively. Describing these three pictures as showing rays or energy going in the directions of the arrows, she asked the participants to choose the picture that demonstrated what happens when we see. On all questions, the evidence was unequivocal. When testing both children and adults, she found that extramission beliefs were definitely evident in children and that they declined with age. Since 1992, we have consistently replicated the developmental decline in extramission beliefs, and we have arrived at a number of findings, some anticipated by Cottrell's original work.

We found, first, that extramission beliefs persist across a wide variety of measures. Second, although they decline between childhood and adulthood, the beliefs persist in some adults. In the college population we have tested, we have generally found from 40% to 70% or more of our participants affirming visual extramission. Third is the fact that extramission beliefs persist despite a number of attempts to overcome them through common educational techniques. Fourth, is that people believe that extramissions play a role in vision. Finally, we arrived at several findings about the origins of these beliefs.

Variations in Measures That Do Not Influence Extramission Responses

A reviewer of one of our papers claimed that college students' belief in visual extramissions was so difficult to accept that our papers should be held to higher standards of proof than is typically the case. Other reviewers have also disputed our evidence for extramission beliefs, questioning the validity of our measures. And there is reason for this skepticism. That participants agree something like rays goes out of their eyes when they see might not mean they believe in a functional visual output. It is possible, for example, that what we refer to as "extramission beliefs" do not actually refer to extramissions that are meaningful for vision.

For example, participants might consider "extramission" in our questions as referring to line of sight rather than to something like rays exiting the eye. Or they might be thinking of a nonfunctional extramission, such as a reflection of light rays that, in exiting the eye, plays no role in vision, as would occur, in the photographic phenomenon "redeye." Or participants might simply have misunderstood our questions in some other way. We must confess that we, too, have difficulty accepting the idea that adults who are presumably literate in science believe in visual emissions.

To determine whether participants do indeed hold extramission beliefs, we have employed a number of different measures across a multitude of studies (see also Winer and Cottrell, 1996a). Although, as might be expected, the number of extramissionists varies somewhat as a function of the testing or the content of our questions, we have consistently found strong evidence of these beliefs.

In our initial research, for example, we asked some purely verbal questions and some questions that referred to diagrams, as in Cottrell, 1992. More recently, however, we have used computer representations of vision. The computer is useful because it can show simultaneously the movement both of rays going toward and into the eye and of those going out of and away from the eye. Moreover, it can show combinations of input and output that are difficult to represent statically such as rays first entering and then leaving the eye or, conversely, first leaving the eye and then returning to the eye from an object of regard.

Figure 5.1 shows three representations of vision, similar to those that have appeared on our computer screen. All three images show a profile of a face on the left side of the screen, with the profiles vertically aligned, each staring directly across the screen at its own separate rectangle. In the representation of visual input, dots appear to move in linear paths from the rectangle toward the eye. The movement is depicted in the figure by arrows, but on the computer screen it is shown by lines of dots appearing to move between the rectangle and the eye. In the representation of pure output the dots move away from the eye toward the rectangle. The third representation depicts rays simultaneously entering and leaving the eye. Not shown in the figure are two other representations of vision we have used: (1) rays first entering the eye from the object of regard and then returning to the object; and (2) rays leaving the eye, meeting the object of regard, and then returning to the eye.

Because more than four representations appeared to create visual chaos when the program was being developed, our computer program allows only four of the five possible representations of vision to be presented on the screen at one time. Throughout a typical testing sequence, we present eight trials, seven of which involve the computer; each of the seven computer trials presents from two to four representations of vision at one time. Always included is the correct choice, pure input. We also always include pure output as a choice, because we thought it important to have more than one representation presented consistently across the trials. A final, eighth trial is purely verbal and asks the participant to select from

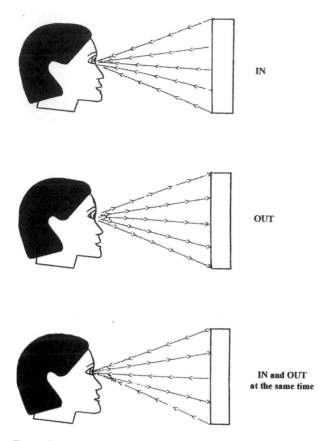

IN

OUT

IN and OUT
at the same time

Figure 5.1
Illustration of three-choice computer problem.

among all five choices: (1) input; (2) output; (3) first input then output; (4) first output then input; and (5) simultaneous input and output.

The computer presentation was designed to eliminate any ambiguity: it clearly shows the movement of elements that might constitute rays going toward and away from the eye. Static figures using arrows to represent movement might be misinterpreted. For example, arrows pointing in an outward direction from the eye, as in Cottrell, 1992, might be interpreted to signify visual orientation or line of sight, as opposed to rays exiting the eye, no matter how explicit the verbal description provided by the experimenter. Computer representations also eliminate or minimize other kinds of errors. For example, because the extramissions demonstrated on the computer screen move in a path directed toward the object of sight, it would be difficult to interpret them as random or stray reflections from the eye. Thus it is perhaps impressive that, in using the computer representations, we have consistently found a minimum of 40% of our adult population affirming extramission beliefs, and sometimes as much as 70 or 80%. These same studies also show that not all extramission interpretations are equally preferred. The two favored extramission interpretations are those demonstrating simultaneous input and output (choice 5 above) and input followed by output (choice 3).

Although we have hypothesized that the extramission beliefs revealed on the computer trials might be due to any one of a number of problems associated with the test, we have found no support for these hypotheses. For example, we hypothesized that extramissionists were not being sufficiently analytical in interpreting the computer representations and were responding "off the cuff," and that, given time to reflect and think before responding, they might be less inclined to give extramission answers. We predicted that, if we specifically warned people that the upcoming trials were going to ask them about input and output during the course of vision, extramission responses would decline. However, warning participants in advance that they were going to be asked about visual input and output made no difference. We also hypothesized that participants might have thought that something could exit the eye, but not that it would go back to the object of regard. We predicted that, if we specifically described the rays as going from the eye back to the object, we would prompt a decrease in extramission responses. But, again, there was no support for the hypothesis.

In a more recent unpublished study designed to examine the validity of our computer tests, we compared two renditions of a computer task. In one, we described the various computer graphics and asked participants to select, as we had in our past research, the graphic that represents vision and how we see. In two other cases, however, instead of having participants select the computer graphic that represents how we see, we used vignettes with different characters describing what was occurring in the representations. Thus in reference to one representation, character A said, "I think it is only something coming into the eyes. Nothing goes out of your eyes when you see." In reference to another choice, character B said, "I think it is the choice that shows something coming in and going out. When you see something first comes in and then goes out." Character C selected and described the computer graphic showing rays simultaneously going into and out of the eye. Participants were asked to choose the character with whom they most agreed. We found no differences between responses to the vignette test and responses to the more standard test in which we asked participants to select the computer representation demonstrating how we see. Moreover, in follow-up work using the vignette test we varied cues, such as inclusion or exclusion of the statements "Nothing has to go out of the eyes in order to see" and "What goes in must come out." These variations in wording had no effect.

One extensive investigation studied the possibility that extramissionists might have been referring to visual output that was not essential for vision. The study attempted to eliminate that interpretation by extensive training. Thus in his master's thesis, Aaron Rader (see Winer et al., 2003) trained participants specifically on the meaning of necessity, correcting them if they did not understand the concept. He then compared two groups of participants who received the "necessity training": one tested and trained on biological examples that might be viewed as somewhat related to extramission; the other trained and tested on nonbiological examples. For instance, on a biological example, participants were asked whether it was necessary for anything to exit the nose in order for someone to smell. On a nonbiological example, they were asked whether a ball must fall if it were released in front of them.

Experimental participants were both trained on the concept of necessity and asked about necessity on the main intromission-extramission (I-E) test questions. Thus, when given a choice of input, output, and simultaneous input and output, participants trained on the concept of necessity were asked, "Is it absolutely necessary for vision that something come into the eye, go out of the eye or come in and then go out at the same time?" In contrast, people in the control group, who were not trained on necessity, were asked only to indicate which computer representation shows how we see (our standard question). Training participants on the concept of necessity and asking them about necessity in the main test trials had absolutely no effect. In fact, the mean for the condition that was supposed to produce the highest number of correct responses, necessity training on biological examples, was actually slightly lower than the corresponding mean for the control group. One additional finding in this study was pertinent. A considerable number of participants who denied that it was necessary for anything to exit the nose in order for olfaction to occur then went on to affirm visual extramission. In other words, people can maintain extramission beliefs for one modality, while denying them for another. (However, it should also be noted that Cottrell and Winer, 1994, indicated that, although college students also hold extramission beliefs about olfaction and hearing, they are more inclined to affirm extramission for the visual than the nonvisual senses.)

In a follow-up study that involved no training, we directly informed experimental participants that, although some people believe in visual input and output, we were concerned only with input and output that were important for vision; moreover, we specifically emphasized that we were not concerned with visual input and output that would not influence how we see, such as stray rays that might enter the eye or reflections that might come from the eye and be insignificant for vision. Participants were required to repeat the instructions and identify what we were and were not interested in. Again, there was no evidence supporting what can be described as the "necessity" hypothesis (although the word *necessity* was not used in this study). In one experimental group two of twelve experimental participants had perfect scores (five of five test items correct), whereas nine of the remaining ten had fewer than three test items correct. In the control group, two of ten participants had perfect scores, whereas all of the other eight had fewer than three correct. When we repeated this study, with a much larger sample, using only two verbal I-E items (a two-choice question pitting input against output and a five-choice item), we again failed to find any evidence in favor of the idea that extramissionists are merely referring to incidental and nonfunctional emissions.

Up to this point, we have focused on the presence of extramission beliefs across many forms of questioning. Before concluding this section, we should mention one case in which we obtained no explicit evidence of extramission beliefs. When we asked participants spontaneously to describe what occurs in vision, not one mentioned "extramission," and only about 40% of our participants mentioned "intromission." Of course, just because people fail to mention "extramission" when giving spontaneous explanations of vision does not mean they have no extramission beliefs. Consider the following example. If we were to ask college students participating in an experiment to explain a strange phenomenon, say, hearing footsteps upstairs when they know nobody is home, we could assume very few would refer to ghosts in their explanation. Yet we know from unpublished research in our laboratory (Winer et al., 2001) that approximately 50% of participants from our group of introductory psychology students believe in ghosts. If, however, we were to take these same students and present another question, "Do you think that hearing strange footsteps above you might be caused by ghosts?" they might very well agree with the supernatural explanation. That they did not use that explanation when given the open-ended question, then, would not mean they did not entertain it, but rather that it might not have been the most salient response in their hierarchy of explanations at that moment. We are currently testing this hypothesis in our laboratory. This example suggests that people might entertain a multiplicity of beliefs, some in accordance with scientific principles, others opposed to them.

Some Variables That Influence Responses

We have found that some variables affect the number of extramission responses. For example, in one study (Winer et al., 1996a) we asked I-E questions about a lit bulb, the same bulb when unlit, and a Styrofoam ball that approximated the unlit bulb in size and physical appearance. As predicted, we found that asking people about the lit bulb, compared to the other choices, diminished the number of extramission responses, although, when tested with the lit bulb, some participants of all ages gave extramission responses. However, when the participants who were first asked about the lit bulb were then asked about an unlit bulb, their extramission responses increased, relative to other conditions, as if turning off the bulb provided a greater opportunity for visual extramission to occur.

We also compared computer, noncomputer, and drawing questions (Winer and Cottrell, 1996b). We predicted, and found, slightly more errors on the computer than the noncomputer version of the questions in one study that involved only simple choices. However, when we used many choices this difference was eliminated. In fact, assuming that purely verbal forms of the question would be less difficult than pictorial ones, we varied the order of these two types of question in an unpublished study with college students, predicting that there would be transfer among the questions. There were no differences between the two types of items.

Another variable that influences responses is sex. For whatever reason, we have often found that females give more extramission responses than males. As is the case with most sex differences, there are no easy explanations for the effect.

Finally, we have compared I-E questions about vision with similar questions about audition and olfaction, in both computer and noncomputer tests, and have tested the influence of answering questions of one type on answering questions of the other type. Three points can be made. First, on noncomputer questions, there is evidence for fewer extramission responses to questions about hearing and smelling than in questions about seeing (Cottrell and Winer, 1994). Second, no matter what the form of the question, there is evidence for extramission beliefs about audition and olfaction, even among adults. Third, we have found evidence that responses to the vision question might be slightly influenced by responses to questions involving the other senses although the effects are not always what we expected. In one unpublished study, we found that on noncomputer items there were fewer extramission responses to questions about hearing than to questions about seeing. Participants (college students) were given two questions, one about vision, one about audition, with the order balanced. Of 127 people tested, 27 had higher scores on the hearing questions, whereas 11 had higher scores on the vision questions, a difference that was statistically significant, χ^2 (1, $N = 38$) = 6.74, $p <$ .02. Moreover, there were higher scores on the vision item when the hearing item preceded the vision item than vice versa, χ^2 (1, $N = 127$) = 3.47, $p < .07$, suggesting there was positive transfer from the less difficult hearing question to the more difficult seeing question.

But, interestingly, there is evidence for something that appears to be nearly the opposite of positive transfer. In an additional unpublished study, college students were given a total of twenty-four computer questions in three blocks of eight. One group received three sets of questions about vision while another group received three sets of questions about olfaction that were identical to the vision questions except that they asked about computer representations of something like odorous rays going into and out of the nose.

Two other groups of students received three sets of questions in which each set referred to a different sense. In one group, eight audition and eight olfaction items preceded eight items on vision. In the other group, eight vision and eight audition items preceded eight items on olfaction. Thus, across all groups, for some participants, the last set of questions was about olfaction, while for others the last set was about vision. In one analysis of variance, we examined the number of intromission responses out of a total of eight, and found a statistically significant condition effect, F (3, 109) = 2.79, $p < .05$, in comparing responses to the last set of eight questions. In this instance, scores for the last set of vision questions were lower ($M =$ 3.8) when they were preceded by the olfaction and audition questions than when they were preceded by two sets of vision questions ($M = 5.2$). The prior appearance of the olfaction and audition questions, then, caused a decrease in correct vision scores, that is, an increase in extramission responses. We assume that many participants might have been uncertain about extramission on the initial smelling and hearing questions, and that, by contrast, they became more certain about extramission when they subsequently encountered the seeing questions. A similar finding, supporting the same interpretation, occurred when we examined responses to the questions about olfaction. Here we found higher scores on the last set of olfaction questions ($M = 5.7$) when they were preceded by vision and audition questions than when they were preceded by other olfaction questions ($M = 4.1$). In this case, we assume that the prior I-E questions made the participants more certain about intromission on the subsequent olfaction questions. Also, there were significantly more intromission responses to the last olfaction questions ($M = 5.7$) than to the last vision questions ($M = 3.8$), when the questions in each set were preceded by questions about different senses. However, additional analyses comparing responses to questions about the three senses showed no differences on responses to the initial set of eight questions that participants received.

The Impact of Learning

What Seems to Be Ineffective

We were alerted, early on, to the futility of most common forms of education in diminishing extramission responses. This observation first occurred when we tested adults whom we assumed had experienced introductory psychology instruction in visual perception—which included classroom instruction, textbook readings, and tests on vision—as well as elementary school children who had received instruction about the eye. We found that large numbers of participants in these samples failed our tests.

Nevertheless, we specifically set out to test the importance of college course instruction in several studies, first simply comparing different students, some tested before and some tested after they had received introductory classroom experiences (see table 5.1). As we had predicted from our initial observations, these common learning experiences generally had no effect. Our college students were seemingly immune to the impact of common educational experiences on understanding visual perception.

We then reasoned that perhaps the college students were erring because they were failing to access the information they had presumably learned. According to this line of thinking, prompting the students by giving them pertinent readings on vision immediately prior to I-E tests should improve their performance. We thus compared students given vision readings with those given no vision readings, and sampled from students who had and had not experienced their introductory psychology class units. The results validated what we had originally suspected. Again, neither testing the students before or after their classroom units,

Table 5.1
Learning variables that are ineffective or effective in diminishing extramission responses

---

Ineffective Variables

1. Testing participants after versus before psychology introductory test/lecture/assignment on vision
2. Testing participants immediately after they read college text material on vision
    a. Simplified or not simplified
    b. With or without figure of eye and object of regard
    c. With warning, prior to reading that participants will be tested
3. Putting participants in groups to discuss extramission
4. Simply repeating questions

Effective Variables

1. Readings or videotapes giving highly simplified lesson stressing input
2. Refutational messages on videotape or readings
3. Fostering a comparison between vision reading and responses to I-E tests
4. Explaining extramission

---

vision readings nor the readings themselves had any effect (some of these studies are reported in Gregg et al., 2001).

One might object that perhaps the readings were at fault. However, they clearly described the process of vision. Furthermore, in separate studies we used readings from different textbooks, simplified the content in the text, added information to stress the idea of visual input, and presented the readings with and without pictures. Overall, in more than ten studies, most of which are unpublished, no gains could be attributed to the readings.

One other ineffective learning variable should be noted. As was indicated, when using the computer items, we typically give multiple trials, and across all of these trials there are always two choices in each question: input and output. Most participants do not favor the pure output choice. Thus one would assume that if these two choices appear across a variety of questions, they would be noticed and a participant might infer that the input choice was the correct answer. However, very few participants switch from consistent extramission to consistent intromission responses over the course of eight trials. There is, in short, no solid evidence of learning because of mere exposure to a relatively large number of trials in which the correct answer repeatedly appears with an incorrect, but nonpreferred, choice.

In summary, a large body of experimental research demonstrates the intractability of extramission beliefs to common forms of college educational experience and practice. These observations mesh well with anecdotal evidence. For example, while in the hospital, one of us (Winer) described our I-E research to a nurse, mentioning to her, incidentally, that of course nothing has to exit the eye during the course of vision. Her response was, "You mean all those diagrams we had on the eye were incorrect"? An even more telling example occurred with one of our female undergraduate students who was experienced in testing our research participants and who had been told the correct answer on numerous occasions. One day, when leading a discussion in the research group, we asked the students whether they thought that rays exit the eye during vision. The student in question proceeded to affirm her belief in extramissions. And these failures are not necessarily restricted to undergraduate students. One year, our computer I-E tests were presented to three high-scoring students who were applying to our graduate program. All three gave evidence of extramission beliefs.

Effective Short-Term Learning Experiences
In one series of studies, we did find some compelling improvements due to learning, although these were transitory for older participants. In her dissertation study, Virginia Gregg (see Gregg et al., 2001) presented fifth graders, eighth graders, and college students with videotaped learning experiences. One experimental group received a simplified message on vision in which visual input was mentioned about twenty times, and a second experimental group received the same message on vision, but accompanied with direct statements that refuted the idea of extramission. This refutational group was explicitly told, both at the beginning and end of the videotaped message that, although some people think that something exits the eye during vision, nothing leaves the eye when we see. Reference was also made to Superman and other such fictitious characters in statements denying extramission. A control group received a message basically irrelevant to vision. Both immediate and deferred posttests were given, the deferred test appearing from three to five months after the initial training and test trials.

As might be expected, virtually all of the college students and most older children receiving the refutational message were correct on almost all of the items in the immediate posttest. Interestingly, whereas we had never had an effect due to a traditional reading on vision, our nonrefutational message, which simply presented straightforward facts about vision, was also effective for college students in the immediate posttest.

However, when we analyzed the results of the delayed posttests, we found that the college students and eighth graders in the experimental conditions had regressed: their scores no longer differed from those of the control group. Take the college students, for example, presumably the most cognitively advanced group in our study. On the immediate posttest, 100% of the students in the refutational group had five or more of eight items correct, whereas, on the delayed posttest, only 59% of those students scored at the same level. Interestingly, among the fifth graders, there was no interaction between time of testing and condition, with both learning conditions yielding higher scores than were found in the control group.

Gregg's dissertation study yielded three findings of interest. The first is that the nonrefutational learning condition succeeded in diminishing college students' extramission responses, whereas seemingly countless presentations of a standard explanation of vision to college students had never done so. It might appear that the mode of presentation might have had an impact because in our previous studies we had never presented videotaped lessons but had only used readings. However, we eliminated mode of presentation as a factor when we replicated the short-term effects with college students using the same script in written form that had appeared on the videotapes.

Two factors might have been responsible for the short-term gain of the college students given the nonrefutational reading on vision: the simplicity of the message, and the fact that we repeatedly emphasized input (about twenty times) in the presentation. There is no way of determining which of these variables accounted for the results, although we favor the explanation based on stressing input, for two reasons. First, we have repeatedly tried to improve performance by simplifying the written presentation of textbook information to no avail, although admittedly we have never altered it so that it would be understandable to fifth graders. Second, in an additional, unpublished study, we found that stressing input could weaken the extramission bias. Thus, when we accompanied the reading on the nature of visual perception with a diagram that had arrows pointing toward the eye, there were fewer extramission responses than when we presented the same reading either without the diagram or with a diagram that had no arrows.

The second significant finding from Gregg's dissertation study is that among the older participants the gain was only transitory. This finding attests to the robustness and strength of the extramission belief, and is all the more surprising because there is evidence for long-term effects of refutational readings in overcoming misconceptions in science (see Guzzetti et al., 1993). This second finding, however, does not signify that extramission beliefs are impossible to overcome through training, only that in one training situation in which there was a powerful short-term effect, the effect dissipated over time. We have no doubt, for example, that if we repeatedly instructed a group of college students that there is no necessary reason for visual output during the act of perception, the students would permanently improve on our tests.

Another potentially effective teaching technique would be to incorporate a refutational message during a typical college lecture, before administering a graded test. We have obtained some informal evidence that such a technique is in fact effective. Some of the graduate students teaching introductory psychology have learned about visual extramission beliefs from participating in graduate courses, and they have counteracted extramission ideas in their classroom instruction on vision. Table 5.2 shows the results of a recent study in which we compared students who admitted that their instructors explicitly counteracted extramission ideas with those who did not. The gain, although small, was statistically significant, but whether such gains would endure remains to be determined.

Table 5.2
Frequency of college students correct or incorrect on three-choice problem depending on whether extramission notions were explicitly refuted in introductory psychology

Intro Psych Experience	Responses	
	Incorrect	Correct
Refuted	3	14
Not refuted	72	83

x^2 (1, N = 172) = 5.17, p < .03.

The third finding of interest from Gregg's research was that, for fifth graders, the condition effect did not interact with the time of testing. The demonstration that the learning about vision endured in the young children but not in the older children or college students should be replicated, but it suggests that with increasing age, the extramission belief becomes more firmly entrenched and less amenable to the influences of education.

The results from the Gregg study were absolutely astounding to us and remain some of the most unusual findings from our laboratory. Yet so strong is the resistance to publishing null results that we had great difficulty in having the study, which we coupled with research showing the futility of traditional introductory psychology course instruction in visual perception, accepted for publication. To make the article acceptable, we ultimately chose not to include some of the studies that yielded null results.

There is one additional series of studies in which we have shown a decrease in extramission responses because of learning experiences. We discovered the effect in an experiment that involved a design different from the ones we had previously used. In all our previous research, we had used either a quasi-experimental or an independent groups design, in which control and experimental participants were randomly assigned to treatments and then, after the treatments, were administered the I-E test. In the new research, we used a repeated measures, pretest-training-posttest design. The pre- and posttests consisted of computer I-E items. The training in the experimental groups consisted of giving the students vision readings that had been used unsuccessfully before and asking them to compare the content of the reading with their previous responses to the pretest; in the words of the instructions: "I want you to think back about the questions you answered about vision. Did the answers you gave to the questions about how we see agree completely with the explanation of vision that you just read? Think before you answer this question. Did your answers to the questions on seeing agree completely with the explanation of vision that you just read?"

The experimental participants were not corrected in any way. They were merely asked about the consistency between their responses on the initial test and what they had just read. Thus not only was there an implied comparison that would have been fostered by the sequence of the pretest, reading, and posttest items; there was also a request for an explicit comparison. In this study, every group but the control group (which read a passage about John Watson) showed a gain from pre- to posttests.

It was unclear in this study whether the gains were due to the fact that a reading on vision intervened between pre- and posttests, or to the explicit request that participants compare the reading with their responses to the initial I-E test. A follow-up study suggested that both variables could improve performance.

These were the only instances in which we have found substantial learning from asking students to read college-level textbook material. The study shows that the difficulty in our prior research was not with the reading material: the same reading used in the successful studies was employed unsuccessfully in countless other investigations. Nor was the difficulty with remembering the information. What was critical was the active processing that involved comparing the reading with one's beliefs.

On the other hand, not every attempt to improve performance through encouraging active processing seems to be effective. For example, we have found no overall gains from giving students initial readings on vision and telling them that they will later be tested on what they read, or telling them that they should restrict their answers to what they have read.

Finally, one other finding has suggested that students might be able to profit from the active processing of information. In a study to determine whether the mere act of being extensively questioned on the meaning of extramission responses would induce the students to improve, we gave experimental students an initial I-E pretest question, followed by an extensive series of questions on the meaning of their extramission responses (an analysis of responses to these questions will be presented below), followed by a repetition of the pretest. A control group of students received an initial I-E pretest item and were questioned, not about the meaning of their extramission responses, but instead about psychology facts that did not involve vision. We predicted that the extensive questioning on visual extramissions would induce the extramissionists in the experimental group to think about their initial responses and thus improve. In Piagetian terms, we predicted there would be an equilibration process, or a process of conflict resolution. Table 5.3 shows the number of students improving, regressing, or remaining the same in the two groups. As can be seen, there was a slight, but statistically significant, benefit among participants in the group that received the extensive questioning.

Table 5.3
Changes across two I-E test trials due to requesting detailed extramission explanation

	Condition	
Change	Explanation Request	No Explanation
Regress	3	10
No change	43	44
Improve	15	6

x^2, $(2, N = 121) = 7.6$, $p < .03$.

Even though, overall, people's beliefs in visual extramission decline with increasing age and education, some people learn and others do not. What, then, differentiates the successful expert in vision from the nonexpert? What accounts for the expert in vision who at times finds it almost impossible, as we do, even to entertain the prospect that anyone could hold extramission ideas?

The Role of Extramissions

What role do emissions play in vision, according to our extramissionists? In our most recent study, stimulated by a skeptic who simply did not believe our findings, we have more extensively examined our student-participants' interpretations. In this study, we initially presented a single computer item that gave a four-choice problem requiring participants to select among (1) input; (2) output or output followed by input, depending on the condition; (3) input followed by output; and (4) simultaneous input and output. Following their response to the question, we asked extramissionists an open-ended question and a series of yes-or-no questions on the meaning of their responses. The open-ended question yielded little information. More promising, however, were responses to the forced-choice, yes-or-no questions.

Table 5.4 presents the questions and the frequencies of yes and no responses. From the data presented in the table and analyses conducted on these data, there is reason to conclude that many if not most extramissionists believe that extramissions (1) help us focus; (2) reverse projected images; (3) project images outward; (4) make our vision better, or (5) are just necessary for vision. Notice that, for three questions listed on the table there was more than a two-to-one ratio of yes to no responses: the belief that extramissions reverse projected images (question 2; point 2); that they project images (question 4; point 3); and that they are necessary for vision (question 7; point 5). Notice also that, to a fourth question (no. 8 on the table: If nothing left the eye, could we see?), nearly 60% of participants responded no, in rough agreement with the predominant yes responses to question 7 (point 5). Thus there is considerable evidence that extramissionists believe that emissions from the eye play a significant role in vision.

Table 5.4
Frequency of extramissionists admitting what extramissions do to help us see and whether extramission help or are necessary for vision

Question	Responses	
	Yes	No
Help focus?	17	16
Reverse images?	23	10
Illuminate?	14	18
Project images outward?	23	10
Sharpen vision?	16	17
Make vision better?	18	15
Just necessary for vision?	26	6
If nothing out, can we see?	14	20

Responses to the remaining four questions on table 5.4 appear to be what could be expected by chance. If participants were actually responding by chance, however, we would not expect responses to those questions to correlate significantly with responses to others. Yet the results generally show significant correlations among responses to the various questions, even those which appear to generate chance responses. Take, for example, the question whether emissions illuminate things, which hardly seems likely. Responses to this question (no. 3 on the table) are at about chance level, with nearly half the people agreeing and half disagreeing. But responses to the illumination question correlated with those to the question whether emissions are necessary for vision (question 7), $r (32) = .43$, $p < .02$, and with those to the question whether, if nothing came out of the eye, we could see (question 8), $r (33) = -.48$, $p < .005$. Another seemingly implausible role of emissions, that they help us focus better, also had endorsements at about chance level, and yet responses to the question on focusing (question 1) strongly correlated with responses to the question whether extramissions help us see better (question 6), $r (33) = .58$, $p < .001$. In fact, there was only one case in which responses to a question were nearly evenly split yet did *not* correlate with responses to any other question, namely, those to the question whether emissions sharpen our vision (question 5). Thus it appears that, even when there were apparently chance levels of responding, most participants were not answering in an haphazard fashion.

The correlational analyses were also useful in helping us to interpret the responses. Take, for example, the question whether outgoing rays help us focus (question 1 on table 5.4). What does that mean? Participants apparently treated that question in a global fashion, because, as noted, positive responses to it correlated significantly with positive responses to another global question, whether emissions make us see better (question 6), and it correlated significantly with responses to the question whether we could see if nothing left the eye (question 8), r (33) $= -.42$, $p < .02$. Moreover, there is consistency between the notions that outgoing rays reverse projected images and that rays are projected outward, r (33) $= .43$, $p < .02$.

Even though the correlational analyses give us some insight into what people believe about the emissions, we should be cautious about them. It is possible, for example, that participants recognized the similarity between questions and thus responded similarly for the sake of wanting to appear to be consistent, rather than because the questions were tapping related beliefs. Nevertheless, that people even admit to some of these functions of extramission is surprising to us.

The Origins of Extramission Beliefs

A particularly knotty, indeed, insoluble problem for us concerns the origins of extramission beliefs. Why should anyone believe in such emissions in the first place? Among the several hypotheses, we have tested, few have been supported.

In a study dedicated to testing three hypothetical explanations, we obtained no significant results in support of any of them. One hypothesis was that extramission beliefs stem from a faulty ontology of light. Perhaps, we reasoned, our participants believed that light has substance, that it ultimately fills up the eyeball and then must spill out. We predicted that informing participants that light is "used up" after it enters the eye—a statement that is of course in error—should decrease extramission responses. Our second hypothesis was that our participants failed to reason analogically and thus did not recognize the similarity between the eye and a camera. We predicted that emphasizing the similarity between the eye and a camera would cause a decrease in extramission responses. And our third hypothesis was that our participants failed to realize the role of the brain in vision. We predicted that if we emphasized the role of the brain in interpreting visual input, participants would have no need to assume that there was output.

To test these hypotheses, we assigned our college student–participants to one of five groups. Participants in all groups were given a reading and then our standard array of tests on vision. The "standard" group was given a brief explanation of vision from a introductory psychology text, but simplified so as to stress visual input. Other participant groups were given the same vision reading, but altered so as to stress information that would presumably be effective in overcoming their extramission beliefs. Thus in the "ontology" group (hypothesis 1), participants read that light was used up after it entered the eye and struck the retina; in the "camera" group (hypothesis 2), an analogy was drawn between the camera and the eye, including statement that in a camera the shutter opens briefly to let light enter and then closes; and in the "brain" group (hypothesis 3), the role of the brain in visual processing was emphasized. The control ("Watson") group was given a reading on John Watson from a introductory psychology text.

The results of this study are presented in table 5.5, where they are grouped by score. As can be seen, there were absolutely no differences among the conditions. (The frequencies of scores represent a profile of the levels of extramission we have found in our other research, as well). Of course, it might be argued that the conditions were insufficient to test the hypotheses. Recall that the vision readings from college texts have generally been ineffective, and perhaps the problem was the inherent difficulty college students have in connecting the readings to the I-E tests. But we know from the results of Gregg et al., 2001, that readings can overcome the extramission belief. Furthermore, in an additional study testing the various interpretations of the origins of the extramission belief, we coupled the same conditions (e.g., "ontology," "camera analogy") with a manipulation that did enhance the learning: fostering a comparison between reading and responses. Again there was no evidence of any improvement except for the comparison conditions.

One explanation for which we have some support is based on the work of diSessa (1993), who has proposed a general theory on the nature of scientific misconceptions. diSessa believes that underlying such misconceptions are core phenomenologically primitive experiences, small, intuitive knowledge structures he calls "p-prims." For example, in thinking about moving a weight, we can conceptualize the process in terms of an agent exerting some impetus, which meets some resistance and then has a result. At first blush, diSessa's theory is difficult to accept as an explanation for extramission beliefs: we are all aware of phenomenological experiences that even the most extreme extramissionist would admit were intromissions. Thus, when entering a lighted area after having adapted to the dark, we are all aware of the dazzle of light pouring into our eyes, as we are when we look directly at an exceptionally bright light, say a flash bulb or the sun itself.

Nevertheless, despite these experiences, we must also admit that in most typical acts of vision there is no experience of visual input. When we see an object, say a wall or a picture, we do not phenomenologically experience light reflecting off the object and entering into our eyes. What we experience is something out there, something that is external to our self. We are obviously completely unaware

Table 5.5
Frequency of college students having different numbers of intromission scores on eight-item I-E test, by experimental conditions involving different reading

Number Correct	Reading Condition				
	Standard	Ontology	Camera	Brain	Watson
0–2	5	5	6	6	8
3–5	6	6	8	5	7
6–8	15	11	12	15	11

of anything at all transpiring between our eyes and the object of our visual regard.

Moreover, there are phenomenological experiences that are consistent with the idea of visual extramission. When we "look out" a dirty window or "through" dirty eyeglasses and find our vision impeded, our experience is not that light, reflecting from objects external to us, fails to penetrate the clouded glass, but rather that we cannot see out of or through things, that our vision is blocked. Vision is also dependent on visual orientation. We have to "look at" objects and direct our eyes at things in order to see them. Finally, there are cultural-linguistic expressions that suggest emanations from the eye, such as "cutting stares" and "piercing glances." Indeed, throughout history, many cultures have accepted the idea of the "evil eye" (Elworthy, 1895), which suggests some power emanating from the eyes.

Although diSessa's theory is extremely difficult to support, we have predicted and obtained some results consistent with it. For example, we predicted that when we had participants draw responses to our vision questions, the act of drawing, involving an outer-directed behavior, would support the phenomenological outgoing experience of vision and hence produce more extramission responses than would occur on a nondrawing task (Winer and Cottrell, 1996b). We also predicted that a computer presentation showing rays going out of the eye would match participants' phenomenology of vision better than a purely verbal description of the same event. And, indeed, we have found that, to some questions, the computer presentation does produce an increase in extramission responses compared to purely verbal tests (Winer et al., 1996b).

But we have also obtained results that do not support diSessa's theory. For example, in one study, we had participants either point or not point at various objects in the room before they were tested, and we also asked them to point to the screen while they were being tested. We predicted more extramission responses in the pointing condition than in the no-pointing (control) condition. There were no differences between the two conditions. We also predicted that belief in extramission would be related to belief that one can feel the unseen stare of another person, as when a person behind you stares at your back. Titchener (1898) had reported that approximately 90% of the adult population he tested believed that they could feel the stare of a person looking at them from behind, as if a magical power emanated from that person's eyes. But when we replicated this effect and studied it developmentally (Cottrell, Winer, and Smith, 1996), we found, not only that there was no connection between the two beliefs, but also that the developmental course of belief in the palpable power of a stare was just the opposite of that of belief in extramission: it increased, rather than decreased, with age.

We have also obtained some support for the hypothesis that extramission beliefs arise from errors in reasoning, such as it is logical for something to leave the eye if it enters the eye on the grounds that "what goes up must come down," or "what goes around comes around." Recently, we presented our student-participants with an I-E test; after they failed it, we explained that there are two theories of vision, one claiming visual output, the other stating that only visual input is involved. We then told the participants that the intromission theory is correct: "Only the intromission theory is correct. . . . Science tells us that in order to see, nothing has to go out of the eyes." We further informed the extramissionists that they were wrong and asked why they had reasoned as they did: "You indicated that you believe that something goes out of the eye when we see. That is an incorrect belief, and it is shared by many college students. I would . . . like to ask you why . . . ?"

We predicted that few people would answer that they were taught the notions of extramission, and we further predicted that many people were erroneously reasoning that, because something came in, something must also go out. We also predicted that some people would admit that they were guessing and that they really did not know why they answered the way they did.

Although the results of an opened-ended question were disappointing and not particularly revealing, we struck pay dirt when we followed up with a series of "yes-or-no" questions, to which participants could give as many yes or no answers as they wished: "Remember I am interested in why you indicated that something goes out of the eyes when we see. You can give as many yes or no answers as you want."

The questions and the percentages of the people agreeing or disagreeing appear in table 5.6. There are several conclusions that can be drawn from the results. First, approximately half the people agreed that they might have been taught about extramissions and that they had read or heard about them somewhere. Although responses to these items were at about chance level, again there was a significant correlation between them, r (76) = .25, p < .04, suggesting that the respondents were not answering randomly. It is also somewhat puzzling that people gave these particular responses after having just been informed that extramission theories of

Table 5.6
Percentages of extramissionists agreeing or disagreeing to various reasons for giving erroneous extramission response

Question	Responses	
	Yes	No
You thought you might have been taught it somewhere	45%	55%
You believed that what goes in must come out	73%	27%
It seems logical or stands to reason	86%	14%
You thought you might have read or heard it somewhere	55%	45%
You were guessing	78%	22%
You really didn't know	77%	23%
Something else that I haven't asked you about	2%	98%

n = 77 except for read or heard, where n = 76.

perception are not scientifically acceptable (and thus, presumably, would *not* have been taught to them). Second, as expected, a large percentage of people agreed that extramission seemed logical, and that what comes in must go out. Interestingly, the correlation between these two responses, although statistically significant, was small, r (77) = .25, $p < .04$. Third, many people admitted that they were guessing and that they did not know. The correlation between these responses was strong, r (77) = .67, $p < .0001$. This finding is not surprising because they did not have correct knowledge about visual processing and, on some level, had to be guessing.

Summary

After more than ten years, we are concluding our research on extramission beliefs. We have documented that extramission beliefs decline across age, that they are present across a wide variety of measures, that they cannot be easily changed by common forms of education, and that many people view extramissions as playing a significant role in vision. We have been less successful in explaining the origins of these beliefs, quite possibly because they are so difficult to alter by experimental intervention. We do have some evidence, however, that the beliefs stem from the believers' phenomenology of vision and possibly their erroneous reasoning.

Although our research began with an analysis of developmental trends, certainly the most outstanding result we have obtained is that extramission beliefs persist in some adults and that common forms of education in introductory psychology classes have failed to eliminate them. Students are leaving our introductory psychology courses with a misunderstanding of one of the most basic processes in psychology (Winer et al., 2002). As Marcel Proust (1913, p. 162) wrote, "facts . . . do not penetrate to the world in which our beliefs flourish; they did not engender those beliefs, and they are powerless to destroy them."

It is clear that there is a misconception about the psychological world—about seeing—that is as difficult for experts to comprehend as any misconceptions about the physical world (McCloskey, Caramazza, and Green, 1980; McCloskey, Washburn and Felch, 1983; Novak, 1987). We also know that similar misconceptions exist with respect to hearing and smelling, albeit apparently to a lesser extent. What remains to be seen is how many other psychological misconceptions can be found. In any event, the visual extramission beliefs of ancient philosophers, long ago discredited by science, are still alive and well among many of our educated adults.

References

Ackerman, J. S. (1978). Leonardo's eye. *Journal of the Warburg and Courtauld Institutes, 41,* 108–146.

Alberti, L. B. (1950). *Della pittura.* Edited by L. Malle. Florence: G. C. Sansoni.

Cottrell, J. E. (1992). The development of theories of visual perception: Implicit and explicit extramission beliefs. Ph.D. diss. Ohio State University.

Cottrell, J. E., and Winer, G. A. (1994). Development in the understanding of perception: The decline of extramission beliefs. *Developmental Psychology*, *30*, 218–228.

Cottrell, J. E., Winer, G. A., and Smith, M. C. (1996). Beliefs of children and adults about feeling stares of unseen others. *Developmental Psychology*, *32*, 50–61.

diSessa, A. A. (1993). Toward an epistemology of physics. *Cognition and Instruction*, *10*, 105–225.

Elworthy, F. T. (1895). *The evil eye: An account of this ancient and widespread superstition*. Reprint, New York: Bell, 1989.

Gregg, V. R., Winer, G. A., Cottrell, J. E., Hedman, K. E., and Fournier, J. S. (2001). The persistence of a misconception about vision after educational interventions. *Psychonomic Bulletin and Review*, *8*, 622–626.

Gross, C. G. (1999). The fire that comes from the eye. *Neuroscientist*, *5*, 1–7.

Guesne, E. (1985). Light. In R. Driver, E. Guesne, and A. Tiberghien (Eds.), *Children's ideas in science* (pp. 10–32). Philadelphia: Open University Press.

Guzzetti, B. J., Snyder, T. E., Glass, G. V., and Gamas, W. S. (1993). Promoting conceptual change in science: A comparative meta-analysis of instructional interventions for reading education and science education. *Reading Research Quarterly*, *28*, 117–154.

Lindberg, D. C. (1976). *Theories of vision from al-Kindi to Kepler*. Chicago: University of Chicago Press.

Lindberg, D. C. (1992). *The beginnings of Western science: The European scientific tradition in philosophical, religious and institutional context, 600 B.C. to A.D. 1450*. Chicago: University of Chicago Press.

McCloskey, M., Caramazza, A., and Green, B. (1980). Curvilinear motion in the absence of external forces: Naive beliefs about the motion of objects. *Science*, *210*, 1139–1141.

McCloskey, M., Washburn, A., and Felch, L. (1983). Intuitive physics: The straight-down belief and its origin. *Journal of Experimental Psychology: Learning, Memory and Cognition*, *9*, 639–649.

Meyering, T. C. (1989). *Historical roots of cognitive science: The rise of a cognitive theory of perception from antiquity to the nineteenth century*. Dordrecht: Kluwer Academic.

Novak, J. D. (1987). *Proceedings of the Second International Seminar: Misconceptions and educational strategies in science and mathematics*. Vol. 3. Ithaca, NY: Cornell University.

Piaget, J. (1929). *The child's conception of the world*. Totowa, NJ: Littlefield, Adams.

Piaget, J. (1974). *Understanding causality*. New York: Norton.

Proust, M. (1913). *Remembrance of things past: Swann's way and Within a budding grove*. Vol. 1. Translated by C. K. S. Moncrieff and T. Kilmartin. Reprint, New York: Random House, 1982.

Strauss, S. (1988). Introduction. In S. Strauss E. (Ed.), *Ontogeny, phylogeny and historical development* (pp. vii–xxi). Norwood, NJ: Able.

Summers, D. (1987). *The judgment of sense: Renaissance naturalism and the rise of aesthetics*. Cambridge: Cambridge University Press.

Titchener, E. B. (1898). The feeling of being stared at. *Science*, *8*, 895–897.

Winer, G. A. (1991). Children's understanding of perception and perceptual processes. In R. Vasta (Ed.), *Annals of Child Development*. Vol. 8 (pp. 177–213). London: Jessica Kingley.

Winer, G. A., and Cottrell, J. E. (1996a). Does anything leave the eye when we see? Extramission beliefs of children and adults. *Current Directions in Psychological Science*, *5*, 137–142.

Winer, G. A., and Cottrell, J. E. (1996b). Effects of drawing on directional representations of the process of vision. *Journal of Educational Psychology*, *88*, 704–714.

Winer, G. A., Cottrell, J. E., Gregg, V. R., Fournier, J. S., and Bica, L. A. (2002). Fundamentally misunderstanding perception: Failing to grasp the basics. *American Psychologist*, *57*, 417–424.

Winer, G. A., Cottrell, J. E., Karefilaki, K. D., and Chronister, M. (1996a). Conditions affecting beliefs about visual perception among children and adults. *Journal of Experimental Child Psychology*, *61*, 93–115.

Winer, G. A., Cottrell, J. E., Karefilaki, K., and Gregg, V. R. (1996b). Images, words and questions: Variables that influence beliefs about vision in children and adults. *Journal of Experimental Child Psychology*; *63*, 499–525.

Winer, G. A., Roder, A. W., and Cottrell, J. E. (2003). Testing different interpretations for the mistaken belief that rays exit the eyes during vision. *The Journal of Psychology* , *137*, 243–261.

Winer, G. A., Raman, L., Cottrell, J., Fournier, J. S., and Bica, L. A. (2001). Increases in non-scientific beliefs between childhood and adulthood: A challenge for developmental Theory. Paper presented at the biennial meetings of the Society for Research in Child Development, Minneapolis.

Chapter 6

Thinking about Seeing: Spanning the Difference between Metacognitive Failure and Success

Daniel T. Levin and Melissa R. Beck

Recent research has documented a series of striking failures of vision in which subjects fail to detect large visual changes in natural and artificial scenes, even when they are attending directly to the changing object. This phenomenon, referred to as "change blindness," is potentially important not only because it informs us about the nature of seeing and the representations that underlie visual experience, but also for what it tells us about the accuracy of people's beliefs about vision. At the most simple level, change blindness strongly contradicts people's intuitions about what they should be able to see, and we feel that this fact, on its own, makes it worthwhile to develop a systematic account of visual metacognition. However, this conflict between predicted and actual visual performance may reflect a deeper problem as well. People may have difficulty reasoning about the relationship between internal representations and seeing, a difficulty all the more interesting in light of research showing that even young children can effectively reason about some visual representations and processes. Thus the question arises, if these early-developing understandings are available to adults, what, specifically, goes wrong when they predict their performance in change detection tasks? In describing research on the metacognitions that accompany change blindness, this chapter attempts to sketch a broader account of visual metacognition, one that encompasses not only misestimates of change detection, but also the more basic understandings of representation and memory that underlie reasoning about vision.

Change Blindness, Inattention Blindness, and Other Limits to Visual Awareness

The link between visual attention and awareness has been central to scientific psychology since its inception. From William James on, most psychologists would agree that there is a close link between attending to a stimulus and becoming aware of it. Accordingly, understanding limits to attentional capacity has been critical to delimiting visual awareness.

However, the extent of the link between attention and awareness has recently resulted in a series of surprising empirical phenomena. For example, in a fascinating series of experiments Mack and Rock (1998) asked subjects to discriminate whether the horizontal or vertical line in a cross was longer. While they fixated on the cross, another stimulus appeared on the screen (e.g., a black square) in one of the quadrants defined by the cross (see figure 6.1). Even though this second stimulus ought to count as an onset which one would think should draw attention (see Jonides and Yantis, 1988), subjects often did not detect it. This effect is very robust—subjects also missed the appearance of color singletons, spontaneous groupings, and even meaningful stimuli such as words. Also, in strong contrast to intuition, they were even more likely to miss the second stimulus when they fixated on the exact location where it appeared (so long as their attention was focused on the cross; see figure 6.1).

This kind of effect is not limited to artificial stimuli such as Mack and Rock's. In a classic experiment, Neisser and Becklen (1975) showed subjects a video of a simple basketball game between two teams of players (one wearing black shirts and one wearing white shirts) as they passed a basketball among themselves. Subjects were given the task of counting one team's passes, which demanded considerable visual focus. While subjects were attending to one of the teams, a woman carrying an umbrella walked right through the scene. Even though this would surely count as a novel event, most subjects did not detect it. This effect has recently been replicated using a person dressed in a gorilla outfit (Simons and Chabris, 1999), and even a woman who audibly scratched a chalkboard with her fingers (Wayand and Levin, 2001). Thus, in these natural scenes, there appears to be no bottom-up alert that something new has appeared—if subjects are attending to something else, they exhibit inattentional blindness and do not become aware of salient, bizarre, or even highly noxious new stimuli.

A related finding is that people have great difficulty detecting visual changes in a wide variety of displays. A compelling early demonstration of this phenomenon was achieved by carefully tracking subjects' fixation point while they read sentences on a computer screen (for other antecedents of change blindess research see, Simons and Levin, 2003). McConkie and Zola (1979) made changes to the sentences while the subjects were engaged in a saccade, and observed that subjects would miss large changes. In one experiment subjects read sentences in

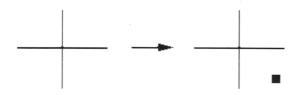

Figure 6.1
Inattentional blindness paradigm used by Mack and Rock (1998). Subjects study the display at left, judging the relative lengths of the horizontal and vertical lines. During one of the judgment trials, a new stimulus unexpectedly appears for 200–800 msec (as illustrated on the right), and subjects are asked if they detected it.

which EaCh LeTtEr AlTeRnAtEd from uppercase to lowercase. During some saccades, the computer changed the case of every letter (thus "EaCh" would change to "eAcH"). But even when the case of every letter in a sentence was changing, subjects rarely detected the changes, and read the sentence as if nothing were different. The actual experience thus powerfully conflicted with intuition and the phenomenal impression that the texts were being fully experienced not as bits, isolated in time and space by saccades, but as wholes. In a particularly compelling example of this conflict, Grimes (1996) describes an incident in which McConkie and Zola were first testing their complex saccade-contingent change apparatus. Zola was fitted with the eye tracker, and was sitting in front of the rapidly changing display while others in the laboratory were standing behind him watching the sentences as they shimmered on the screen, changing over and over again. While the observers were no doubt congratulating themselves on their technological achievement, Zola shook his head with disappointment and began to insist that the apparatus was not working. Surely, if all those changes had actually been happening he would have seen them!

Extending the saccade contingent technique to natural scenes, Grimes (1996) found that even quite dramatic changes to full color images of objects typically went unnoticed. Several other laboratories devised techniques for masking the changes by displacing the pre- and postchange images or by flickering them in alternation, interspersed with a brief (80 msec) blank field (Blackmore et al., 1995; Rensink, O'Regan, and Clark, 1997). All of these techniques rely on masking the perceptual transient (akin to apparent motion) that might call attention to an immediate change by using a blank-screen interstimulus interval, or by adding a more global transient associated with changing the retinal position of the pre- and postchange images (see also O'Regan, Rensink, and Clark, 1999, for a clever way of masking transients that does not depend on shifting the entire image). Rensink's flicker paradigm has been especially influential, partly because it provides such a striking illustration of change blindness as subjects are exposed to many repetitions of a change before finally detecting it.

Levin and Simons (1997) added to these techniques by making changes during the cuts in motion pictures. In our initial experiment, we created a short film of two actresses having a conversation in which a visual change occurred on every cut. For example, in one cut an actress's scarf disappears (see figure 6.2), and in another the plates on the table change from red to white. When subjects were told to view the video carefully but were not told to be on the lookout for changes, only one of our ten initial subjects was able to report any of the changes, and that single "success" was a vague mention of changing body position. Even when they were told to watch for changes, subjects saw an average of only two out of the nine changes.

Based on these results, one might reasonably conclude that attention to a changing object is necessary to detect the anomaly. Although this conclusion is supported by the straightforward observation that changes to objects relatively central

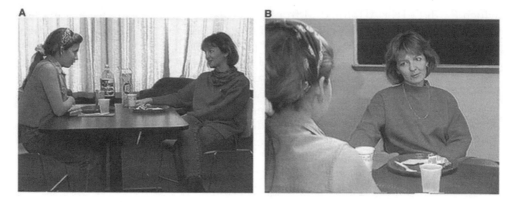

Figure 6.2
Stills from a video in which the right-hand actor's scarf has disappeared across a cut.

to a scene (as defined by judges' inclusion of the changing objects in verbal descriptions of the scenes) are more easily detected (Rensink, O'Regan, and Clark, 1997), we wondered whether attention to a changing object was really sufficient for detecting a change. Our initial intuitions were based on research suggesting that infants do not seem to notice changes to attended objects until they know the words for those objects (Xu and Carey, 1996). Accordingly, one might conclude that labeling might play a large role in detecting changes to attended objects. On the other hand, it seemed to us that labeling was not the kind of thing that anyone, infant or adult, typically does when attending to objects in natural circumstances. This is particularly true of object properties—it is at least conceivable that we generate basic-level classifications for attended objects (Rosch et al., 1976), but any more specific verbalization, explicit reflection, or other conscious manipulation of object properties seemed unlikely unless one were to be forced to focus on this information by some specific task constraint (see Jolicoeur, Gluck, and Kosslyn, 1984; Archambault, O'Donnell and Schyns, 1999). In the absence of such constraint, we thought it might be possible that people would miss changes even in attended objects.

We first tested this hypothesis by making videos in which the sole actor in a scene changed from one person into another. For example, in some of our films, one actor began an action (stepping into the hall to answer a phone) and another completed it. Even though the first actor in the film changed into another person right before their eyes, two-thirds of our subjects failed to detect the change when they were not on the lookout for it (Levin and Simons, 1997). One might argue that this occurred because people do not typically pay much attention to videos, or that some other specific aspect of the experiment led our subjects to miss the changes, but the same thing occurs in the real world. In a follow-up to these initial findings, we created a variety of situations where subjects were exposed to a quick substitution of their conversation partner and we still found that about half failed to detect this change. In one case, an initial experimenter approached a subject on a college campus and asked for directions to a building on campus. Midconversation, two other experimenters carrying a door walked between the subject and the first experimenter. While the subject's view was briefly blocked, one of the experimenters carrying the door traded places with the first experimenter, who walked off behind the door. Thus the subject's conversation partner suddenly changed from one person into another. Yet, even though the change occurred right in front of them, about half of the subjects missed it, continued the conversation as if nothing had happened, and were later quite surprised to find that the person who finished the conversation with them was not the same person who had started it (Simons and Levin, 1998; see figure 6.3). In replicating this effect using a number of different scenarios, we have found that subjects also missed substitutions both when they were photographing the experimenters and when they were receiving consent forms from them (Levin et al., 2002).

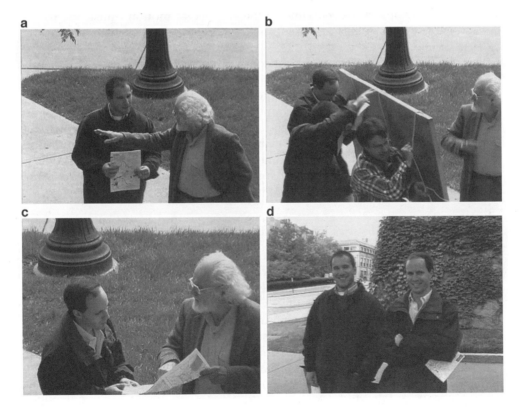

Figure 6.3
Real-world substitution of a conversation partner (from Simons and Levin, 1998).

These experiments demonstrate an important visual limit, and suggest that visual experience is not what we think it is. First, change blindness suggests that attention is more active and selective than previously thought. To understand what people see, we need to know, not only which object, but also which specific features or aspects they have focused on (Simons and Levin, 1998; O'Regan et al., 2000). In addition, the effects of attending may be very transitory. We may not get much benefit from attending to something, then reattending it. Instead, attending may bring objects, features, or both into a coherence for only the moments they are within focus, and when attention leaves them, that coherence is lost, and there may remain only limited benefits from having attended (Wolfe, 1998; Rensink, 2000). More important for present purposes, these findings suggest that our phenomenal experience of a rich, detailed visual percept is somehow illusory. In particular, our sense of inhabiting a visual world that is continuous may not arise in the way we think it does. The perceptual basis of visual experience might be aptly characterized as a montage of impressions and features that, though organized in the moment by complex perceptual processes, are integrated at only a highly abstract level. Thus, in the absence of motion transients, we do not integrate visual details across views, fixations, or over even the briefest of delays.

The illusion of feature-based visual continuity has been discussed frequently (Dennett, 1991; O'Regan, 1992; Blackmore et al., 1995; Rensink, 2000; Noë, Pessoa, and Thompson, 2000; Levin and Simons, 2000; Noë, 2002), is only now being approached empirically. Indeed, so counterintuitive is the change blindness effect that, despite mounting evidence, even researchers confirming it remain incredulous. Thus, every time Simons and Levin set up an experiment to test this effect they world be quite certain that this time they had gone too far. We would nervously present the new stimuli to their subjects, who world amaze them yet again by missing changes they believed were impossible to miss.

Change Blindness Blindness as Visual Metacognition

We have completed a variety of experiments confirming that change blindness does, in fact, run strongly counter to people's intuitions about what they should be able to see. In the most basic of these experiments, we used a postdiction methodology (see Brigham and Bothwell, 1983; Wells, 1984) in which subjects read scenarios describing the original experiments demonstrating change blindness. For example, in our initial experiment, subjects read a scenario describing Levin and Simons, 1997, experiment 1. The subjects were told to imagine that they were watching a movie in which an actor's scarf disappeared across a cut from one shot to the next. They were then shown an illustration including the two relevant shots (see figure 6.2), and the disappearing scarf was pointed out to them. Based on this information (and a reminder that they were not on the lookout for changes), subjects judged whether they would see the change if they had experienced the event.

In experiments of this kind, subjects radically overpredicted their change detection success. For example, in the scarf scenario, up to 90% of the subjects predicted that they would detect a change that none in the actual experiments detected. In another scenario, subjects estimated the likelihood that they would detect the real-world person change described above. This time, 98% of the subjects predicted they would detect a change that was actually detected by only 46%. As is clear from table 6.1, this overoptimism is consistent across scenarios. Also, the confidence ratings in the table make clear that many subjects are highly confident of their incorrect predictions, suggesting that they are not simply taking uncommitted guesses in the absence of any strong conviction.

We refer to this error as "change blindness blindness" (CBB) because people are effectively blind to their change blindness, and it is robust across a wide variety of situations. Subjects show equivalent CBB for predictions about themselves and others' performance (Levin et al., 2000), and they show it when their predictions are based on the actual videos used in the original experiments (instead of stills; Levin et al., 2002). In addition, subjects show CBB even when the pre- and postchange views are separated in time. In these experiments, subjects were asked to imagine that the critical change event was interrupted. For example, in the scarf scenario, they imagined the following. They would be watching a video when the telephone would ring midscene; they would stop their VCR during a shot showing an actor wearing a scarf and get up to answer the phone. After a phone conversation (lasting up to an hour), they would return to the TV and restart their video on the next shot, showing the actor from a different angle without the scarf. Despite the delay, subjects again predicted they would notice the change and showed no overall reduction in CBB for delay scenarios across the three experiments reported in Levin et al., 2002.

This latter finding is important because it refutes the hypothesis that subjects have simply misconstrued the perceptual experience associated with changes.

Table 6.1
Predicted and actual success at detecting changes

Scenario	Predicted Success	Confidence	Actual Success
Plate	76.3%	3.88	0%
Scarf	90.5%	3.98	0%
Actor	69.5%	3.83	0%
Live/Person	97.6%	4.43	46%

Source: Levin et al., 2000. Base rates for "Plate," "Scarf," and "Actor" scenarios are from Levin and Simons, 1997; base rate for "Live/Person" scenario is from Simons and Levin, 1998.
Notes: In "Plate" scenario, plates on table change from red to white; in "Scarf," actor's scarf disappears; in "Actor," sole actor in two-shot video changes from one person into another; and in "Live/Person," one real-world conversation partner is substituted for another. Confidence was rated on scale from 1 ("not confident") to 5 ("very confident").

Otherwise, predictions of success might be based on the belief that the changes would cause perceptual transients akin to apparent motion (see O'Regan, Rensink, and Clark, 1999). According to this hypothesis, change blindness blindness reflects subjects' misunderstanding of a set of fairly narrow and unfamiliar circumstances under which transients occur. Instead, it seems that these demonstrations of CBB do not depend on confounding subjects' intuitions with unfamiliar situations; rather, CBB reflects misjudgments in situations that subjects are generally familiar with, such as viewing a video or having a conversation. Moreover, many people are familiar with the occurrence of between-shot errors in films, and that these can be difficult to detect. Indeed, numerous books and Web sites, some quite popular, are devoted to cataloging such errors.

What, then, causes change blindness blindness? Before proposing a general framework for understanding this phenomenon, it is important to eliminate two alternative explanations. The most intuitive explanation for CBB is that people recruit their beliefs about memory, and conclude that if they remember a few visual details over a short period, then they can remember many over a very short period. Combined with the assumption of a rich visual representation, this might easily lead to CBB. A similar explanation is that the ease with which we can sample visual information from the environment leads us to believe that visual detail is represented internally (see, for example, Rensink, 2000). However, delayed-change CBB runs counter to both of these explanations: lengthening the delay over which details must be remembered does not significantly reduce CBB, and it apparently does not lead people to consider the need for representations in detecting changes. In response justifications for delayed-change scenarios, subjects rarely mention memory, in stark contrast to those for delayed–digit span scenarios, where they almost always do (Levin et al., 2002).

Another alternative explanation for change blindness blindness is that subjects simply do not understand perceptual inference in general, and assume that everything they see is based in a continuous perceptual contact with the targets of attention. A related proposal is that CBB is a straightforward case of our expectation that we should "notice what takes place before our eyes" (Noë, Pessoa, and Thompson, 2000, p. 103). That is, subjects expect to see salient events and are surprised when they do not.

Although both explanations might be correct in a sense, neither is sufficiently articulated to help us understand where and when people are likely to misconstrue visual experience, an important limitation because change blindness blindness is not part of a blanket overestimate of all visual capabilities. For example, Beck and Levin (in review) found that subjects could accurately predict change detection performance for an intentional change detection task where the number of objects in real-world scenes varied from trial to trial. We suspect that subjects were accurate in this instance for two reasons. First, subjects may be far more accurate in estimating their performance on intentional change detection tasks where detecting changes is their primary focus and not incidental to some other task. Second, because scenes were repeated with different numbers of objects, subjects may have focused explicitly on set size and based their decision on the assumption that they would have to search the display for changes. However, neither of these factors alone eliminate CBB: subjects in Levin and Beck's study showed CBB for arraylike scenes in the incidental conditions, and in Scholl, Simons, and Levin's study (chapter 7, this volume), they show it for an intentional change blindness task. The challenge, therefore, is to develop a systematic understanding of visual metacognition in adults that can make sense of this kind of evidence (something we begin to do below).

Before doing so, we would also like to point out that although it is probably accurate to suggest that change blindness blindness occurs because people believe that they should see salient events, this explanation begs the question of what is to count as a salient event. Clearly, if we cannot explain the difference between unsurprising failures to detect "small" visual changes and shocking failures to detect "large" ones, we will not have a useful understanding of visual metacognition (for additional discussion, see Levin, 2002). The next sections ask whether a careful comparison between the tasks at which children succeed and those at which adults fail can help us develop a more general explanation of visual metacognition that encompasses both.

Change Blindness Blindness and Children's Success in Reasoning about Representations

When we began this project, we were surprised to discover just how little research explored adults' understanding of vision. The exceptions to this rule have been research exploring people's incorrect belief that seeing depends on extramissions from the eye, as opposed to intromissions of reflected and emitted light into the eye (see Winer and Cottrell, chapter 5, this volume, for review), and a small number of studies on appearance-reality conflations in adults (Taylor and Mitchell, 1997). It is interesting to note that in the former case, the research was initiated as an attempt to understand the development of concepts about seeing and that the authors initially assumed that only children would hold extramissionist beliefs. As we will review below, other developmental research has explored beliefs about visual attention, and although adults' understandings are more correct than children's, it may be that here as well, the developmental process does not include an end point of successful understanding. On the other hand, a vast tradition of research in cognitive development clearly shows that by the age of 4, children can reason effectively about representations, especially in circumstances where representations conflict with the real world (e.g., Wimmer and Perner, 1983; Baren-Cohen, 1995; see Wellman, Cross, and Watson, 2001, for review). Therefore, one of the most basic questions that needs answering about change blindness blindness and other visual metacognition errors is, how do people make such big mistakes when we know that they must understand something about the representational process?

This question is particularly compelling because of the conceptual similarity between the false-belief task, used to test children's understanding of representation, and the change detection task. In both cases, the subject is asked whether they or someone else will become aware of a change in the visual world. In a typical false-belief task, a child might witness an object being hidden in one of two hiding places in the company of a puppet. Then, with the puppet out of the room, the scene is changed—the object is moved from its original hiding place to the other location. The key question is whether the child will realize that the puppet has a belief that does not match the changed state of the real world because the puppet was out of the room when the object was moved. Three-year-olds appear not to understand this, and will consistently predict that the puppet will look in the new hiding place; they cannot appreciate that the puppet has an internal representation that is now out of date because the object was moved in its absence. By age 4, however, children begin to consistently predict that the puppet will look in the old hiding place, demonstrating the critical understanding that representations of the world are not simply copies of it. In developing a "representational theory of mind" these children have achieved the understanding that mental contents refer to the world and can be different from it. This achievement is assumed to underlie a wide array of skills, ranging from word learning (Doherty and Perner, 1998; Jenkins and Astington, 1996; Ricard, Girouard, and Gouin Decarie, 1999) to the ability to integrate local information into global meaning (Jarrold et al., 2000).

It is important to emphasize that this developmental shift occurs both for understandings of representations in other people, and those in oneself. In a first-person analogue to the false-belief task above, children's understanding that their own representations of the world had previously been at odds with reality can be demonstrated. In one such task, children might be shown a cereal box and be asked what they believe it to contain. Naturally, they claim it contains cereal. Once they report this belief, they are shown that the box contains unexpected contents, such as rocks. Now, once the box is closed again, they correctly report that it contains rocks, but they also claim they knew the box contained rocks all along and will even insist that this is what they said in response to the initial questioning. Finally, they will predict that someone who had not seen the contents of the box would believe it contained rocks. By the time they are 5, however, children correctly report their own previously false beliefs, and realize that their understanding of the world can depart significantly from reality (see, for example, Hogrefe, Wimmer, and Perner, 1986; Perner, Leekham, and Wimmer, 1987; Gopnik and Astington, 1988).

Taken together, these findings suggest that even kindergarteners have a substantive understanding of the difference between their representation of reality and the real world. Related research suggests that this understanding extends into the visual domain as well, and that even children considerably younger than 4 understand how representations refer to things in the world: they have a fundamental "aboutness." Young children overcome appearance-reality conflicts, begin to understand the perceptual consequences of differing viewpoints, and realize that people who have only partial perceptual access to an object may be unaware of its identity (see Flavell, chapter 1, this volume). As a number of authors have noted, an intentional theory of mind may have a perceptual basis in vision (Gopnik, Slaughter, and Meltzhoff, 1994; Flavell, Green, and Flavell, 1990). One line of evidence suggests that perception of gaze targets constitutes the basis for understanding that people refer to things when they talk, and may eventually become the basis for decoding their intentions. The primary purpose for this visual coding of intention is probably word learning, a task for which it is clearly necessary to have a good understanding of what people are referring to when they make an utterance. As reviewed by Flavell (chapter 1, this volume), these developments may be allied with an emerging understanding of attentional focus—in several experiments, children have demonstrated an understanding of limits to the spatial extent of the attentional spotlight by age 8; they also appear to have some understanding of the necessity of focusing on a subset of visual information for the purpose of remembering it. Flavell, Green, and Flavell's (1995) experiment is particularly important for present purposes (see also Pillow, 1989; Miller and Weiss, 1982). They asked children if they would see one thing while focusing their attention on another thing at the same time. For example, children were asked if, while looking at a painting, they would see the frame it is in. Young children were more likely to respond affirmatively than older children. Based on these findings, Flavell, Green, and Flavell argue that children think of visual attention as more of a lamp than a spotlight: once one directs attention to a scene, it is completely illuminated, and one can "see" everything that is in the room.

It is, however, interesting to note that despite a developmental trend for improvement, adults' intuitions about visual attention are by no means unanimous, a finding hinted at in the diversity of opinion about attentional limits in Flavell, Green, and Flavell's older children and in the results of recent work in our laboratory on adult intuition about attentional focus. We have consistently found that adults give a wide range of responses to these questions. For example, in one series of experiments, we asked subjects to imagine that they were looking across the street at their friend. Subjects were then asked whether they could see a fire hydrant while looking at their friend, and were almost evenly split into those who predicted they probably or definitely would see the hydrant, those who predicted there was a 50% probability of seeing the hydrant, and those who predicted they probably or definitely would not see the hydrant. In addition, in open-ended response justifications for change blindness blindness scenarios in Levin et al. (2002), adults give hints that they hold something of a lamplike theory of visual attention. For example, when asked if paying attention directly to the changing object is necessary to see a change, one subject wrote, "I think you could see the change without paying direct attention to the objects because the changes often affected the whole scene," and another wrote, "I would often notice the change without paying direct attention to the object, but to the entire scene itself." More recent experiments have also shown that responses to the kind of "attentional breadth" questions described above predict CBB; subjects who think they have a particularly broad spotlight also think they will see more changes. In addition, subjects who think that they typically attend to a large proportion of the objects in a scene show more CBB (Levin, 2001).

Although at first blush it appears that people develop a basic understanding of representation early on, as embodied by a representational/intentional theory of mind, something may prevent people from accurately reasoning through the entailments of this theory. Thus the failure implicated in change blindness blindness is that people may not consider the degree to which visual representations are necessary for change detection even though they understand the degree to which representations are necessary for other, closely related tasks such as the false-belief task. Clearly, then, it would appear necessary to delimit how the foundational metaknowledge that drives children's early reasoning successes leaves even adults without accurate guidance in specific situations. One possibility is that visual experience overrides adults understanding of representation by sometimes obscuring the need to consider the role of representation in seeing, and the need to explicitly focus on specific aspects of the visual world to be aware of them.

Intentional Representations in an Intentional Loop
To think through these metacognitive errors, it is helpful to consider more broadly the interaction between representations and the visual world. For our present purposes, we will refer to this interaction as an "intentional loop" in which an organism forms intentions, interacts with the environment, and modifies intentions based on this interaction. Although this interaction can be described at a variety of levels of complexity, for now, we would like to limit our focus to four cyclic steps. First are intentions—the beliefs, desires, and other representations *about* the world that drive interactions with the world (see, for example, Dennett, 1997). Second are plans to explore the world, which we form based on intentions. These could include plans to sample the world visually or to interact with it physically by reaching. Third are perceptions of the world, and fourth is the information sampled from the world, which we must evaluated to determine the degree to which beliefs are verified and our desires satisfied. If more information is needed, the loop continues to operate and new plans are made to continue exploring the world. It is important to note right away that this model is really a simple description of endogenous attention because it starts and ends with intentions. Therefore, much visually guided behavior might not be aptly described by this kind of cognitively elaborate visual exploration.

A basic intentional theory of mind affords at least the possibility of reasoning effectively about each step in this process. Children understand that the puppet in the false-belief task has a distinct belief about the world (that the candy is in box A), will engage in action to test that belief (by opening box A), will update that belief if it is wrong (by deciding that the candy must be in box B), and then will interact with the world again to test this updated belief (by opening box B). The same holds for the first-person intentionality tested in the cereal box task. Again, by age 4, children understand that they have a distinct belief about the presence of cereal in the box, that they must do something to test that hypothesis, and that they must revise their belief if they find out there are rocks in the box. (It is important to note that the foundations of an intentional theory of mind might emerge earlier than age 4, and that the false-belief task should be considered a particularly rigorous means of demonstrating an intentional theory of mind, but not the sole means of demonstrating it; see Flavell, chapter 1, this volume, for review).

Thus, to understand why the early-developing understanding of representation does not allow consistently effective reasoning about vision, one might focus on how the false-belief task allows subjects effective access to its representational underpinnings, whereas the change blindness task does not. In the latter case, an intentional loop is a similarly useful means for understanding more basic interactions with the visual world. When viewing the typical scene, one has a set of beliefs about it, which are tested by continuously sampling the scene, and by developing new representations that are used to update one's beliefs about the visual world. If there is one thing that change blindness suggests, it is that this kind of goal-directed, search-and-abstract process underlies a large share of perceptual experience relative to more exogenous perceptual alerting. This comparison is particularly compelling given that recent theorizing about visual attention has even described attention as a hand that reaches into a scene, affording perceptual organization to only a small number of objects or features at a given time (Rensink, 2000).

The question is, if perceptual experience is a representationally mediated intentional search through complex visual information, why do people not realize this? As mentioned above, a number of authors have suggested that people mistake the ease with which visual information can be accessed for rich internal representations of that information. Because it is so easy to look at something, and because visual information quickly springs into awareness the moment we focus our attention on something, it is easy to make the small mistake of conflating the external world for an internal representation. One problem with this particular formulation is that people do not seem to have much by way of explicit beliefs that they represent anything in particular. As mentioned above, subjects rarely mention "knowing" or "remembering" the changing features, even when the pre- and postchange objects are separated by long delays (Levin et al., forthcoming). It seems more apt to suggest that the whole notion of representation has been dropped from the equation entirely, that the thinking part of the look-think-look cycle has been enfolded into the experience of seeing. In this sense, one might suggest that the intentional loop has collapsed into a pure perceptual experience.

The notion that an intentional loop might collapse in this way is consistent with a number of discussions about vision, especially visual expertise. For example, Gopnik (1993) suggests that perceptual inference becomes less salient as expertise causes tasks to become compiled and more automatic. Experts think they can "see" things that novices have to search effortfully for. Research exploring the development of expertise in radiological diagnosis suggests that novices detect distinctive features at a consistent rate over the minute or so they might search an image. In contrast, expert radiologists detect features quickly at the onset of the search, then detect fewer over the remainder of the search. Although Christensen and colleagues (1981) concluded that the task was more perceptual for experts, they may have taken their subjects' reports too seriously. Experts' initial glances at a slide may be more automatic than those of novices, but this does not preclude the kinds of abstraction inherent to an intentional loop. More generally, the expertise effect might simply rely on the fact that the efficiency afforded by familiarity is mistaken for a rich perceptual experience, when the richness is, in fact, more abstract and grounded in the rich representational experience.

It seems plausible that intentional collapse can have a number of different causes: it can be structural or more social and focused on perceiving intentions. In the former case, the organization inherent to many natural scenes allows a unitization that can have a perceptual feel to it, even though it is entirely conceptual. So, one might see a complex scene of a table, some people, some plates, some cups, a rug, and some curtains, represent it as two people talking at a cafe, thus giving a disparate array of information a simple coherence. This coherence allows the scene to be processed efficiently at a conceptual level and is probably associated with a set of perceptual expectations that allows it to be searched efficiently as well (a key role for the quickly coded "gists" discussed by many authors; see, for example, Friedman, 1979). Coupled with an efficient search experience, this conceptual organization, could cause intentional collapse and the failure to realize that detecting changes relies on a kind of representation that is not available. Gaze-directed attention may also play an organizing role. As discussed above, much developmental research has demonstrated that joint attention is critical for language learning, and a number of authors have argued that it is the perceptual basis for an intentional theory of mind. In adults, following a look probably serves as an automatic means of guiding fixations around a scene. In many cases, this may closely mirror a third-person intentional loop in which percepts are organized around codings of relations among objects and people.

One nice illustration of this process comes from descriptions of film editing. A number of editors describe the editing process as akin to asking and answering questions (see, for example, Pudovkin, 1929). The most commonly used example is a close-up of an actor looking off screen, which is conceptualized as a question that needs to be answered in the next shot. Thus the editor, having induced the viewers to ask, "What is it?," answers the question by cutting in a shot of the actor's gaze target, and often also by cutting back to the actor, who reacts to what they have seen. In this way, the editor organizes a series of percepts into an intentional event. This is probably a specific instance of the more general editing principles that interact with, sometimes guiding, sometimes following, the viewers' train of visual thought. The key to these principles is to make the editing disappear—to create a seamless impression of settings and events without awareness of the degree to which that impression is constructed from a series of partial (and often inconsistent; Levin and Simons 2000) views. An experiment by Kraft (1986) supports this by showing that film viewers are largely unaware of the presence of edits when viewing films.

It is important to note that the notion of intentional collapse is not a description of visual cognition, but rather of visual metacognition. Change blindness demonstrates that, even when scene perception is fluid and efficient, people still rely on abstraction to understand scenes and guide attention. Because it does not seem that way, however, the role of representation and the fact of abstraction are not apparent: people believe that they will see things in detail that are only represented in the abstract. Thus change blindness blindness may reflect, not an explicit belief in visual detail representation, but rather the belief that one will see significant visual events, on the one hand, and the failure to consider the need for a representationally intensive process to bridge the gap between pre- and postchange views, on the other.

If visual organization and intentional collapse lead people to incorrectly short-circuit the need for reasoning about representations, then how do theory-of-mind and appearance-reality tasks differ from tasks that illustrate CBB, in allowing people to effectively reason about representations? The key factor that probably allows effective reasoning is that the typical false-belief task stops the intentional loop cold, and allows subjects a moment for some real introspection about the mind of the observer who was out of the room when the situation changed. As mentioned above, the standard false-belief task is similar to a change detection task in that there is a prechange scene (candy in box A), a postchange scene (candy in box B), and the need to determine whether someone will notice the difference between the two and behave appropriately. Even children get it right, and realize that someone will not notice the change because they have represented scene A and have had no opportunity to observe scene B. In this situation, perception cannot overwhelm representation, and the intentional loop is laid bare. The critical junction between intention and perception has been cut, and the subject must consider an intention that cannot guide an interaction with the perceptual world.

One advantage of organizing visual metacognition around the idea of an intentional loop is that this idea may encompass not only overestimates of visual performance but underestimates as well. For example, what if perceptual fluency is effectively disrupted and subjects are forced to focus on perceptual complexity while at the same time they fail to consider the utility of the representational part of the loop. One situation that might satisfy these conditions is picture memory. Several experiments have shown that recognition memory for pictures is surprisingly good (Nickerson, 1965; Shepard, 1967; Standing, 1973). Subjects viewing inspection sets of 50, 100, 1,000, and even 10,000 pictures were found to accurately distinguish these pictures from new ones. One means of reconciling this success with the failures inherent to change blindness is to assume that gists, or long-term abstract categorical descriptions of visual scenes, are efficiently coded and remembered for each scene we encounter. Although not detailed and therefore not useful in distinguishing between similar scenes with different details (charge detection), gists are highly useful in distinguishing between scenes that have different meanings and visual organizations.

From a metacognitive standpoint, then, a picture memory experiment is associated with a mass of perceptual detail and with the need to code or organize individual samples from the perceptual world ad infinitum. Because no scene is associated with any particular belief or desire, this coding or organization occurs in the absence of a recognizable representational process. In a sense, the intentional loop has exploded into an apparently undifferentiated mass of perceptual experience, and unrelated intentions. In this case, it is the powerful representational process that is metacognitively transparent, and therefore ignored because it is not part of the subject's theory of mind. Because gists may be coded automatically (Friedman, 1979), their ability to effectively differentiate targets and nontargets in the picture memory task may be underappreciated by perceivers. Accordingly, people may underestimate their ability to perform this task. We will be the first to admit that, given the enormous number of pictures people can remember, this is hardly a bold hypothesis. However, nobody had done this experiment, and when we did, we found that not only did subjects underestimate their ability to remember large numbers of pictures, but they also were not at all certain of their ability to remember comparatively small inspection sets. For example, in one of our initial experiments, we described a picture memory task to subjects, and illustrated it with an inspection set of widely disparate images. As is clear from figure 6.4, subjects did not consistently predict full success for even ten-image sets, and their predicted performance fell off sharply for any larger sets until their predictions diverged almost as far as possible from performance as measured in the original research.

One issue we have not touched on thus far is perhaps the most basic. That is, is the intentional loop explicitly *intentional*? Are representational understandings specific to an intentional level of analysis, and to a specific set of knowledge or processes necessary for reasoning about beliefs, desires, and their mapping onto the external world? A number of authors argue that a distinct cognitive subsystem underlies reasoning about theory-of-mind problems. One line of research supports this hypothesis by showing that children who have difficulty with a false-belief task can reason effectively about a formally similar "false photograph"

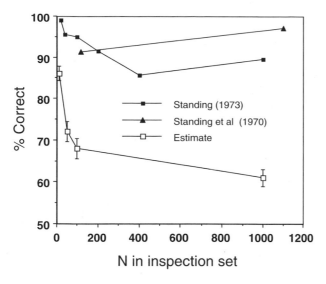

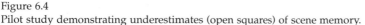

Figure 6.4
Pilot study demonstrating underestimates (open squares) of scene memory.

task in which a photograph of the prechange situation becomes outdated by a change. For example, using Zaitchick's paradigm (1990), Slaughter (1998) placed a toy frog on a chair adjacent to his 3-year-old subjects, took a Polaroid picture of it, then placed the picture facedown on a table. With the picture developing on the table, the frog was replaced by a white teddy bear, and the children were asked whether the picture had the frog or the bear in it. Not only did the 3-year-olds perform considerably better on this task than on the standard false-belief task, but they also showed task-specific training effects: training on the photograph task improved performance on that task, but not the false-belief task. The converse was true for false-belief training (Slaughter, 1998). Research with autistic children supports a similar conclusion, demonstrating a dissociation between false-representation tasks with intentional and mechanical surface structures. These children could reason much more effectively about false photographs than false beliefs despite their advanced chronological and mental ages. Leslie (2000) goes so far as to argue for a functionally dissociable theory-of-mind module (see also Sabbagh and Taylor, 2000).

If there really is a distinct process for reasoning about the mind, and if visual metacognition draws upon it, then it should be possible to create a situation where subjects can effectively reason about visual representations outside the context of the mind. The most obvious example of the need for this kind of reasoning is in understanding how computers function. Computers are, or at least can be described as, nonintentional in that their representations usually refer to the world in an arbitrary way (see Dennett, 1997). And, as inanimate objects, they can hardly be said to have beliefs and desires in the same way that people do. (However, it is important to point out that computers have many "cognitive" characteristics that subjects seem to understand, and therefore might be considered a hybrid between intentional and nonintentional systems; see Scaife and van Duren, 1995). Thus it should be possible to describe a computerized visual system that manipulates abstract visual representations and to have subjects effectively reason about its limits. In a recent series of experiments Levin (in prep), we have attempted to manipulate a scenario describing a computerized vision algorithm that leads subjects to avoid intentional reasoning in one condition and to engage in it in another.

In the nonintentional condition, subjects read about a computer vision program called "SOCAR" (Scene and Object Collation and Recognition) that searches scenes for "unusual events." The program was described as having two distinct stages. In the first, an object-processing system codes the features of each object in the scene, focusing on one at a time, and uses property information to identify each object in the scene. The key to the first stage is that its output is a one-word label for each object (in the actual scenarios this is illustrated with a "mug"). Also important is that the first stage is explicitly described as "resetting" and clearing this property information for each new object it processes. Thus the system has essentially no visual memory that survives different views, although this is something subjects must infer, based on the labeling-reset cycle. The first stage identifications are then sent to a second stage, which places the identifications in a list, and, once all the objects in the scene have been labeled, the program continues to identify objects, and the second stage checks each label with the list to determine whether the object has been added to the scene since the initial coding. If a label is not in the list, the program generates an alert that a human operator is to follow up on. For the intentional condition, the same program is renamed "OSCAR" (Object and Scene Collation and Recognition) and described in intentional, anthropomorphic terms. Thus OSCAR is referred to as "he," described as having goals, and said to "see" and "notice" things.

Once they have read one of these descriptions, subjects are asked whether "the program" would generate an alert, or whether "OSCAR" would see various changes to a hypothetical scene. These include property changes to an object, substitutions of one object for another, appearances of new and duplicate objects, and disappearances. In addition, subjects are asked to predict both the performance of the program in a picture memory task and details of its operation. The first result of interest is that subjects clearly understand that this representational system does not track visual details across views. In the nonintentional condition, very few of the subjects predicted that the program would detect a salient property change. Subjects also understood that the system would detect changes that involved the addition of a new object to the scene so long as it would be associated with a label that was not in the list. These results clearly suggest that the visual metacognitive errors we observed above are not the result of some basic limit to subjects ability to reason about even fairly complex representational systems (see also Zaitchick, 1990).

In addition, changing the surface structure of the problem had a number of effects on subjects responses. First, on two of the change detection questions, subjects were more likely to predict success for the intentional agent than for the "program." When asked whether the addition of another object sharing a name with an object previously in the scene (in this case, another mug was added to a scene that already had a mug in it) would be detected, significantly more subjects believed that "OSCAR" would see the change than that "the program" would. Similarly, more subjects thought that OSCAR would see the disappearance of an object than that the program would, although this result was nonsignificant. In contrast, subjects appeared to believe that OSCAR was less likely than the program to remember large numbers of scenes.

Taken together, the results of the above experiments suggest that many visual metacognition errors may result from an interaction between a default to reason about representations using an intentional framework and specific situations that can confound this kind of reasoning. In situations where perception is effortless and transparent, subjects may fail to consider the role of any representations, on the one hand, and to make use of their understanding that representations are distinct from the things represented and can diverge from the current state of the real world, on the other. However, when the intentional loop is stopped and subjects are forced to consider the role of representations in guiding behavior, they can reason effectively, as demonstrated by successful reasoning about false beliefs. Finally, when representations are made salient as a confusing mass of unrelated intentions, subjects demonstrate a metacognitive error opposite to change blindness blindness—they underestimate performance on a task testing picture memory.

Underlying these specific theory-task interactions is the question of why people do not adapt their reasoning more fully to each of these specific situations. Clearly, experience affords at least some opportunities to understand how difficult it can be to countenance detailed visual information, and how easy it can be to remember the gist of a place we have visited or a picture we have looked at. When people consider whether they can detect a specific change, however, or remember some set of pictures, they may fall back on a heuristic approach, or a basic theory of representation even where it does not give effective guidance. Because a default to reasoning about intentional representations may reflect the foundational status of an intentional theory of mind, intentional reasoning may color much of folk psychology, and even more general problem solving about representations, as demonstrated in the above experiment on reasoning about a computer vision system.

A critical challenge for future research on visual metacognition and on meta-cognition more generally is to develop a systematic theory coordinating the extensive body of research on the developing theory of mind with the legion of successes and failures of adults when they attempt to make sense of their own limits and those of others. After all, our metacognitions are probably accurate and well adapted to many natural circumstances (see Levin, 2002; Diana and Reder, chapter 8, this volume), whereas in other situations they can be wildly inaccurate. Some systematic means of delimiting when metacognitions are accurate is therefore necessary, especially in light of recently documented perceptual failures such as change blindness and inattention blindness. In both of these cases, not only does the failure to understand perceptual limits lay open the possibility that people will be ineffective at allocating visual resources, but it also makes the objective evaluation of others' perceptual experience extraordinarily prone to error. Examples of this kind of failure abound (see Levin, 2002, for review), ranging from legal settings where people must consider what another person "should have seen" to industrial settings where complex human-machine interfaces are constantly designed based on folk psychology understandings of perceptual limits.

Acknowledgments

We would like to thank Saul Levin and Maria Zaragoza for commenting on previous versions of this chapter, whose preparation was supported by National Science Foundation grant SES-0214969 to Daniel Levin.

References

Archambault, A., O'Donnell, C., and Schyns, P. G. (1999). Blind to object changes: When learning the same object at different levels of categorization modifies its perception, *Psychological Science, 10*, 249–255.

Baron-Cohen, S. (1995). Mindblindness: An essay on autism and theory of mind. Cambridge, MA: MIT Press.

Beck, M. R., and Levin, D. T. (in review). Understanding the active process of vision.

Blackmore, S. J., Brelstaff, G., Nelson, K., and Troscianko, T. (1995). Is the richness of our visual world an illusion? Transsacadic memory for complex scenes. *Perception, 24*, 1075–1081.

Brigham, J. C., and Bothwell, R. K. (1983). The ability of prospective jurors to estimate the accuracy of eyewitness identifications. *Law and Human Behavior, 7*, 19–30.

Christensen, E. E., Murry, R. C., Holland, K., Reynolds, J., Landay, M. J., and Moore, J. G. (1981). The effect of search time on perception. *Diagnostic Radiology, 138*, 361–365.

Dennett, D. C. (1991). *Consciousness explained.* New York: Little, Brown.

Dennett, D. C. (1997). True believers: The intentional strategy and why it works. In Haugeland, John (Ed.), *Mind design 2: Philosophy, psychology, artificial intelligence.* 2nd ed. (pp. 57–79). Cambridge, MA: MIT Press.

Doherty, M., and Perner, J. (1998). Metalinguistic awareness and theory of mind: Just two words for the same thing? *Cognitive Development, 13*, 279–305.

Flavell, J. H., Green, F. L., and Flavell, E. R. (1990). Developmental changes in young children's knowledge about the mind. *Cognitive Development, 5*(1), 1–27.

Flavell, J. H., Green, F. L., and Flavell, E. R. (1995). The development of children's knowledge about attentional focus. *Developmental Psychology*, *31*, 706–712.

Friedman, A. (1979). Framing pictures: The role of knowledge in automatized encoding and memory for gist. *Journal of Experimental Psychology: General*, *108*, 316–355.

Gopnik, A. (1993). How we know are minds: The illusion of first-person knowledge of intentionality. *Behavioral and Brain Sciences*, *16*, 1–14.

Gopnik, A., and Astington, J. W. (1988). Children's understanding of representational change and its relation to the understanding of false belief and the appearance-reality distinction. *Child Development*, *59*, 26–37.

Gopnik, A., Slaughter, V., and Meltzoff, A. (1994). Changing your views: How understanding visual perception can lead to a new theory of the mind. In C. Lewis and P. Mitchell (Eds.), *Origins of an understanding of mind* (pp. 157–181). Hillsdale, NJ: Erlbaum.

Grimes, J. (1996). On the failure to detect changes in scenes across saccades. In K. Akins (Ed.), *Perception*. Vancouver Studies in Cognitive Science. Vol. 2 (pp. 89–110). New York: Oxford University Press.

Hogrefe, G. J., Wimmer, H., and Perner, J. (1986). Ignorance versus false-belief: A developmental lag in attribution of epistemic states. *Child Development*, *57*, 567–582.

Jarrold, C., Butler, D. W., Cottington, E. M., and Jimenez, F. (2000). Linking theory of mind and central coherence bias in autism and in the general population. *Developmental Psychology*, *36*, 126–138.

Jenkins, J. M., and Astington, J. W. (1996). Cognitive factors and family structure associated with theory of mind development in young children. *Developmental Psychology*, *32*, 70–78.

Jolicoeur, P., Gluck, M. A., and Kosslyn, S. M. (1984). Pictures and names: Making the connection. *Cognitive Psychology*, *16*, 243–275.

Jonides, J., and Yantis, S. (1988). Uniqueness of abrupt visual onset in capturing attention. *Perception and Psychophysics*, *43*, 346–354.

Kraft, R. N. (1986). The role of cutting in the evaluation and retention of film. *Journal of Experimental Psychology: Learning, Memory, and Cognition*, *12*, 155–163.

Leslie, A. M. (2000). "Theory of mind" as a mechanism of selective attention. In M. Gazzaniga (Ed.), *The new cognitive neurosciences* (pp. 1235–1247). Cambridge, MA: MIT Press.

Levin, D. T. (2001). Visual metacognitions underlying change blindness blindness and estimates of picture memory. Poster presented at the Vision Sciences Conference, Sarasota.

Levin, D. T. (2002). Change blindness blindness as visual metacognition. *Journal of Consciousness Studies*, *9*, 111–130.

Levin, D. T., Drivdahl, S. B., Momen, N., and Beck, M. R. (2002). False predictions about the detectability of unexpected visual changes: The role of metamemory and beliefs about attention in causing change blindness blindness. *Consciousness and Cognition*, *11*, 507–527.

Levin, D. T., Momen, N., Drivdahl, S. B., and Simons, D. J. (2000). Change blindness blindness: The metacognitive error of overestimating change-detection ability. *Visual Cognition*.

Levin, D. T., and Simons, D. J. (1997). Failure to detect changes to attended objects in motion pictures. *Psychonomic Bulletin and Review*, *4*, 501–506.

Levin, D. T. (in prep). Visual metacognition and intentional theory of mind.

Levin, D. T., and Simons, D. J. (2000). Perceiving stability in a changing world: Combining shots and integrating views in motion pictures and the real world. *Media Psychology*, *2*, 357–380.

Levin, D. T., Simons, D. J., Angelone, B. L., and Chabris, C. F. (2002). Memory for centrally attended changing objects in an incidental real-world change detection paradigm. *British Journal of Psychology*, *93*, 289–302.

Mack, A., and Rock, I. (1998). *Inattentional blindness*. Cambidge, MA: MIT Press.

McConkie, G. W., and Zola, D. (1979). Is visual information integrated across successive fixations in reading? *Perception and Psychophysics*, *25*, 221–224.

Miller, P. H., and Weiss, M. G. (1982). Children's and adults' knowledge about what variables affect selective attention. *Child Development*, *53*, 543–549.

Nickerson, R. S. (1965). Short-term memory for complex meaningful visual configurations: A demonstration of capacity. *Canadian Journal of Psychology*, *19*, 155–160.

Neisser, U., and Becklen, R. (1975). Selective looking: Attending to visually specified events. *Cognitive Psychology*, *7*, 480–494.

Noë, A., Ed. (2002). Is the visual world a grand illusion? *Journal of Consciousness Studies*, *9*, 5–6. (Special issue.)

Noë, A., Passoa, L., and Thompson, E. (2000). Beyond the grand illusion: What change blindness really teaches us about vision. *Visual Cognition*, *7*, 93–106.

O'Regan, J. K. (1992). Solving the "real" mysteries of visual perception: The world as an outside memory. *Canadian Journal of Psychology*, *46*, 461–488.

O'Regan, J. K., Deubel, K., and Clark, J. J. (2000). Picture changes during blinks: Looking without seeing and seeing without looking. *Visual Cognition*, *7*, 191–211.

O'Regan, J. K., Rensink, R. A., and Clark, J. J. (1999). Change-blindness as a result of "mudsplashes." *Nature*, *398*, 34.

Perner, J. Leekman, S., and Wimmer, H. (1987). Three-year-olds' difficulty with false belief: The case for a conceptual deficit. *British Journal of Developmental Psychology*, *5*, 125–137.

Pillow, B. H. (1989). The development of beliefs about selective attention. *Merrill-Palmer Quarterly*, *35*, 421–443.

Pudovkin, V. I. (1929). *Film technique*. Reprint, New York: Random House, 1970.

Rensink, R. A. (2000). The dynamic representation of scenes. *Visual Cognition*, *7*, 17–42.

Rensink, R. A., O'Regan, J. K., and Clark, J. J. (1997). To see or not to see: The need for attention to perceive changes in scenes. *Psychological Science*, *8*, 368–373.

Ricard, M., Girouard, P. C., and Gouin Decarie, T. (1999). Personal pronouns and perspective taking in toddlers. *Journal of Child Language*, *26*, 681–697.

Rosch, E., Mervis, C. B., Gray, W. D., Johnson, D., and Boyes-Braem, P. (1976). Basic objects in natural categories. *Cognitive Psychology*, *8*, 382–439.

Sabbagh, M. A., and Taylor, M. (2000). Neural correlates of theory of mind reasoning: An event-related potential study. *Psychological Science*, *11*, 46–50.

Scaife, M., and van Duren, M. (1995). Do computers have brains? What children believe about intelligent systems. *British Journal of Psychology*, *13*, 367–377.

Shepard, R. N. (1967). Recognition memory for words, sentences, and pictures. *Journal of Verbal Learning and Verbal Behavior*, *6*, 156–163.

Simons, D. J., and Chabris, C. F. (1999). Gorillas in our midst: Sustained inattentional blindness for dynamic events. *Perception*, *28*, 1059–1074.

Simons, D. J., and Levin, D. T. (1998). Failure to detect changes to people in a real-world interaction. *Psychonomic Bulletin and Review*, *5*, 644–649.

Simons, D. J., and Levin, D. T. (2003). What makes change blindness interesting? In D. E. Irwin and B. H. Ross (Eds.), *The Psychology & Learning and Motivation*, Vol. 42 (pp. 295–322). San Diego, CA: Academic Press.

Slaughter, V. (1998). Children's understanding of pictorial and mental representations. *Child Development*, *69*, 321–332.

Standing, L. (1973). Learning 10,000 pictures. *Journal of Experimental Psychology*, *25*, 207–222.

Taylor, L. M., and Mitchell, P. (1997). Judgments of apparent shape contaminated by knowledge of reality: Viewing circles obliquely. *British Journal of Psychology*, *88*, 653–670.

Wayand, J., and Levin, D.T. (2001). Ignoring a merciless act. Poster presented at the Vision Sciences Conference, Sarasota.

Wellman, H. M., Cross, D., and Watson, J. (2001). Meta-analysis of theory-of-mind development: The truth about false belief. *Child Development*, *72*, 655–684.

Wells, G. L. (1984). How adequate is human intuition for judging eyewitness testimony? In G. L. Wells and E. F. Loftus (Eds.), *Eyewitness testimony* (pp. 256–272). Cambridge: Cambridge University Press.

Wimmer, H., and Perner, J. (1983). Beliefs about beliefs: Representation and constraining function of wrong beliefs in young children's understanding of deception. *Cognition, 13,* 103–128.

Wolfe, J. M. (1998). Inattentional amnesia. In V. Coltheart (Ed.), *Fleeting memories: Cognition of brief visual stimuli* (pp. 71–94). Cambridge, MA: MIT Press.

Xu, F., and Carey, S. (1996). Infants' metaphysics: The case of numerical identity. *Cognitive Psychology, 30,* 111–153.

Zaitchick, D. (1990). When representations conflict with reality: The preschooler's problem with false beliefs and the "false" photograph task. *Cognition, 35,* 41–68.

Chapter 7

"Change Blindness" Blindness: An Implicit Measure of a Metacognitive Error

Brian J. Scholl, Daniel J. Simons, and Daniel T. Levin

Most people have strong but mistaken intuitions about how perception and cognition work. Such intuitions can give rise to especially pernicious 'metacognitive errors', which are directly fueled by visual experience. Here we explore one such metacognitive error, which infects our intuitions about visual awareness and the perception of change. In the phenomenon called "change blindness," observers fail to notice large changes made to scenes when they are viewing, but typically not attending, the changed regions. This phenomenon has been the focus of much recent research, largely because it is so surprising: people vastly overestimate their change detection ability. In this chapter, we demonstrate and quantify an implicit effect of this metacognitive error, and explore some of the factors that mediate it. In a series of experiments we conducted, observers viewed an original and a changed photograph that repeatedly alternated, separated by a brief blank interval. They were told that the change could be added to the "flickering" display at any time. In reality, the change was added either immediately (experiment 1) or after 4 sec (experiment 2). Upon detecting the change, observers were informed of their response time and were then asked to estimate when the change had been added. Observers underestimated the degree to which they were change-blind, typically inferring that the change had been added much later than it actually was. Average estimates ranged up to 31 sec after the "flickering" began—over 85 times the correct value. Such effects were further magnified in an additional study (experiment 3), which employed natural scenes and changes specifically designed to induce a high degree of this change blindness blindness (CBB). These experiments collectively demonstrate that CBB can persist across many trials in an actual change detection task and provide a new way to quantify and explore the factors that mediate CBB. This research highlights the extent to which we can overestimate the fidelity of some aspects of visual processing.

Metacognitive Errors and Visual Awareness

Under the grip of incorrect theories about how aspects of their minds work, people often fail to accurately predict their own behavior. Several of the most pernicious of these metacognitive errors involve the nature of visual awareness. Recent research on inattentional blindness, for example, has shown that, when engaged in an attentionally demanding task, many people will completely fail to perceive a novel salient object that enters their visual field, even if it differs in salient ways from all other objects in the display (Mack and Rock, 1998; Most et al., 2001). For example, subjects in one experiment watched a group of people passing basketballs back and forth as they moved around and had to keep a count of the number of times that the white-shirted players—but not the black-shirted players—made such passes. While engaged in this attentionally demanding task, many of the subjects failed to notice when another person in a gorilla suit walked through the scene. In contrast, all subjects saw the intruder when they simply watched the scene, without counting the ball passes (Simons and Chabris, 1999; see also Neisser and Becklen, 1975).

Such results are important not only because they reveal a lack of visual awareness, but because such effects are *surprising*: we intuitively think that under almost any circumstances we would see a novel salient object when it entered a relatively un-crowded scene. Moreover, metacognitive errors of this type are not mere academic curiosities, but can have a real-world impact. Recent research using a computerized version of the "gorilla" task, for example, showed that the incidence of inattentional blindness can increase by more than 50% when subjects are simultaneously talking on a cellular phone (Scholl et al., 2003; Scholl et al., under review). The danger that such effects could pose in real-world driving situations is only compounded by the fact that inattentional blindness is not an intuitively obvious phenomenon: without awareness of such effects, we will typically not work to monitor and prevent them (Strayer and Johnston, 2001).

Change Blindness and Change Blindness Blindness

Here we explore a related metacognitive error, which infects our intuitions about visual awareness and the perception of change. Our visual experience of the world typically seems *complete*. As long as a salient object or region of a scene is currently within our field of view, we readily assume that we will be visually aware of it. It thus seems natural to predict that we would immediately detect large changes in an actively viewed scene—for instance, an object repeatedly disappearing and reappearing. In contrast, observers are surprisingly poor at detecting changes to visual displays so long as the change does not call attention to itself by causing a large motion transient. Such *change blindness* (CB) typically occurs when the changes are obscured by a more global disruption such as a brief blank field, an eye movement, an eye blink, a film cut, or the coinciding abrupt appearance of another object (for recent reviews see Rensink, 2002; Simons, 2000a). However, CB can also occur when the visible transient introduced by the change is not masked, but is simply too slow to capture attention (Simons, Franconeri, and Reimer, 2000). Such phenomena have been the focus of much recent research (see Simons, 2000b), largely because they are so surprising: Despite the pervasiveness of CB, people greatly overestimate their change detection abilities (Levin et al., 2000). This overestimation, termed *change blindness blindness,* is our focus here. This counterintuitive aspect of CB is crucial (Simons and Levin, 1998): after all, it would not be of much interest to find that observers failed to detect changes that nobody thought they could detect in the first place (e.g., a single pixel that changed slightly in luminance during a visual disruption). Change blindness demonstrations are striking in part because once a change is finally seen, it seems almost inconceivable that it could have been missed only moments before.

Empirical Demonstrations of "Change Blindness" Blindness

The term *change blindness blindness* (CBB) refers to the fact that observers don't intuitively predict the existence of change blindness (Levin et al., 2000). Consider the following experimental scenario (from Simons and Levin, 1998): a person walking on a college campus is stopped by another person (the "questioner"), who asks for directions to a nearby building. While the person is giving directions to the questioner, their conversation is rudely interrupted by two other persons carrying a large door between them. During this interruption, the questioner and one of the door carriers surreptitiously switch places, so that the unwitting subject ends up continuing the conversation with a completely new person. As Simons and Levin (1998) demonstrated, more than half of such subjects (59%, averaging across several conditions) do not realize that this change has taken place! But is this really surprising? Would most people actually predict that they would notice such a change? The answer to this question determines whether such situations engender change blindness blindness in addition to change blindness.

Levin and colleagues (2000) demonstrated the existence of CBB for both person and object changes. In their first experiment, 300 students in a classroom listened to descriptions of the person change study just described (Simons and Levin, 1998) and of a second similar study involving film cuts, where observers failed to detect large changes made to actors and objects across sudden changes in camera views (Levin and Simons, 1997). For each study, the students were told the relevant procedures and were shown static images of the stimuli, with the change pointed out to them. They were then asked whether they thought they would have noticed the changes and rated their confidence in that judgment. Whereas only a minority of subjects in the two previous studies actually detected the changes (46% detected the person change in the real-world study described above; 0% detected the object changes in the film cut study), a large percentage of the students nevertheless thought, with high confidence, that they would have detected such changes (98% thought they would have detected the person change; 83% thought they would have detected the object changes made during film-cuts). A second experiment obtained similar evidence for CBB when subjects were tested individually on these and other control tasks; more recent work has found similar magnitudes of CBB even when observers viewed the actual videos, instead of still frames (Levin et al., 2002). The subjects in these studies thus committed the metacognitive error of overestimating their change detection ability.

The Present Study

This study has four main goals:

1. *An Implicit Measure of CBB.* First, we attempt to demonstrate and measure *implicit* effects of CBB, which do not require subjects to make explicit judgments about the likelihood of change detection. This is important given that such explicit judgments may be contaminated by extraneous beliefs—e.g. about the likelihood of the "obvious" answers to such questions being correct in the context of psychology experiments—which could impact the observed levels of CBB.

2. *CBB in an Actual Change Detection Task.* Second, we attempt to demonstrate effects of CBB in actual change-detection experiments, rather than in situations wherein such experiments are only described and demonstrated, as in Levin et al. (2000). Note that this would not be possible to test via explicit questioning using most paradigms, since when the subject missed the change, they would thereby be made aware of change blindness, and this awareness would by definition pollute any latent CBB.

3. *The Persistence of CBB.* Third, we attempt to see whether CBB will persist across many trials in actual change-detection tasks, or if increasing experience with change detection will attenuate CBB over time.

4. *Quantification of CBB.* Finally, we seek to test the limits of CBB by finding a way to measure it (without direct questioning), and then to explore how various manipulations will affect the observed magnitudes of CBB.

In sum, the experiments reported below attempt to assess the nature and robustness of CBB, and to identify some of the factors that mediate it. We address all of these issues using an indirect test of CBB. Observers viewed change detection trials employing the "flicker" paradigm (Rensink, O'Regan, and Clark, 1997): two photographs of natural scenes—an original and a changed version—alternated back and forth repeatedly, always separated by a gray mask. Observers freely viewed this "flickering" display until they detected the change. (Detecting such changes is difficult, and observers often require many alternations to notice even large changes; Rensink, O'Regan, and Clark, 1997.) Crucially, observers were told that the change could be added to the flickering at any point, and that before the change was introduced, a single scene would just be presented over and over, interspersed temporally with the gray mask. In reality, the change was added either immediately (experiments 1 and 3) or after 4 sec (experiment 2). Upon detecting the change, observers were informed of their response time, and were then asked to estimate when the change had been added. Figure 7.1 summarizes this sequence of events.

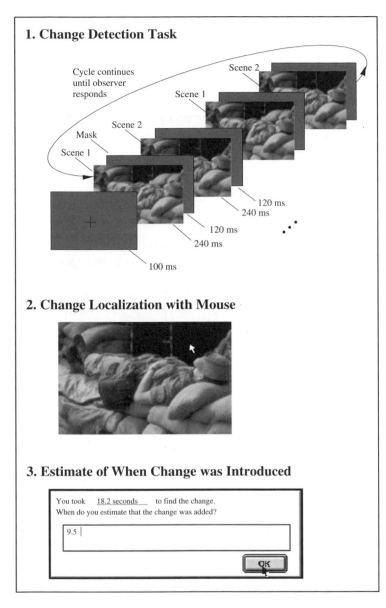

Figure 7.1
Sequence of a single trial in experiments 1 and 3.

In essence, this task forced observers to *estimate* how long they were blind to the change. Note that a correct estimate (that the change had been introduced after 360 msec) in the context of a long change detection response time (say, 18 sec) is in essence an acknowledgment of the existence of change blindness—of the fact that salient repeated changes can fail to be detected for long periods of time. In this case, the estimated change blindness and the actual change blindness are of similar magnitudes. On the other hand, an incorrect estimate (say, 14 sec) in the context of an 18 sec change detection response time is essentially an estimate of 4 sec of change blindness, which is radically lower than the actual degree of change blindness (more than 17 sec). If subjects do not experience change blindness blindness in these experiments, then they should answer accurately. If subjects do suffer from CBB, then they should estimate that the change was added long after its actual introduction: if the change had been added earlier, they would presumably have seen it much earlier.

Experiment 1 provides the basic test of change blindness blindness, using the implicit measure described above: on each trial subjects must detect the change in the flicker paradigm, then estimate when the change was added (when in reality it was added immediately). In experiment 2, we replicate the essential findings from experiment 1 in a situation where the change is not actually added until more than 4 seconds have elapsed—thereby giving subjects the opportunity to overestimate as well as underestimate their change blindness. Finally, in experiment 3, we test the limits of this metacognitive error by employing scenes and changes explicitly designed to induce high degrees of CBB.

Experiment 1: Immediate Changes

Method

Participants   Ten naive observers participated in one 25 min session. All observers had normal or corrected-to-normal acuity and had not previously participated in (or heard of) similar experiments.

Materials   The displays were presented on the monitor of an iMac computer. Observers were positioned approximately 42 cm from the monitor, without head restraint. At this distance, the images subtended approximately 37° by 28° of visual angle. The displays were generated by custom software written using the VisionShell graphics libraries (Comtois, 2002). The experiment involved 64 image pairs. Each pair consisted of a color photograph of a natural scene and a counterpart constructed by removing or adding one of the objects in the scene using Adobe Photoshop. All changes were large, easily seen once noticed, and readily seen when the two images were not separated by an intervening mask (Simons, Franconeri, and Reimer 2000).

Procedure   A single trial proceeded as follows (see figure 7.1). Observers initiated the trial by pressing a key, which blanked the screen. After 100 msec, the "flickering" began, repeatedly displaying the following sequence: (1) the first scene for 240 msec; (2) a uniform gray mask for 120 msec; (3) the second (changed) scene for 240 msec; and (4) a uniform gray mask again for 120 msec. This sequence was repeated until the observers pressed a key to indicate that the change had been detected. Following this keypress, the observers clicked the mouse, which controlled a small colored probe, to indicate the location of the change (this response ensured that observers had detected the change). Following this mouse click, a small window appeared on the screen to inform observers of their response time (RT), measured from the very beginning of the trial until the keypress when they detected the change. This window might say, for instance, "You took 18.2 seconds." With this RT in mind, observers used the keyboard to estimate when the change had been introduced into the display (this estimate was always expressed, as was their change detection RT as a certain number of decimal seconds from the beginning of the trial). Following their entry of this "time stamp," observers pressed another key to initiate the next trial.

At the beginning of the experimental session, observers were told what types of changes were possible, and that: "At some point during the flickering, the image that appears will be slightly changed (something will be added to or deleted from the scene), and from that point forward, the original and modified version of the scene will alternate." Before the experimental trials, observers completed 5 practice trials with a different set of images.

Results and Discussion

Because observers knew that a change was made on each trial, errors in change detection consisted of clicking the mouse outside of the changed object or region (defined for this purpose as the rectangle of minimal area that encompassed all changed pixels). As in other change blindness studies employing the "flicker" paradigm, these error rates were extremely low—no more than 2 errors (out of 64 trials) per subject (with a mean error rate of 1.6%; SD = 1.28%). These error trials were not included in the analyses. The image set used in this experiment engendered a considerable amount of change blindness: on average, observers took 6.35 sec (17.64 alternations) to detect the change, a value comparable to that in previous flicker experiments with other natural scenes (e.g., Rensink, O'Regan, and Clark, 1997).

An analysis of the magnitude of change blindness blindness in these experiments requires several steps. On every trial, we first compute the magnitude of actual change blindness, namely, the change detection RT (which was 6.35 sec on average) minus the duration of the trial that proceeded with no change (which, in this experiment, was always 360 msec—one display and one blank). To facilitate comparisons across analyses and experiments, we express this and most other values as percentages of total trial durations rather than as raw times (which are meaningful only in the context of the actual detection RTs). Thus 5.67% of each trial had elapsed, on average, before the change was added; subjects, on average, were change-blind (i.e., were looking for the change) for 94.3% of the duration of a trial. On average, subjects estimated that 26.7% of a trial had elapsed before the change was introduced. The difference between this value and the actual change introduction time is the magnitude of change blindness blindness, the degree to which subjects overestimated when the change had been added. Thus, on average, observers incorrectly estimated that 21% of the duration of each trial did not involve change, when in fact it did.

These mean values, represented graphically in the leftmost bar of figure 7.2, are for all trials, however—including those with short change detection times (and thus minimal change blindness), which leave no room for the possibility of change blindness blindness. When we restricted the analysis of change blindness blindness to those trials engendering maximal change blindness, analyzing only trials that fell above the average change detection RT of 6.35 sec (an average of 16.6 trials per observer, with a mean change detection RT of 16.36 sec), the observers estimated that 45.6% of a trial had elapsed before the change was added, whereas in fact the changes were added, on average, after only 2.2% of a trial had elapsed. Observers on these trials thus suffered from change blindness blindness for 43.4% of the total trial duration: the estimated change blindness for these trials was only 54.4% of a trial's duration, whereas the *actual* change blindness was on average 97.8% of a trial's duration. (See figure 7.2 for depictions of all of these values.)

Another way to characterize the possible extent of change blindness blindness is simply to look at the largest single estimated "time stamp" per observer; this average value was 31.02 sec—over 85 times the correct value of 360 msec. (There was also especially high variance here, of course; the standard deviation in these values was 24.91 sec.) Overall, we take the pattern of results obtained in this experiment as an indication of the robustness of CBB: even averaged over 64 trials, observers greatly overestimated the duration of flickering without change in this paradigm, presumably because they thought they would have been quicker to detect changes that had been introduced earlier.

One goal of this study was to see if CBB would persist throughout many trials of an actual change detection experiment. We can also ask whether the magnitude of CBB increased or decreased as the experiment progressed. When we compared the first 21 trials with the last 21 trials, we found that the change introduction estimates (again, expressed as percentages of the actual change detection RTs) were almost identical (27.7% versus 26.4%; $t(9) = .38$, $p = .71$). The actual change detection RTs decreased nonsignificantly from the first 21 trials (8,173 msec) to the last 21 trials (5,221 msec), $t(9) = 1.90$, $p = .09$. Thus it seems that the large degree of CBB observed in this experiment is not diminished even after 64 trials.

Mean CB and CBB Statistics Expressed as
Percentages of Total Trial Durations

Experiment 1

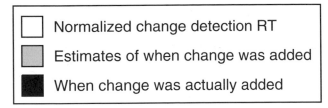

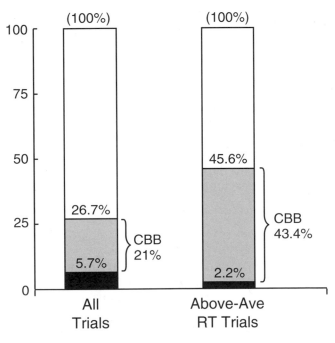

Figure 7.2

Results from experiment 1 are presented as percentages of normalized total trial durations to facilitate comparison across analyses and across experiments. The overall height of the white bars (measured from the horizontal axis) represents the normalized change detection RT (the actual raw detection RTs were always much higher when only the above-average detection trials were considered). The height of the black bars represents the percentage of a trial that had elapsed, on average, when the actual change first appeared. The height of the gray bars (measured from the horizontal axis) represents the percentage of the trial the observer *estimated* had elapsed, on average, when the change first appeared. The difference between the heights of the gray and black bars thus represents the degree of "change blindness" blindness—the degree to which observers overestimated their change detection ability.

Experiment 2: Delayed Changes

Experiment 1 demonstrated that change blindness blindness can be observed via an implicit measure, even in the context of an actual change detection task involving many trials. Recall, however, that one of our concerns with the original demonstrations of change blindness blindness (Levin et al., 2000) was the possibility of task demands contaminating the estimates of change blindness. The results of experiment 1, it might be argued, could also be due to a similar task demand: because subjects are explicitly informed that the change could be added at any time, it would be unnatural for them to then respond that all the changes were added immediately. Perhaps, given the chance to respond in the other direction— to estimate that the changes were in fact added *earlier* than their actual introductions—they would do so, and thus exhibit less CBB. To test whether the CBB observed in experiment 1 was due in part to this potential task demand, we added the change in experiment 2 after 4.32 sec (6 full cycles). This gave subjects the opportunity to underestimate the change introduction time, and should result in decreased CBB if the task demand discussed above contributed to the CBB observed in experiment 1.

Method

Ten naive observers, none of whom had participated in experiment 1, participated in one 25 min session. All observers had normal or corrected-to-normal acuity and had not previously participated in (or heard of) similar experiments. This experiment was identical to experiment 1, except that the change was now added after 4.32 sec of "flickering" had elapsed—for the first 4.32 sec (12 alternations) of each trial, the first image of each pair alternated with the gray mask alone.

Results and Discussion

The average error rate in the change detection portion of the task was again 1.6% (SD = 2.44%); as in experiment 1, error trials were excluded from the analyses. Observers took, on average, 9.47 sec (26.31 alternations) to find the changes, measured from the beginning of the trial, or 5.15 sec (14.3 alternations), measured from the beginning of the actual changes. Considered this last way, changes were detected slightly faster than those in experiment 1, though this trend was not significant ($t(9) = 1.79$, $p = .09$). The analysis of change blindness blindness in this experiment proceeded exactly as in experiment 1, and the relevant values are summarized in figure 7.3. One major difference between the results of experiments 1 and 2 lies in the percentage of a trial that had actually elapsed before the change was added: because of the extra 4.32 sec of no change, these values were much larger in experiment 2. Over all trials, 45.6% of a trial had elapsed before the change was actually introduced; considering only those trials on which change detection RTs were above average (there were, on average, 19.3 such trials per

Mean CB and CBB Statistics Expressed as Percentages of Total Trial Durations

Experiment 2

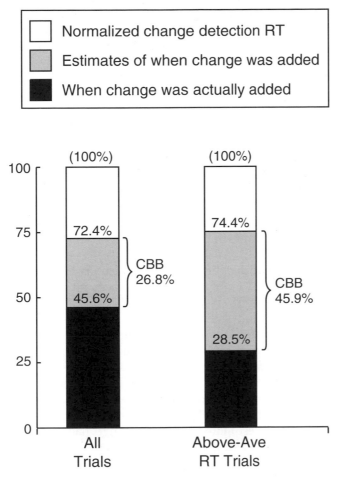

Figure 7.3
Results from experiment 2, presented as percentages of normalized total trial durations. See caption to figure 7.2 for details.

observer, with an average detection RT of 15.16 sec), 28.5% of a trial had elapsed before the change appeared.

Intriguingly, these radically greater percentages for the actual change introductions did not affect the magnitude of change blindness blindness. Over all trials, subjects estimated that, on average, 72.4% of a trial had elapsed before the change was added, for a CBB magnitude of 26.8%. Averaged over only those trials on which change detection RTs were above average, observers estimated that 74.4% of a trial had elapsed before the change was added, for a CBB magnitude of 45.9% (see figure 7.3). These CBB values did not differ significantly from those in experiment 1, either for all trials ($t(9) = .98$, $p = .34$) or for the subset of trials with above-average change detection RTs ($t(9) = .31$, $p = .76$). We also again compared these values on the first 21 and last 21 trials for experiment 2. Though observers were quicker to detect changes in the final 21 trials (8.83 sec) than in the first 21 trials (10.35 sec); ($t(9) = 2.50$, $p = .034$), no such differences were observed in the CBB estimates (25.5% for the first 21 trials versus 24.9% for the last 21 trials; $t(9) = .21$, $p = .83$). Observers also still produced exceedingly high estimates of when the changes were introduced: the single largest raw estimate of when the change was added in experiment 2 was on average 24.98 sec (factoring out the 4.32 sec that actually had no change; SD = 15.02 sec). This value did not differ from the corresponding value in experiment 1 (31.02 sec); $t(9) = .66$, $p = .52$).

The fact that none of these CBB measures differed between experiments 1 and 2 shows that observers took the extra 4.32 sec of no change into account when estimating their ability to detect changes. As expressed in figures 7.2 and 7.3, it is clear that observers ascribed the same magnitudes of CBB to themselves across the two experiments, rather than basing their estimates of change blindness on a constant offset from either the beginning or end of the trial. The results of experiment 1 thus seem not to have been due to the fact that observers could not underestimate the change introduction time. Even when the change was added 4.32 sec into the flickering in this experiment, observers still estimated that the change was added over half of the way into the actual duration of flickering with change, and in some extreme change blindness trials estimated that the change had not been added until after more than 20 sec of changing scenes had elapsed.

Finally, it is interesting to note in comparing experiments 1 and 2 that each is in some ways the more compelling demonstration. Experiment 2 has the advantage that it allows subjects to underestimate change blindness, but in experiment 1 change blindness blindness persisted even in the face of evidence that the changes were probably being introduced early. In experiment 1, subjects never had the experience of looking at an object or feature, noting that it did not change, then seeing it change later as would be expected had changes been putatively clearly visible and been introduced late in the trial. It appears as though subjects in experiment 2 did note that objects went from stable to changing because they adjusted their estimates to be proportionally later than those of subjects in experiment 1. Thus, even in the face of discernible evidence to the contrary, subjects in experiment 1 still demonstrated strong CBB.

Experiment 3: Increasing the Magnitude of Change Blindness Blindness

Experiments 1 and 2 explored the extent of change blindness blindness using a set of natural scene images that were originally created to study other aspects change blindness (e.g., Simons, Franconeri, and Reimer, 2000), and the resulting magnitude of CBB varied depending on the particular images and changes being analyzed. In particular, as noted above, some trials did not provide even the opportunity for CBB, since they did not engender much change blindness in the first place. (In other words, the changes in certain image pairs were easily and quickly detected by most observers.) Thus the magnitudes of CBB observed in experiments 1 and 2 were considerably increased by analyzing only those "above-average-RT" trials that engendered above-average change blindness.

Even for images that do result in high levels of change blindness, however, we have noticed informally that there can be massive differences in the resulting CBB. In particular, in the context of a standard change blindness experiment (i.e., where subjects know that the changes are always occurring), some changes can be very difficult to find, and yet seem extremely large and salient once they are discovered. (These are the demonstrations we often show in our introductory classes, which result in the loudest exclamations of surprise.) Such changes seem to engender a high degree of CBB, simply because it seems so intuitively unlikely that large and salient changes could go undetected for so long. Other changes, however, can seem almost disappointing when found. For example, a change involving only a few nonsalient pixels may also be difficult to detect, yet engender a relatively low level of CBB—we are not intuitively surprised, given the insignificance of the change. In this experiment, we follow the same method used in experiment 1, but we now use a smaller set of images specifically designed to engender a high level of CBB. In particular, pilot testing suggests that these changes are reasonably difficult to detect, despite their intuitive salience.[1] As a result, this experiment may help to determine whether the magnitudes of CBB observed in experiments 1 and 2 represent an upper bound on the limits of CBB, or whether the extent of this metacognitive error can be even greater with particular images and changes.

Method

Ten naive observers, none of whom had participated in the previous experiments, participated in one 10 min session. All observers had normal or corrected-to-normal acuity and had not previously participated in or heard of similar experiments. This experiment was identical to experiment 1, except that a new set of 17 image pairs was employed, designed to produce a high degree of CBB. All images were color photographs of natural scenes, and the changes consisted of objects and areas of the scenes that disappeared, or local image regions whose texture was replaced with another. Again, all changes were quite large, were easy to see once noticed, and were seen immediately when the two images were not separated by an intervening mask (for sample trials using this image set, see <www.yale.edu/perception/cbb/>.

Results

The average number of errors per subject in change detection performance (as assessed by the probe positions of the mouse clicks) was less than 1 of the 17 trials (mean error rate = 5.4%; SD = 5.5%); error trials were excluded from the analyses. Observers took, on average, 22.47 sec (62.42 alternations) to find the changes, measured from the beginning of the trial—a value more than 3.5 times greater than the corresponding change detection latencies of 6.35 sec in experiment 1 ($t(9) = 3.72$, $p < .01$) or 5.14 sec in experiment 2 ($t(9) = 4.00$, $p < .005$). This high degree of change blindness confirms that our images and changes at least provided for the possibility of a high degree of CBB, which is assessed in the remainder of the analyses.

The analysis of CBB in this experiment proceeded exactly as in experiment 1, and the relevant values are summarized in figure 7.4 (because this experiment involves many fewer images than experiments 1 and 2, we do not break down these data by "above-average RTs"; thus figure 7.4 has only a single bar). Over all trials, an average of only 1.6% of the trial had elapsed before the change was actually introduced. In contrast, observers now estimated that, on average, 61.86% of a trial had elapsed before the change was added. The difference between these values—60.26%—constitutes the magnitude of CBB, and this value is significantly greater than all values observed in experiments 1 and 2, including the value of 21% for all trials in experiment 1 ($t(9) = 5.25$, $p < .001$); the above-average-RT value of 43.4% in experiment 1 ($t(9) = 2.15$, $p < .05$); the value for all trials of 26.8% in experiment 2 ($t(9) = 4.9$, $p < .001$); and the above-average-RT value of 45.9% in experiment 2 ($t(9) = 2.2$, $p < .05$). In other words, observers in this experiment incorrectly estimated that more than 60% of the duration of each trial did not involve change, when in fact it did.

We can also again assess the magnitude of CBB by looking at the average of each subject's single largest raw estimate of when the change was introduced: in experiment 3 this value was 43.5 sec—more than 120 times the correct value of 360 msec—greater than the corresponding values of 31.02 sec in experiment 1 or 24.98 sec in experiment 2. (Neither of these comparisons is significant, however, because of the extremely high variances involved, experiment 1: SD = 24.91 sec ($t(9) = 1.12$, $p = .277$); experiment 2: SD = 15.02 sec ($t(9) = 2.01$, $p = .063$); experiment 3: SD = 24.9.)

Discussion

The primary goal of experiment 3 was to see if the magnitude of change blindness blindness observed using our implicit measure could be pushed even higher

Mean CB and CBB Statistics Expressed as Percentages of Total Trial Durations

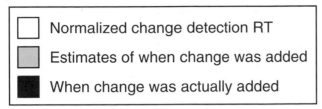

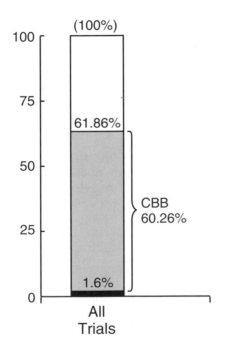

Figure 7.4
Results from experiment 3, presented as percentages of normalized total trial durations. See caption to figure 7.2 for details.

by employing sets of images and changes specifically designed to induce high levels of CBB. In this we succeeded, more than doubling the magnitude of CBB observed with the entire image set used in experiments 1 and 2. In this experiment, subjects actually estimated that well over half of each trial, on average, had elapsed before the change was introduced, when in reality less than 2% of the trial had elapsed. This increased CBB—now covering the majority of each trial, on average—confirms that the magnitude of CBB can grow to be quite large, and that it depends on the nature of the particular images and changes used. These results suggest that the metacognitive error of CBB will be particularly strong when the changes are perceptually large and salient, yet are hard to detect in practice.

That the magnitude of change blindness blindness depends on the nature of the images and changes used is perhaps worth emphasizing in a more general context. Many researchers have argued that the phenomenon of change blindness itself suggests that our visual memory for detailed scene information is much sparser than has been previously assumed (e.g., Rensink, 2000; Rensink, O'Regan and Clark, 1997; Scholl, 2000). However, other recent researchers have argued that visual memory can actually be quite good, as indexed by more direct recognition tests (e.g., Hollingworth and Henderson, 2002; Hollingworth, Williams, and Henderson, 2001).

It seems to us, however, that a good deal of this debate may rest on the particular images and changes that are used in each study—a methodological factor that is rarely discussed. In most change blindness studies, the changes are typically designed haphazardly (e.g., using Photoshop) to induce high levels of change blindness, and thus will typically involve relatively nonsalient regions of background objects, etc. In contrast, some recent studies which demonstrate better visual memory seem to involve changes that are easier to detect—e.g. changes that involve one of only a few salient foreground objects in each scene (e.g., Hollingworth and Henderson, 2002). In other words, the particular changes used in such experiments often seemed designed to show what the authors want to show—a strategy we explicitly made use of in this experiment. It is difficult to assess this hypothesis in practice, since the precise nature of the changes is rarely reported in these studies in any detail. In the future, however, it might be worth remembering that any such global claims (about the magnitude of change blindness or the fidelity of visual memory) will likely depend on the details of the particular images and changes that are used.[2]

General Discussion

In the three experiments reported here, observers estimated that the changes in the "flicker" displays had been added much later than they really were—misestimating that up to 60% of the trials, on average, had proceeded changeless, when in reality the change was added in immediately. We interpret these radical overestimates as consistent with the existence of change blindness blindness—the metacognitive error of overestimating change detection ability. To give a correct (i.e., early) change introduction estimate in this experimental situation on a trial engendering a long change detection RT would in essence be to acknowledge the existence of change blindness, namely, that changes can go undetected for long periods of time. We suggest that our observers did not think that the changes had been added sooner because they mistakenly inferred that they would have then detected them much sooner. In short, our experiments provide evidence for the existence of CBB using an implicit measure, extending earlier demonstrations and showing that CBB occurs even in the context of actual change detection tasks, and can persist unattenuated for many trials.[3]

One advantage of using an implicit measure of CBB, as we have done here, is that it may provide a link between visual metaknowledge and metacognitive control over visual processes. Most of the research described in this volume is focused specifically on the content of people's beliefs about vision, and leaves the relationship between these beliefs and performance on actual visual tasks unexplored (see Levin, 2002, for more discussion). However, in these experiments, the knowledge implicated by CBB is closely linked to the possibility of adapting to a specific visual task. It is likely that the best way of improving one's performance in a change blindness task may well be to gradually learn the degree to which intentional search is necessary for change detection, and to realize that checking a location once might not be sufficient to see a change in that location. However, in the current experiments, the subjects were unable to moderate their understanding of the conditions that led to change blindness across many trials, and therefore may have sacrificed improvements that otherwise would have been possible. An intriguing research project would be to explore the extent to which improvement in change detection across trials in different complex search tasks is affected by the degree to which those tasks confound subjects' beliefs about the detectability of different kinds of search targets.

In everyday life, we rarely think about the possibility that salient details in the world go unrepresented by our visual systems: we enjoy a phenomenological sense that we are constantly representing the visible world in all of its detail. Part of this sense is surely due to the fidelity of the computations employed by the visual system to recover the structure of the world, but another part of this sense may be due to the fact that we overestimate the fidelity of visual processing. Such metacognitive errors have long gone undetected simply because we do not normally have the opportunity to uncover them. In the experiments reported here, however, the magnitude and robustness of one such error are made plain.

Acknowledgments

We thank Nicholaus Noles, Vanya Pasheva, Rachel Sussman, and Joe Vuckovich for assistance with data collection and for helping to create the images used in experiment 3; Steve Mitroff for computing the change detection errors in experiments 1 and 2; and Adriane Seiffert for helpful conversation. Portions of this work were reported at the 2000 meeting of the Psychonomic Society. Brian Scholl was supported by National Science Foundation grant BCS-0132444 and by National Institutes of Mental Health grant 1-R03-MH63808. Daniel Simons was supported by National Science Foundation grant 9905578 and by a fellowship from the Alfred P. Sloan Foundation.

Notes

1. These images and changes were constructed largely unsystematically, using the experimenters' intuitions about what types of changes would give rise to high degrees of CBB, and then confirming these intuitions in pilot testing. Two of these types of changes were: (1) changes involving the disappearance and reappearance an entire large object in the scene which is nevertheless naturally parsed as being in the background of the image—e.g., a building in a skyline, or a large tree in a forest scene; and (2) changes wherein the surface characteristics of a large area of the scene disappeared or changed, without affecting the overall manner in which the scene was parsed into objects—e.g., completely changing the texture on the street in a street scene, or removing half of the windows from every building in an urban scene. Some sample trials using the images from this experiment are available for inspection on the internet at http://www.yale.edu/perception/cbb/.
2. To assess these ideas, it would perhaps be useful if researchers always tested their stimuli on a standard set of tasks, such as the standard "flicker" task of change blindness, Hollingworth and Henderson's more direct test (2002) of visual memory, and the change blindness blindness task employed here. The ideas discussed above predict, for instance, that higher levels of change blindness will be observed using the stimuli from the original change blindness studies (e.g., Rensink, O'Regan, and Clark, 1997), compared to the rendered scenes of more recent studies showing intact visual memory (e.g., Hollingworth and Henderson, 2002; Hollingworth, Williams, and Henderson, 2001)—and vice versa for the more direct recognition tests of visual memory.
3. Indeed, the original idea for these experiments came from the observation that subjects in an unmodified "flicker" task (Scholl, 2000) often refused to believe that the changes they were being asked to detect were always present. That is, those subjects were essentially assuming, *spontaneously*, that the slight deception explicitly employed here was correct.

References

Comtois, R. (2002). *VisionShell PPC.* (Software libraries.) Cambridge, MA: Author.

Hollingworth, A., and Henderson, J. M. (2002). Accurate visual memory for previously attended objects in natural scenes. *Journal of Experimental Psychology: Human Perception and Performance, 28,* 113–136.

Hollingworth, A., Williams, C. C., and Henderson, J. M. (2001). To see and remember: Visually specific information is retained in memory from previously attended objects in natural scenes. *Psychonomic Bulletin and Review, 8,* 761–768.

Levin, D. T. (2002). Change blindness blindness as visual metacognition. *Journal of Consciousness Studies, 9,* 111–130.

Levin, D. T., and Simons, D. J. (1997). Failure to detect changes to attended objects in motion pictures. *Psychonomic Bulletin and Review, 4,* 501–506.

Levin, D. T., Drivdahl, S., Momen, N., and Beck, M. R. (2002). False predictions about the detectability of unexpected visual changes: The role of beliefs about attention, memory, and continuity of attended objects in causing change blindness blindness. *Consciousness and Cognition, 11,* 507–527.

Levin, D. T., Momen, N, Drivdahl, S. B., and Simons, D. J. (2000). Change blindness blindness: The metacognitive error of overestimating change-detection ability. *Visual Cognition, 7*, 397–412.

Mack, A., and Rock, I. (1998). *Inattentional blindness.* Cambridge, MA: MIT Press.

Most, S. B., Simons, D. J., Scholl, B. J., Jiminez, R., Clifford, E., and Chabris, C. F. (2001). How not to be seen: The contribution of similarity and selective ignoring to sustained inattentional blindness. *Psychological Science, 12*, 9–17.

Neisser, U., and Becklen, R. (1975). Selective looking: Attending to visually specified events. *Cognitive Psychology, 7*, 480–494.

Rensink, R. A. (2000). Seeing, sensing, and scrutinizing. *Vision Research, 40*, 1469–1487.

Rensink, R. A. (2002). Change detection. *Annual Review of Psychology, 53*, 245–277.

Rensink, R. A., O'Regan, J. K., and Clark, J. J. (1997). To see or not to see: The need for attention to perceive changes in scenes. *Psychological Science, 8*, 368–373.

Scholl, B. J. (2000). Attenuated change blindness for exogenously attended items in a flicker paradigm. *Visual Cognition, 7*, 377–396.

Scholl, B. J., Noles, N. S., Pasheva, V., and Sussman, R. (2003). Talking on a cellular telephone dramatically increases "sustained inattentional blindness." Paper read at the annual meeting of the Vision Sciences Society, 5/13/03, Sarasota, FL. [Abstract published in Journal of Vision, 3(9), 156a, *http://journalofvisionl.org/3/9/156/*]

Scholl, B. J., Noles, N., Pasheva, V., and Sussman, R. (under review). Driving blind: Talking on a cellphone dramatically increases inattentional blindness.

Simons, D. J. (2000a). Current approaches to change blindness. *Visual Cognition, 7*, 1–15.

Simons, D. J., Ed. (2000b). *Change blindness and visual memory.* Psychology Press.

Simons, D. J., and Chabris, C. (1999). Gorillas in our midst: Sustained inattentional blindness for dynamic events. *Perception, 28*, 1059–1074.

Simons, D. J., Franconeri, S. L., and Reimer, R. L. (2000). Change blindness in the absence of a visual disruption. *Perception, 29*, 1143–1154.

Simons, D. J., and Levin, D. T. (1998). Failure to detect changes to people in a real-world interaction. *Psychonomic Bulletin and Review, 5*, 644–649.

Strayer, D. L., and Johnson, W. A. (2001). Driven to distraction: Dual-task studies of simulated driving and conversing on a cellular telephone. *Psychological Science, 12*, 462–466.

Chapter 8

Individual Differences in the Visual Representation of Scenes

Heather L. Pringle, Arthur F. Kramer, and David E. Irwin

Whether one is a surgeon performing an operation, a pilot landing an aircraft, or a driver navigating a car through rush hour traffic, accurately perceiving details and changes in the environment is fundamental to one's ability to fully comprehend the current situation, anticipate the future, and plan appropriate actions. For example, automobile drivers need to notice important road signs, to perceive the position of pedestrians and other vehicles, and to anticipate changes in the trajectories to safely navigate and control their vehicles. In recent years, however, research has demonstrated that when environmental change coincides with an interruption to ongoing visual processing (e.g., eye movements, blinks), we are surprisingly slow to detect changes (if we detect them at all), suggesting that we often lack a detailed representation of the environment.

Change detection is poor under a variety of circumstances, such as during saccadic eye movements (Grimes, 1996; Hollingworth, Schrock and Henderson, 2001; Irwin, 1991; Zelinsky, 2001), simulated saccadic suppression (Rensink, O'Regan and Clark, 1997), blinks (O'Regan, Deubel, Clark and Rensink, 2000), "mud splashes" (O'Regan, Rensink and Clark, 1999), dynamic simulated scenes (Wallis and Bulthoff, 2000), movie clips (Levin and Simons, 1997) and even real-world interactions (Simons and Levin, 1998). This phenomenon has been referred to as "change blindness." Indeed, perceptual change detection is less than perfect for a variety of changes, for example, transformations of object features (e.g., color) and objects themselves (e.g., substituting or deleting objects), when these are accompanied by an interruption in visual processing (Mondy and Coltheart, 2000). While detecting changes during interruptions is indeed difficult, it is not impossible. This implies that some (apparently limited) representation of a scene must be constructed and maintained. Otherwise, successful change detection could not occur.

Recent research on perceptual representation and change detection has focused on the role of attention in the successful detection of environmental changes. For example, Rensink, O'Regan, and Clark (1997) showed that changes to items of "central interest" in scenes were detected faster than changes to items of "marginal interest," even though marginal interest changes tended to be larger on average. Such data might be interpreted to suggest that individuals are more likely to detect changes in areas of scenes on which they focus their attention. Consistent with this, Scholl (2000) showed that change blindness could be attenuated by precueing areas of the visual field in which changes were likely to occur. Furthermore, Hollingworth, Schrock and Henderson (2001) had observers scan displays of detailed scenes to look for changes and found that fixation on the changed object generally drove change detection although particularly salient changes could be detected in the periphery.

Other research has suggested that memory for objects and object relations also contributes to scene representation and change detection. For example, research on transaccadic memory has suggested that humans can retain the details of three to four objects across eye movements (Irwin, 1992). Other researchers (e.g., Rensink, 2000) have estimated that memory capacity in free viewing situations varies as a function of the nature of the changes that have to be detected and retained. Finally, recent studies have also shown that individuals can, with relative accuracy, detect changes to an object, when that object has been fixated previously but is no longer within the focus of attention when the changes occur. Accurate performance in these studies was obtained on both short- and long-term memory tests (Hollingworth and Henderson, 2002; Hollingworth, Williams, and Henderson, 2001). In summary, these findings emphasize the importance of memory in the representation and retention of meaningful aspects of visual scenes, even though we may not retain a highly detailed representation of those scenes (Hollingworth and Henderson, 2000; Pringle et al., 2001).

Adopting an individual differences approach to scene representation and change detection, we examined the extent to which change detection performance could be predicted from observers' performance on tests of visual attention, verbal and visuospatial memory, perceptual speed, executive control, and inhibition. The individual differences approach has been successfully employed in the study of cognitive processes such as skill acquisition and automaticity (Ackerman and Cianciolo, 2000), attention (Duncan, 1995; Yee, Laden, and Hunt, 1994), executive control (Miyake et al., 2000), and verbal ability (Zelinski, Gilewski, and Schaie, 1993). In our current study, it provided converging evidence for the role of different perceptual and cognitive processes in perceptual change detection in real-world scenes. Furthermore, because we recorded eye movements during participants' search for changes, we were able to examine the relationship between individual differences in memory, attention, and other cognitive (and metacognitive) processes, on the one hand, and the eye movements that individual participants employed to detect and identify environmental changes, on the other. Finally, we included both young and older adults as participants in our study to increase the magnitude of individual differences on the cognitive tasks.

In our study, observers detected and identified changes in a "flicker" paradigm (Rensink O'Regan, and Clark, 1997), where observers are presented with two different views of a scene separated by a briefly presented gray screen (to mask any apparent motion caused by a change). A change in a specific object is made from one version of the scene to the next; observers are specifically instructed to detect and identify the change as quickly and accurately as possible. We employed high-resolution driving scenes, photographed from the driver's perspective out the front windshield. Scene changes included objects that had been previously rated (by independent judges) as having high or low salience and high or low meaning in the driving context (see Pringle et al., 2001). Specific changes included deleting or adding objects and changing their color or location.

We examined the hypothesis that change detection performance is related to performance on visuospatial working memory tasks and on a test of attentional breadth. Given previous demonstrations (e.g., Salthouse, 1992) of the importance of perceptual speed in a variety of complex tasks, we predicted that performance on tests which entailed perceptual speed would account for a portion of the variance in change detection. And given the importance of systematic search strategies that are at least somewhat immune to disruption by salient stimuli, we also predicted that measures of inhibition would account for a portion of the variance in change detection. We examined, as well, the secondary hypothesis that visuospatial working memory and attentional breadth performance is related to eye movement behavior during change detection. That is, we expected that observers with larger attentional spans and visuospatial working memories would require fewer eye movements to detect and identify changes in the driving scenes. To augment the more explicit measure of change detection provided by observers' verbalization of the changed object, we recorded saccades as an implicit measure of attention strategies and change detection. Because previous studies have found that, under some conditions, eye movements reflect scene changes even in the absence of observer verbalization of changes (Ryan et al., 2000), one might expect eye movement measures might prove more sensitive to change detection than other measures that depend on explicit recognition of the change.

Method

Participants
Sixty-six young adults (19 men and 47 women; mean age = 20.9 years) were recruited from the University of Illinois at Urbana-Champaign; 65 older adults (21 men and 44 women; mean age = 68.3 years) were recruited from the local community. All participants had corrected visual acuity better than 20/40.

Apparatus
Participants were seated on a raised platform approximately 33 inches from a vertical projection-based display, such that the display subtended 90° horizontally, 72° vertically. Eye movements were monitored using an Applied Science Laboratories eye and head tracker (model 501), mounted on the participant's head. The equipment was calibrated for each individual at the beginning of the experiment and as needed thereafter.

Perceptual Change Detection Task
Stimuli Eighty digital photographs of scenes taken from a driver's perspective inside a car were manipulated in the experiment (80 experimental trials). Changes to these photographs involved a single object's color, location, or presence in the scene and were categorized along two dimensions (meaning and salience) by independent judges (see Pringle et al., 2001, for an in-depth discussion). *Meaning* was defined as the relevance or importance of the change to driving performance. For example, changing the color of a restaurant sign was rated as having low meaning, and changing the color of a stoplight was rated as having high meaning. *Salience* was defined in terms of low-level perceptual factors. For example, a large and bright change was rated as having high salience, and a small and dim change was rated as having low salience. For the purpose of analysis, the scene changes were divided into four categories on the basis of the median ratings across raters: low meaning/low salience; low meaning/high salience; high meaning/low salience; and high meaning/high salience.

Procedure The trial sequence began with a bull's-eye displayed in the center of a gray screen, which participants were instructed to fixate. The experimenter manually initiated the trial after ensuring the individual participant's gaze on the center fixation point corresponded to an appropriate value on the eye data output. The bull's-eye then disappeared and the flicker sequence immediately began. The flicker sequence consisted of an original image (A) and a modified version (A'), which were displayed in the sequence A, A', A, A' (in the same fashion as Rensink, O'Regan, and Clark 1997). Gray blank fields were placed between successive images and to eliminate apparent motion across image displays. Each image was displayed for 240 msec and each blank screen (gray field) for 80 msec (see figure 8.1).

Participants were allowed to search freely for the image change for up to 60 sec. On detecting the change, they depressed a handheld button and then verbally described the change. Before beginning the experiment, they were told of the types of changes possible and were given five practice trials, but they were not provided with feedback on their performance. Fast and accurate responding was emphasized in the instructions. Response time was measured from the first presentation of the scene. At the conclusion of the session, participants completed a postexperiment questionnaire to assess the extent to which they believed that salient or meaningful changes influenced their performance (portions of the questionnaire were adapted from Witmer and Singer, 1998).

Psychometric Assessment
In a separate, two-hour session following the perceptual change detection task, participants were assessed in the following areas of cognitive and psychomotor function: attentional breadth, memory, perceptual speed, and the ability to inhibit irrelevant information. A description of each task is provided in table 8.1.

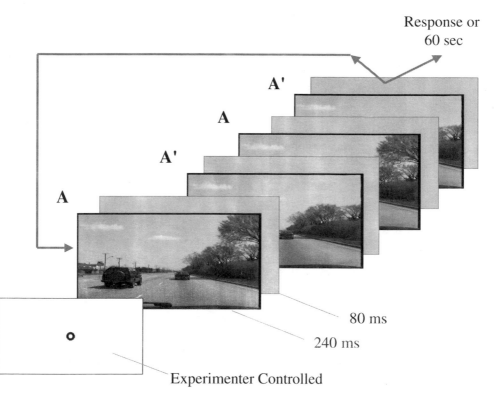

Figure 8.1
Graphical illustration of the perceptual change detection task.

Attentional Breadth   Participants were measured on their ability to localize an oblique peripheral stimulus appearing at one of three eccentricities (10°, 20°, or 30° of visual angle from fixation) in the presence of 11 vertical distractors. Targets appeared at random eccentricities on any given trial, and at least one distractor (but no more than two) appeared on each of the eight meridians. The stimulus display was presented for 250 msec and then terminated. Participants used a mouse to click on the target location. Participants completed two blocks of 144 trials each, with 48 practice trials to become familiar with the task. Each individual's functional field of view (FFOV) was defined as the eccentricity at which 50% accuracy was achieved (chance performance was 4%, given 25 possible target locations; see table 9.1; see also Ball et al., 1988; Pringle et al., 2001).

Working Memory and Executive Function   Tests were administered to assess two aspects of working memory: visuospatial working memory and verbal working memory (see table 8.1). Visuospatial working memory (which involves spatial

Table 8.1
Description of psychometric measures

Cognitive Measure	Task	Task Description	Dependent Measure
Attention	FFOV Task	Localize 20° oblique target, appearing for 250 msec among 11 vertical distractors, at one of three eccentricities (10°, 20°, 30° from center). Control task: localize oblique target without distractors. (modified stimuli from Ball et al., 1988)	Degree of eccentricity (at 50% accuracy; range 0°–30°)
Perceptual speed	Box completion	Create as many boxes (squares) as possible within 30 sec by drawing the fourth line of an unfinished square. (Salthouse, 1992)	Number of boxes completed (max = 100)
	Digit copying	Copy as many digits (numbers) as possible within 45 sec. (Salthouse, 1992; Wechsler, 1955)	Number of digits copied (max = 100)
	Digit symbol	Write the symbol corresponding to each number until the time limit expired (60 sec). Each number (1–9) was assigned a unique symbol (a key was always available for reference). (Salthouse, 1992; Wechsler, 1955)	Number of digits scored (max = 50)
Visuospatial working memory	Visual retention (modified)	Reproduce figural material. After viewing the stimuli for 10 sec, participants had unlimited time to draw all objects and their features in the proper locations (drawing aptitude was irrelevant). Stimuli consisted of simple shapes (i.e., triangles, squares, lines), but they progressively increased in number and complexity; 12 stimuli were presented. (Modified from Benton, 1963, with more complex combinations of stimuli)	Number of correctly drawn figures (max = 12); Number of features missed (min = 0)
	Memory tiles	Find matching tiles in 6 × 10 grid by flipping over two tiles at a time until all pairs are found. Tiles were initially placed with picture-side down in a random order and participants were allowed to view 2 tiles at a time. If the 2 selected tiles matched, they were removed from the grid. If not, the tiles were returned to picture-side down. Participants continued to flip pairs of tiles until all matches were found and no tiles remained on the grid. Performance was recorded by the time (sec) it took to find all of the matches and by the total number of pairs flipped to find all of the matches. Practice on a 3 × 3 grid, using different pictures on the tiles, was provided.	Number of pairs examined (min = 30); time to find all pairs
	Card rotations test	Determine whether series of simple and complex shapes are the same (but rotated) or different (i.e., mirror image) within 3 min. Two trials, 3 min each. (Ekstrom et al., 1987)	Number of correctly identified shapes each trial (max = 80 each)
	Maze tracing	Draw a continuous line through a series of short mazes within 3 min. (Ekstrom et al., 1987)	Number of completed mazes (max = 24)

Executive function	Sequential and coordinative complexity arithmetic	Solve a series of arithmetic problems until 3 min expires. Each equation had 6 single-digit numbers and 5 operands, either addition or subtraction, which had to be solved in sequential order (i.e., sequential complexity). A second series of arithmetic problems contained brackets or parentheses delineating priority of operations. Equations enclosed by brackets or parentheses had to be solved first, followed by equations enclosed by brackets, and then the remaining unenclosed equation could be solved (i.e., coordinative complexity). All solutions (and all intermediate solutions) were between 1 and 9. (Paper and pencil modification of Verhaeghen, Kliegl, and Mayr, 1997)	Number of correct solutions (max = 46 each series)
	Backward digit span	Immediately recall a sequence of numbers in the reverse order of its presentation. Digit sequences progressively lengthened as participants continued to correctly recall numbers. (Wechsler, 1955)	Number of digits recalled in (max = 14 backward)
Verbal working memory	Rey audio-verbal learning test (AVLT)	Immediately recall a list comprising 15 everyday words after an auditory presentation 5 times (trials 1–5), followed by the immediate recall of a novel list (trial 6). The first list was then recalled an additional time without the auditory presentation (trial 7). (Rey, 1964; Lezak, 1995)	Number of words recalled (max = 15 per trial)
	Wechsler Memory Scale paragraph recall	Immediately recall a story after verbal presentation in which 67 words describe a story with a logical progression. Some paraphrasing is allowed (must meet scoring criteria; Wechsler and Stone, 1973). Two stories presented.	average score of both paragraphs (max = 25)
	Verbal paired associates	Recall easy and difficult word associations for 8 word pairs, presented at a rate of 1 per 3 sec. Then one word from each pair was presented, and the participant had to recall the word that was associated with it. Feedback was provided each time. Easy word pairs were semantically associated (e.g., "fruit" and "apple"), while difficult word pairs were arbitrary (e.g., "obey" and "inch"). Participants had 3 attempts to recall all 8 associations. (Wechsler and Stone, 1973)	Number of words correctly recalled (max = 12 easy, 12 hard)

Table 8.1 (continued)

Cognitive Measure	Task	Task Description	Dependent Measure
Inhibition	Proactive interference	Recall by writing a series of 7 stimuli presented on a computer monitor. Stimuli consisted of 3 characters, either all letters or all numbers, presented on 5 trials. All stimuli on the first 4 trials were letters; all stimuli on the last trial were numbers. Before each trial began, a fixation (+) was displayed (1 sec). The 7 stimuli were then presented at a rate of 1/sec, followed by a 45 sec writing interval during which the word "WRITE" appeared. A 5 sec warning was provided before the next trial automatically began. Participants were instructed to write as many of the stimuli as they could remember. Order of recall was not important, as long as the sequence within a string was correct. (Modified from Wickens et al., 1963)	Number of correctly recalled strings (max = 7 per trial)
	Rey AVLT interference	Immediately recall a list comprising 15 everyday words. The same list was recalled after an auditory presentation 5 times (trials 1–5), followed by the immediate recall of a novel list (trial 6). (Rey, 1964; Lezak, 1995)	Number of words correctly recalled (trial 1–trial 6)
	Stroop	Respond to the hue of the letters on the display as quickly and as accurately as possible. An initial fixation (+) appeared for 750 msec, which was immediately followed by either a neutral letter string/hue (e.g., XXXXX), a congruent word/hue (e.g., RED displayed in red) or an incongruent word/ hue (e.g., RED displayed in blue). Four responses were possible (red, green, blue, yellow). Word/hue congruency was blocked. Observers had 3 sec to respond to the hue, while ignoring the name of the word. There were 24 practice trials followed by 6 blocks of 24 test trials each (i.e., 2 blocks of each condition). Feedback was provided, but instructions emphasized speed and accuracy. (Based on Stroop, 1935)	Cost = RT-incongruent – RT-neutral trials (min = 0 msec)

orientation, scanning, and spatial relations) was defined as the ability to associate object identity and spatial location information immediately after visual presentation; verbal working memory, as the ability to immediately recall verbal material and associations between verbal material; and executive function, as the ability to manipulate information in working memory.

Perceptual Speed   To assess perceptual speed, participants performed three paper-and-pencil tasks (i.e., box completion, digit copying, and digit symbol; Salthouse, 1992; see table 8.1 for descriptions), selected because they emphasized perceptual/motor aspects of processing speed and de-emphasized higher level aspects of cognition.

Inhibition   The ability to inhibit irrelevant information was gauged by performance on three tasks: the Stroop task, a proactive interference (PI) task, and the Rey audio-verbal learning test (AVLT). The Stroop task was selected because it demonstrates a robust interference effect in which the participant is unable to ignore an irrelevant feature of the stimulus (e.g., the meaning of the word) while attending to a relevant one (e.g., the color of the word; based on Stroop, 1935). The primary reason for including the PI task (modified from Wickens, Born, and Allen, 1963) was to measure PI buildup; release from PI was not examined. Finally, the Rey AVLT task was used to measure interference over the course of learning verbal material (Rey, 1964; Lezak, 1995). Together, these tasks provide converging estimates of the ability to inhibit irrelevant verbal and visual stimuli (see table 8.1 for descriptions).

Results

Relationship between Psychometric Performance and Change Detection Response Times
To facilitate comparison across psychometric measures with different means and standard deviations, standard z-scores were computed for each task (excluding the functional field of view measure). Z-scores were based on the overall group mean and standard deviation (i.e., across young and older adults).[1] As needed, the signs of the task z-scores were inverted so that performance across different tasks could be compared (e.g., so that high values on each composite measure corresponded to good performance). Composite scores were then derived from the average of these z-scores, representing a priori defined psychological constructs of perceptual speed, inhibition, and each of the identifiably different working memory constructs.[2] The use of composites can be justified as a means of reducing the data to variance-adjusted figures based on the assumption that each task comprised by the composite measure is equally important (i.e., equal weight; see also Salthouse, 1992). More important, the alignment of tests onto the composite measure was consistent with a factor analysis solution.

Composite measures were entered into regression analyses to predict change detection latency. For the purposes of the regression analyses, change detection response time referred to each individual's average response time across all pictures in which the change was correctly identified, excluding those times exceeding 3 standard deviations beyond the age-respective mean. Response time was considered a reasonable criterion measure of change detection performance because there was no speed-accuracy trade-off (see below for additional details). A summary of the intercorrelations among the measures of interest is provided in table 8.2.

Multiple regressions were performed on the change detection response times, using the factors in table 8.2 as predictors, to examine the hypothesis that perceptual change detection is mediated by attentional breadth, memory, inhibition, and perceptual speed abilities. Thus a forward stepwise regression analysis was conducted to determine if a subset of the factors could explain a significant amount of the variance and the benefit to be gained by adding each subsequent variable to the regression equation. In other words, this analysis started with the "best" factor of the set, and determined the additional variance explained by the second best factor, and so on (i.e., as long as the predefined F-value was exceeded). Results are presented in figure 8.2.

As figure 8.2 shows, three factors were significant (i.e., $p < .05$) in predicting change detection performance. The best predictor was visuospatial working memory (VSWM), followed by attentional breadth, then finally by perceptual speed. Together, they explained 69% of the response time variance, with VSWM accounting for the greatest share (i.e., 24%). Results also indicate that attentional breadth accounted for 6% of the variance, beyond what was already accounted for by VSWM and what was shared between the two factors. Perceptual speed accounted for 1% of the remaining variance.

Table 8.2
Intercorrelations among the measures of interest

	1	2	3	4	5	6	7	8
1. Age	—	.83	−.57	−.34	−.57	−.79	−.40	−.44
2. Change detection response time[a]		—	−.67	−.27	−.51	−.78	−.44	−.39
3. Attention[b]			—	.15	.33	.61	.30	.25
4. Composite inhibition[b]				—	.21	.34	.09	.12
5. Composite perceptual speed[b]					—	.56	.36	.38
6. Composite Visuospatial working memory[b]						—	.52	.48
7. Composite executive function[b]							—	.27
8. Composite verbal working memory[b]								—

Note: Correlations greater than ±0.19 are significant at $p < .05$.
[a] Low values correspond to better performance. [b] High values correspond to better performance.

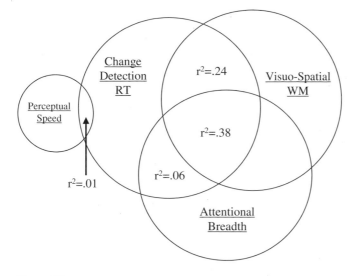

Figure 8.2
Amount of variance in change detection latency accounted for in a forward stepwise regression by attentional breadth, visuospatial working memory, and perceptual speed. Psychometric composites not included in the figure did not account for any significant amount of the variance in change detection performance.

The strong shared variance between attentional breadth and visuospatial working memory ($r^2 = 38\%$) may be related to the spatial components of the tasks underlying these factors. Recall that the functional field of view is a measure of the ability to localize targets in the periphery, whereas the VSWM tasks assess the ability to remember and manipulate objects, their features, and their spatial locations. Thus the shared variance between attentional breadth and VSWM may correspond to the spatial orienting to a (simple or complex) target and remembering its location. Spatial orienting and remembering is required for both the attentional breadth and the VSWM tasks, but not for other tasks, such as verbal working memory tasks. Accordingly, the variance explained by the VSWM alone may be for object memory. An analysis conducted post hoc compared tasks that were "more object/less spatial" (i.e., card rotations and visual reproduction tests) to tasks that were "more spatial/less object" (i.e., maze tracing and memory tiles tests). The analysis suggests that the "more object" tasks share 52% of the variance in response time with attentional breadth, whereas the "more spatial" tasks share slightly more of the variance in response time with attentional breadth (i.e., 61%), which is to say, that the shared variance between attentional breadth and VSWM corresponds to spatially orienting to an object and remembering its location. Additional studies are needed, however, to clarify this relationship.

Although the remaining factors were not significantly associated with performance on change detection, seemed possible that they might, in fact, when considered separately, but not in conjunction with some (or all) of the other measures. That is, these factors might account for small amounts of variance in change detection performance that overlap with attention, visuospatial memory, and perceptual speed.

We examined this issue by performing separate hierarchical regressions for inhibition, executive function, and verbal working memory. Each of these accounted for small but significant amounts of the variance in change detection response time ($p < .002$), but only when considered as the first variable in the regression. In other words, these three factors do not appear to account for performance beyond what is already accounted for by attention and visuospatial working memory; they appear to account for substantially less variance than visuospatial working memory.

Change Detection Response Time Performance
Based on Pringle et al., 2001, we predicted that change meaningfulness would enhance change detection performance for older and younger adults, and that this benefit would be moderated by change salience and observer age. And, indeed, we observed these effects in the response time data for trials where change was correctly detected and identified (see figure 8.3). These results demonstrate how observers explicitly responded to changes in the scenes. Differences were apparent in the overall speed of responding between the two groups of observers. Younger adults were 6 sec faster than older adults in detecting changes ($F(1, 125) = 191.03$, $p < .001$). Additionally, characteristics of the change differentially influenced responding, such that enhanced change detection performance was associated with changes of high meaning ($F(1, 125) = 44.78$, $p < .001$) and of high salience ($F(1, 125) = 582.50$, $p < .001$).

The main effects were mitigated by several significant two-way interactions, which can best be understood in terms of the significant three-way interactions presented in figure 8.3. The meaningfulness of the change did interact with observer age and change salience, as in Pringle et al., 2001. Here, the interaction showed that increased meaning positively influenced change detection across both age groups and across high and low change salience, except for older adults when change salience was also low ($F(1,125) = 6.16$, $p < .01$). Scheffé post hoc analyses indicated that increasing change meaningfulness had no effect on performance for older adults when changes were of low salience ($p > .10$). On the other hand, increasing change meaningfulness aided the performance of older adults when changes were highly salient ($p < .05$), and it generally aided the performance of younger adults for changes of both low and high salience ($p < .05$).

Recall that Pringle et al., 2001, showed that change meaningfulness only influenced change detection performance when change salience was low. There are

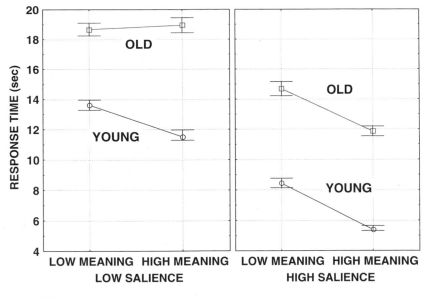

Figure 8.3
Age × meaning × salience interaction for response time (sec).

several reasons why this might be the case. Observers in the high salience condition were performing faster overall in that study than their counterparts in the current study. Their faster responses might have been close to or at ceiling performance; thus a meaning effect would not appear in the high salience condition. In the current study, on the other hand, where responses were relatively slower and further from ceiling performance, meaning could show an effect. These slower responses might be attributed to the larger display size (i.e., 90° × 72° compared with 25° × 20° of visual angle in Pringle et al., 2001); by making the field of view feel more "immersive," the larger display could have enhanced the meaning or context of the scenes, relative to that in Pringle et al., 2001. Finally, it is important to note that the older adults' insensitivity to meaningful changes of low salience in the current study does not mean they did not see them; their response times represent trials where they correctly detected and identified change.

Overall, older adults are slower to detect an inconspicuous change (i.e., one of low salience), regardless of its meaning to the scene context. However, the eye movement data will reveal that older adults are perhaps *initially* sensitive to meaning under low salience conditions, but that the effect is attenuated over the duration of a trial (perhaps indicated by their lower confidence in detecting change). Thus observers' eye movement behaviors were analyzed as a means to elucidate the relationship between their processing of the scene and their response to detecting change.

Relationship between Individual Differences and Eye Movements
A total of 9,306 trials were available for analyses across participants. The observers' point of fixation was used as the basis for eye movement behavior. We hypothesized that a broader attentional breadth would be related to faster change detection performance by decreasing the number of dwells (i.e., sequential fixations in close proximity) needed to scan the scene for change. Our hypothesis was supported by a significant negative correlation between attentional breadth (functional field of view) and the total number of dwells in the scene ($r = -.61$, $p < .001$; see figure 8.4).

We also examined the relationship between visuospatial memory and the total number of dwells needed to find the change, assuming that individuals with larger memory capacity would maintain a better memory representation of the scene and therefore revisit areas less frequently. Indeed, our hypothesis was supported by a significant negative relationship, as illustrated in figure 8.4 ($r = -.71$, $p < .001$).

At this point, to elucidate the extent to which eye movements reflect observers' strategies, let us consider the relationship between eye movements and subjective responses on the postexperiment questionnaire (see table 8.3 for relevant questions). Separate analyses of variance were first conducted on each of the questions, using age as a between-subjects factor. Two questions identified age differences. The younger adults were more likely than the older adults to enjoy viewing the scenes and to have confidence in their ability to detect changes. While it is possible that the enjoyment of the scenes may have been of some benefit to younger adults' behavioral responses (as reflected in their response times), the difference in confidence ratings is not likely to account for a large portion of the variance in the age differences reported. Although one might expect that the young adults' greater confidence would result in riskier responding (i.e., overconfidence), analyses on accuracy data actually indicate a conservative response bias (i.e., lower false alarm rates, higher beta), compared with older adults.

Both age groups reported a similar emphasis in looking for salient change characteristics (as evidenced by the nonsignificant age differences, $p > .70$), although the means for each age group were moderately high (i.e., 5.3 for both younger and older adults). Participants also believed they emphasized looking for salient changes over meaningful ones, consistent with the response time data. A within-subjects analysis on participants' responses to questions whether they were looking for changes that were meaningful versus changes that were salient revealed that participants believed they were attending to salience to a greater extent than they were attending to meaningfulness ($F(1,125) = 4.79$, $p < .03$), but this did not differ across age ($F(1,125) = 0.177$, $p < .68$).

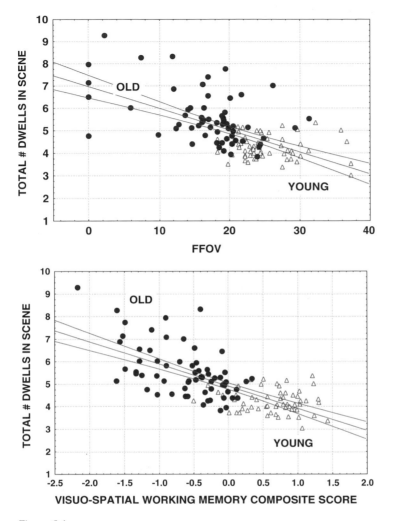

Figure 8.4
Relationship between the total number of dwells in a scene and the attentional breadth measure, functional field of view (FFOV; top), and between the total number of dwells in a scene and the visuospatial working memory composite score (bottom).

Table 8.3
Select postexperiment questions and mean responses from younger and older participants

Question	Young	Old
What was your overall enjoyment viewing these scenes? (1 = not at all enjoyable; 7 = very enjoyable)	5.1*	4.6*
How high was your self-confidence in your ability to detect change? (1 = not at all confident; 7 = completely confident)	5.1*	4.2*
To what extent did you attempt to look for changes related to driving? (1 = not at all; 7 = all the time)	4.9	4.8
To what extent did you attempt to look for changes that were conspicuous or salient? (1 = not at all; 7 = all the time)	5.3	5.3

* $p < .05$.

It is especially interesting to note that older adults believed they looked for meaningful changes to the same extent as younger adults ($p > .70$), when their response times indicated that they did so only when the change was also salient (similar age differences in sensitivity to meaning were observed in Pringle et al., 2001). Thus older adults either are not sensitive to the fact that their actual responses to changes of high meaning but low salience are slower (relative to younger adults), or their subjective responses reflect a different aspect of their search behavior, such as eye movements.

To examine this issue further, we compared age differences in viewing the changing scene. Our primary focus was on the amount of time subjects spent searching the scene before their eyes first fixated on the change, which provides an index of scene processing, or perhaps search strategies, prior to detecting the change. These measures could potentially elucidate links between change meaningfulness, change salience, and observer age. Figure 8.5 depicts the effects of these three factors on the elapsed time searching the scene before the first time the eyes fixated on the change region.

As depicted in figure 8.5, younger adults' eyes generally fixated on changes more quickly than the older adults' eyes did (approximately 1.5 sec earlier), on changes of high salience more quickly than on changes of low salience, and on changes of high meaning more quickly than on changes of low meaning. What is especially interesting is that the age × meaning × salience interaction was not significant ($p > .50$). In the response time data (figure 8.3), results indicated that older adults were not sensitive to meaning when the change was also of low salience. It now seems likely that the measure of overt response to the change was not sensitive enough to detect the effect of scene meaningfulness. In figure 8.5, older adults' eye movements are sensitive to meaningfulness when there is a low salience change. In fact, older adults appear to be as sensitive as younger adults, as indicated in their self-reports of their viewing behavior. Thus it appears that,

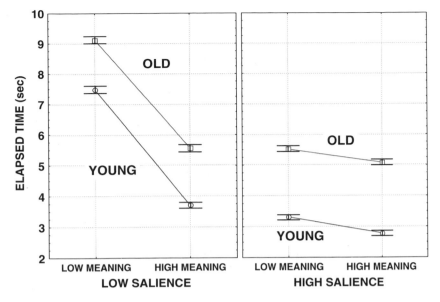

Figure 8.5
Age × meaning × salience interaction for the amount of elapsed time (sec) in scene prior to the initial fixation on the change area.

though older adults fixate on meaningful change, their explicit response to the change is significantly delayed.

Discussion

The current study clarifies the role of multiple processes involved in change detection, and their relative contributions. It not only links change detection and attention (as previously implied by Rensink, O'Regan, and Clark, 1997; Pringle et al., 2001; and others), but it also establishes the relative weight of that link in light of other mediators of change detection latency. Most important, it shows that, in accounting for change detection response time, visuospatial working memory plays a greater role than attentional breadth, and that perceptual speed plays a very small but significant role. Taken together, these findings suggest that change detection is influenced both by the number of attentional samples required to scan the scene and by a representation of what was sampled, specifically, the object-spatial properties of the sample. Thus, a major part of the difficulty in change blindness may be linked to a limited encoding and retrieval ability, consistent with other findings in the literature (e.g., Hollingworth and Henderson, 2002; Irwin, 1996; Zelinsky, 2001).

It was somewhat surprising that some of the other cognitive constructs did not play a greater role in change detection performance. In particular, the relative weakness of perceptual speed as a predictor of change detection performance was unexpected in light of research showing that speed measures often account for substantial variance in complex tasks (Salthouse, 1992). Also unexpected was the finding that proactive interference measures did not account for any unique variance in perceptual change detection performance. One explanation for this might be the nonrepeating nature of the pictures: though contextually similar, they were not identical. Likewise, the specific changes to the pictures in the "flicker" paradigm were all different. Thus proactive interference might only build up when participants are repeatedly exposed to the stimuli (as in Flicker et al., 1989).

The link between visuospatial working memory and change detection performance is consistent with findings that suggest memory plays a role in perceptual change detection. For example, observers may fail to retain identity information about an object, despite having successfully attended to it previously, resulting in the failure to detect a change in the object (e.g., Becker, Pashler, and Anstis, 2000). Furthermore, the findings presented here are consistent with the notion that memory for scenes is not detailed (e.g., McConkie and Currie, 1996; Irwin, 1996; Henderson and Hollingworth, 1999).

The finding that memory is one of several components important for successful change detection suggests that the capacity of visuospatial working memory may limit the number of objects represented in the scene and their spatial relations. Irwin (1996) suggests that the identity and approximate location for three to four objects can be maintained across a single saccade. Thus the greater the number of the objects in the scene represented (associated with greater working memory capacity), the greater the likelihood that one of them corresponds to the item undergoing change.

We do not mean to imply that working memory always plays a stronger role than attention in the representation of scenes and that inhibition and perceptual speed never play a role. Rather, these roles may vary with demands of the task and training on the task. For example, if attentional breadth increases with practice (as observed by Ball et al., 1988), this could result in improved performance in change detection.

Finally, with regard to metacognitive search strategies, either older adults are not sensitive to the fact that their responses to changes of high meaning but low salience are slower (relative to younger adults) or their answers to our questionnaire reflect their initial search in the scene, rather than their overall search. This is supported by the finding that older adults' initial eye movements were just as sensitive as those of the younger adults to the meaning of the changes, although young adults were more successful than older adults at using the information acquired in these eye movements to speed change detection on the basis of meaning. Thus, to fully understand metacognitive abilities in change detection, research needs to consider individual differences as well as indirect measures of change detection.

These findings also have implications for change detection in the real world. Seemingly harmless and routine interruptions, such as blank screens (or blinks and saccades, as in other studies), can significantly delay the detection of changes to objects in complex, real-world scenes. Similar change blindness effects have been observed in the real world. For example, change blindness has been documented in the cockpit of highly automated aircraft (Sarter and Woods, 2000). Pilots sometimes fail to detect and respond to changes in automation configuration, especially when the automation takes an unexpected action or when it fails completely. Coupling this with subjective reports that pilots look where they expect to find changes (Sarter and Woods, 1997), a dangerous pattern emerges. If pilots only look where they expect to find changes, then the potential exists for them to miss valuable information from other sources that may have changed for reasons they could not anticipate. The findings reported here suggest that, although it is important to draw the pilots' attention to the changing displays, it may be more important to enhance their memory (i.e., representation) of the properties of the change, through some combination of display design and training.

Acknowledgments

This research was supported by grant AG14966 from the National Institute on Aging and by cooperative research agreement DAAL01-96-2-0003 with the Army Research Laboratory. We would like to thank Roger Marsh for his assistance in programming, Meg Vais and Shawn Bolin for their assistance in running subjects, and Daniel Levin for his helpful suggestions.

Notes

1. Given that the relationship between performance on the psychometric tests and that on the change detection tests was similar for the young and older adults, we collapsed the data for the two age groups in reporting on our current study.
2. Although we originally considered the visuospatial working memory composite as two separate composites, visual working memory and spatial working memory, because of the high intercorrelation ($r = .75$) of these factors, we instead combined them into a single visuospatial working memory composite.

References

Ackerman, P. L., and Cianciolo, A. T. (2000). Cognitive, perceptual-speed, and psychomotor determinants of individual differences during skill acquisition. *Journal of Experimental Psychology: Applied, 6*, 259–290.

Ball, K., Beard, B. L., Roenker, D. L., Miller, R. L., and Griggs, D. S. (1988). Age and visual search: Expanding the useful field of view. *Journal of the Optical Society of America, A, 5*, 2210–2219.

Becker, M. W., Pashler, H., and Anstis, S. M. (2000). How quickly we forget: Change blindness in a highest digit task shows the volatility of visual representation. Poster presented at ARVO Annual Meeting, April 30–May 5, Fort Lauderdale.

Benton, A. L. (1963). *The revised visual retention test: Clinical and experimental applications*. New York: Psychological Corporation.

Duncan, J. (1995). Attention, intelligence, and the frontal lobes. In M. S. Gazzaniga (Ed). *The cognitive neurosciences* (pp. 721–733). Cambridge, MA: MIT Press.

Ekstrom, R. B., French, J. W., Harman, H. H., and Dermen, D. (1987). *Manual for kit of factor-referenced cognitive tests*. Princeton, NJ: Educational Testing Service.

Flicker, C., Ferris, S. H., Crook, T., and Bartus, T. R. (1989). Age differences in the vulnerability of facial recognition memory to proactive interference. *Experimental Aging Research, 15*, 189–194.

Grimes, J. (1996). On the failure to detect changes in scenes across saccades. In K. A. Akins (Ed.), *Perception: Vancouver studies in cognitive science*. Vol. 5. (pp. 89–110). New York: Oxford University Press.

Henderson, J. M., and Hollingworth, A. (1999). The role of fixation position in detecting scene changes across saccades. *Psychological Science, 10*, 438–443.

Hollingworth, A., and Henderson, J. M. (2000). Semantic in formativeness mediates the detection of changes in natural scenes. *Visual Cognition, 7*, 213–235.

Hollingworth, A., and Henderson, J. M. (2002). Accurate visual memory for previously attended objects in natural scenes. *Journal of Experimental Psychology: Human Perception and Performance, 28*, 113–136.

Hollingworth, A., Schrock, G., and Henderson, J. M. (2001). Change detection in the flicker paradigm: The role of fixation position within the scene. *Memory and Cognition, 29*, 296–304.

Hollingworth, A., Williams, C. C., and Henderson, J. M. (2001). To see and remember: Visually specific information is retained in memory from previously attended objects in natural scenes. *Psychonomic Bulletin and Review, 8*, 761–768.

Irwin, D. E. (1991). Information integration across saccadic eye movements. *Cognitive Psychology, 23*, 420–456.

Irwin, D. E. (1992). Memory for position and identity across eye movements. *Journal of Experimental Psychology: Learning, Memory, and Cognition, 18*, 307–317.

Irwin, D. E. (1996). Integrating information across saccadic eye movements. *Psychological Science, 5*, 94–100.

Levin, D. T., and Simons, D. J. (1997). Failure to detect changes to attended objects in motion pictures. *Psychonomic Bulletin and Review, 4*, 501–506.

Lezak, M. D. (1995). *Neuropsychological assessment*. 3d ed. New York: Oxford University Press.

McConkie, G. W., and Currie, C. B. (1996). Visual stability across saccades while viewing complex pictures. *Journal of Experimental Psychology: Human Perception and Performance, 22*, 563–581.

Miyake, A., Friedman, N. P., Emerson, M. J., Witzki, A. H., and Howerter, A. (2000). The unity and diversity of executive functions and their contributions to complex "frontal lobe" tasks: A latent variable analysis. *Cognitive Psychology, 41*, 49–100.

Mondy, S., and Coltheart, V. (2000). Detection and identification of change in naturalistic scenes. *Visual Cognition, 7*, 281–296.

O'Regan, J. K., Deubel, H., Clark, J. J., and Rensink, R. A. (2000). Picture changes during blinks: Looking without seeing and seeing without looking. *Visual Cognition, 7*, 191–211.

O'Regan, J. K., Rensink, R. A., and Clark, J. J. (1999). Change-blindness as a result of "mudsplashes." *Nature, 398*, 34.

Pringle, H. L., Irwin, D. E., Kramer, A. K., and Atchley, P. (2001). The role of attentional breadth in perceptual change detection. *Psychonomic Bulletin and Review, 8*, 89–95.

Rensink, R. A. (2000). Visual search for change: A probe into the nature of attentional processing. *Visual Cognition, 7*, 345–376.

Rensink, R. A., O'Regan, J. K., and Clark, J. J. (1997). To see or not to see: The need for attention to perceive changes in scenes. *Psychological Science, 8*, 368–373.

Rey, A. (1964). *L'examen clinique en psychologie*. Paris: Presse Universitaire de France.

Ryan, J. D., Althoff, R. R., Whitlow, S., and Cohen, N. J. (2000). Amnesia is a deficit in relational memory. *Psychological Science, 11*, 454–461.

Salthouse, T. A. (1992). *Mechanisms of age-cognition relations in adulthood*. Hillsdale, NJ: Erlbaum.

Sarter, N. B., and Woods, D. D. (1997). Team play with a powerful and independent agent: Operational experiences and automation surprises on the Airbus A-320. *Human Factors, 39*, 553–569.

Sarter, N., and Woods, D. D. (2000). Team play with a powerful and independent agent: A full-mission simulation study. *Human Factors, 42*, 390–402.

Scholl, B. J. (2000). Attenuated change blindness for exogenously attended items in a flicker paradigm. *Visual Cognition, 7*, 377–396.

Simons, D. J., and Levin, D. T. (1998). Failure to detect changes to people during a real-world interaction. *Psychonomic Bulletin & Review, 5*, 644–649.

Stroop, J. R. (1935). Studies of interference in serial verbal reactions. *Journal of Experimental Psychology, 18*, 643–661.

Verhaeghen, P., Kliegl, R., and Mayr, U. (1997). Sequential and coordinative complexity in time-accuracy function for mental arithmetic. *Psychology and Aging, 12*, 555–564.

Wallis, G., and Bulthoff, H. H. (2000). What's scene and not scene: Influences of movement and task upon what we see. *Visual Cognition, 7*, 175–190.

Wechsler, D. (1955). *Manual: Wechsler Adult Intelligence Scale*. New York: Psychological Corporation.

Wechsler, D., and Stone, C. P. (1973). *Manual: Wechsler Memory Scale*. New York: Psychological Corporation.

Wickens, D. D., Born, D. G., and Allen, C. K. (1963). Proactive inhibition and item similarity in short-term memory. *Journal of Verbal Learning and Verbal Behavior, 2*, 440–445.

Witmer, B. G., and Singer, M. J. (1998). Measuring presence in virtual environments: A presence questionnaire. *Presence, 7*, 225–240.

Yee, P. L., Laden, B., and Hunt, E. (1994). The coordination of compensatory tracking and anticipatory timing tasks. *Intelligence, 18*, 259–287.

Zelinski, E. M., Gilewski, M. J., and Schaie, K. W. (1993). Individual differences in cross-sectional and 3-year longitudinal memory performance across the adult life span. *Psychology and Aging, 8*, 176–186.

Zelinsky, G. J. (2001). Eye movements during change detection: Implications for search constraints, memory limitations, and scanning strategies. *Perception and Psychophysics, 63*, 209–225.

Chapter 9

Visual versus Verbal Metacognition: Are They Really Different?

Rachel A. Diana and Lynne M. Reder

In the lead role of his film *That Obscure Object of Desire*, Luis Bunuel uses two different actresses, Carole Bouquet and Angela Molina, alternating between them depending on the mood of the scene. At times, one actress walks into a doorway and the other actress appears on the other side. It is quite possible to be absorbed in watching the entire film without ever noticing that two different people are playing the same character at different times. This finding is not unique. An entire research enterprise has developed surrounding the phenomenon known as "change blindness," where participants are not aware that their conversation partner has been switched with another person during a distraction (e.g., Rensink, O'Regan, and Clark, 1997; Simons and Levin, 1998). It seemed amazing to us that such bold substitutions of actors could occur without awareness, but it is perhaps equally important to ask whether one should be surprised that people fail to notice these changes. Do people typically assume that they would notice such major substitutions in the visual aspects of a display?

The answer to that question is yes; people do assume that they will notice major visual events such as a change in who portrays a character (Levin et al., 2000). In fact, our intuitions about our visual abilities are often incorrect. The military designed a new instrument panel for airplanes to be superimposed on the windshield of the plane, thus allowing the pilot to simultaneously view the area in front of the plane and the instruments of the control panel. The intuition was that placing the control panels on the windshield would improve efficiency and performance because pilots would not be required to move their head and eyes between controls at a lower level and the cockpit window. Tests in flight simulators demonstrated that this "head-up" control panel produced dramatically different performance than that anticipated by its creator (Haines, 1991). Attention to this control panel caused two out of eight pilots to proceed on paths that would have caused them to crash into planes directly in front of them during the landing process.

The examples of the film and aircraft simulator suggest that human perception is far from perfect and that our intuitions or metacognition about our visual processing are not always accurate. Despite a large body of research devoted to people's metacognition concerning factual knowledge (e.g., Metcalfe and Shimamura, 1994; Reder and Schunn, 1996; Yzerbyt, Lories, and Dardenne, 1998), there has been relatively little attention to the metacognitive processes associated with visual processing (for exceptions, see Busey et al., 2000; Chun and Jiang, 1998; Levin et al., 2000; Winer et al., 1996a; Winer et al., 1996b). The dramatic results from change blindness paradigms, such as failing to notice that one's conversation partner has changed identity mid conversation (Simons and Levin, 1998) underscores the need for more appreciation of the mechanisms involved.

Experiments in this area have found that participants are unable to predict their poor performance in change detection scenarios. The metacognitive errors seem to involve a systematic overestimation of human cognitive capacity in processing. Perhaps this overestimation is based on a lifetime of accurate (or seemingly accurate) perception of visual scenes, which results from the adaptive nature of metacognition, as addressed later in the chapter. Is visual metacognition as inaccurate as we have suggested above? If so, why? Can we understand visual metacognition by relating to previous research on metacognition that focused on semantic knowledge? In this chapter, we propose answers to all three questions.

What Is Metacognition?

Noting that the term *metacognition* seems to have different meanings for researchers in different subdisciplines of cognitive science, Reder (1996) asks whether these researchers have simply focused on different aspects of the same concept or whether there is actually a collection of different concepts that have all been labeled with the same term. "Metacognition" has been used to describe theory of mind, cognition about cognition, beliefs, monitoring of cognitive performance, and strategy selection. Although it has often been assumed within these areas that metacognitive functioning involves the conscious awareness of activities within the mind, we will present evidence that strategy selection and monitoring of cognitive performance are not always conscious. If this is so, it would seem that, to keep consciousness as a criterion, we would have to limit metacognition to a far narrower set of activities.

When we assume that metacognition is unconscious in some situations, we leave open the possibility that it may occur automatically, with no prompting from conscious systems. For the purposes of this chapter, we assume that metacognition refers to information about our cognitive state and that it is often associated with the control of behavior and the selection of control procedures to achieve a goal. We believe that such procedures, though sometimes conscious, are often automatic and part of a larger cognitive process (Cary and Reder, forthcoming; Reder and Schunn, 1996).

Feeling of Knowing: An Illustration

Classically defined as the state of believing that a piece of information can be retrieved from memory even though it currently cannot be recalled, feeling of knowing (FOK) is a research paradigm that has led to much debate over the character of metacognition. People often experienced FOK as a tip-of-the-tongue phenomenon, when they are not able to retrieve an item from memory, but feel that they should be. Recent research has suggested that feeling of knowing includes a rapid, automatic process beginning prior to actual memory retrieval and determining the course of the retrieval process (Miner and Reder, 1994). According to this proposal, an FOK judgment often occurs within retrieval, but it becomes consciously available only when retrieval fails (as in the tip-of-the-tongue phenomenon) or when participants are asked to search for and report their judgment. When conceptualized as an automatic process in the procedure of memory retrieval, feeling of knowing can be tested by asking participants to make judgments about their ability to retrieve an item before they actually attempt retrieval. These judgments can then be compared to the participants' actual ability to retrieve and to characteristics of the question or problem itself. Despite evidence presented earlier that metacognition is often inaccurate, FOK ratings are highly related to performance on cued-recall tests, relearning rates, and feature identification. Participants are able to successfully predict correct recognition and recognition failure (Miner and Reder, 1994). Accuracy in this paradigm is well above chance, but not nearly perfect.

Several mechanisms have been proposed to account for the accuracy of feeling of knowing judgments. The trace access hypothesis suggests that, when a question is asked, there is an immediate partial retrieval of the answer, which enables participants to monitor some aspects of the target item and decide whether they will be able to fully retrieve the answer (e.g., Nelson, Gerler, and Narens, 1984). This hypothesis accounts for the ability of someone experiencing the tip-of-the-tongue phenomenon to recount the first letter or number of syllables of the desired word. The cue familiarity hypothesis suggests that FOK judgments are actually based on a feeling of familiarity with the question itself. Cues that are associated with the question or the context provide evidence as to the likelihood of retrieving the answer. This hypothesis predicts that as cue familiarity increases, so should the FOK judgment. For example, frequency of exposure to unfamiliar math problems was correlated with higher FOK judgments, even when only part of the problem was familiar (Reder and Ritter, 1992).

The evidence that feeling of knowing judgments represent a rapid preretrieval stage in memory leads one to ask what purpose FOK is fulfilling in retrieval processing. Research suggests that FOK judgments act as an automatic strategy selection device (Reder, 1988). The automatic determination whether a response can be retrieved allows one to quickly decide whether a memory search is a worthwhile expenditure of resources. If the item is judged to be unfamiliar and thus not retrievable, then one can quickly decide to look for the answer by using another strategy, such as calculating a math problem or researching a question (Reder, 1982, 1987; Reder and Ritter, 1992). This type of judgment could also be used to determine how long to continue a search before conceding that another strategy should be used. If the FOK judgment were strong, one would allow the search to continue for a longer period of time. Research shows that FOK judgment has a positive correlation with duration of search (Gruneberg, Monks, and Sykes, 1977; Nelson, Gerler, and Narens, 1984).

Strategy Selection Can Be Unconscious

A number of experiments have shown that participants can select and use strategies they are unaware of. For example, when experimental designs vary the base rates of the usefulness of various types of problem-solving strategies, participants' results indicate that they adapted their base rates of selecting among these strategies. Interestingly, although the data clearly suggest these adaptations, postexperimental interviews indicate that participants are often unaware of the manipulation of base rates. In an experiment where participants were required to judge the plausibility of statements based on a story they had read, they were unaware of the strategy they used or the likelihood that retrieval would be successful (despite strong adaptation). All participants believed they had used direct retrieval, even when that strategy was not possible (Reder, 1987).

Likewise, strategy selection in verification of math equations was shown to be sensitive to rates of success with the verification strategies. Thus, if many of the equations could be judged as false because they violated the parity rule (where the sum is even when the addends are both even or both odd), participants became more likely to test all equations for parity, although they claimed to be unaware that one strategy was more successful than another (Lemaire and Reder, 1999). On Lovett's "building sticks" task (Lovett and Anderson, 1996), where the probability of a successful "overshoot" versus "undershoot" strategy was varied, the results showed that, although the base rates of strategy success had an effect on strategy selection, participants did not accurately explain their behavior.

Even low-level strategies can be affected implicitly by base rates of success. When participants are asked to respond to a target item in one of several locations while ignoring the distractor item that appeared in one of those same locations, their performance was affected by the frequency with which distractors appeared in specific locations (Reder and Weber, 1997). Over time, participants learned to prefer to examine certain locations and to ignore others, based on the probability of a target or distractor appearing in that location. When questioned at the end of the study about the distribution of distractors over the locations, however, they were unaware of any differential distribution. Chun and Jiang (1998) were able to affect the strategy used to detect a target by providing repeated contexts that predicted the location of the target. Whereas participants detected targets more quickly when the configuration of stimuli was repeated than when it was novel, they were at chance in discriminating repeated from novel configurations. Although we would hesitate to label these low-level tasks "metacognitive," they do provide evidence that search strategies can be affected implicitly.

Why Is Metacognition Sometimes Unconscious?

Thus, as we have shown, people are sometimes unaware of what causes them to select one strategy over another, and even of what strategy they may be using. We propose (see Reder and Schunn, 1996) that people are unlikely to be aware of the resulting strategy when the process requires rapid execution; that metacognition, in general, may be unconscious when the time course of processing is short; that cognitive monitoring, typically assumed to be a conscious process, may actually operate without much awareness; and that control of cognitive processing may be governed by implicit learning and memory.

There is a reason why metacognitive processes should be automatic and unconscious. When conscious control of metacognitive activity is not required, other cognitive resources are released and can be used in cognitive processing. Furthermore, metacognitive processes are less likely to interfere with regular cognitive processing if they are unconscious. For example, during a task that requires quick and accurate responses, the mind is able to monitor target location probabilities and adjust strategies without interfering in the rapid response to targets we are consciously aware of. Koriat (2000) has proposed that metacognitive feelings are an interface between automatic processing and consciously controlled processing and that experience-based metacognitive processing, which consists of a transition from low-level experience to high-level experience, may be implicit, whereas information-based metacognitive processing, involving analysis of higher-level experiences, is always explicit. Koriat allows for the possibility that these automatic cognitions can influence behavior and that "consciousness is not the sole gateway to action."

Other theorists have also supported the idea that metacognition may be unconscious under certain conditions. Defining *metacognition* as beliefs and opinions about our beliefs and opinions, Graham and Neisser (2000) maintain that, because our first level of beliefs and opinions (such as thoughts about "family and friends, Mahler's Fifth, and avocados") can be implicit, it is unreasonable to assume that our second level (our opinions about those earlier thoughts) must never be. Based on their work with a blindsight patient, Kentridge and Heywood (2000) make the argument that metacognition is not inherently conscious, that awareness might not always be necessary for changes in automatic processing to occur. Their patient could not see in certain regions of the visual field; this failure of an automatic process (vision) led to its replacement with another, unconscious strategy, outside the patient's awareness. The blindsight patient was able to orient his attention within the field of vision loss such that his reaction time to stimuli he could not consciously see was sped up by cues he could not consciously report.

When and Why Is Metacognition Inaccurate?

Using conscious processing in a task that is normally automatic can interfere with performance. For example, within the field of implicit learning, it has been established that strategy use is optimal when there is no conscious awareness of the strategy (Berry and Broadbent, 1984; Lewicki, Hill, and Bizot, 1988; Reber, 1989). When subjects are asked to consciously access and verbalize their experience in implicit learning tasks (e.g., Berry and Broadbent, 1984) or are otherwise given information that distorts an automatic process such as perception (Smith et al., 1976), their performance is significantly worse. In another example, verbalizing a description of a specialized stimulus (such as a face) produces a deficit in ability to recognize that face later on (Dodson, Johnson, and Schooler, 1997; Meissner and Brigham, 2001; Schooler and Engstler-Schooler, 1990; Westerman and Larsen, 1997). Some have proposed (Dodson et al., 1997; Westerman and Larsen, 1997) that this effect is due to a general shift in the processes involved in face recognition, rather than impairment for the stimulus face alone. Thus consciously analyzing and verbalizing an automatic process (such as storage of a face in memory) is detrimental to its outcome.

The difference in performance between novices and experts also provides evidence that conscious processing harms performance on automatic tasks. Research shows that expert golfers do not apply step-by-step attentional control to their putts (Beilock and Carr, 2001). This finding reflects an overall consensus that practice on a particular task will lead to its becoming automatic (Anderson, 1982; Logan, 1985, 1988; MacLeod and Dunbar, 1988; Regan, 1981). Expert golfers were found to putt more accurately when their attention was distracted ("distracted condition") than when they were told to pay step-by-step attention to their putting performance ("skill-focused condition"; Beilock et al., 2002). Expert soccer players were more successful when dribbling with their dominant foot in the distracted than in the skill-focused condition—and more successful when dribbling with their *non*dominant foot in the skill-focused than in the distracted condition. In contrast, novice soccer players performed better in the skill-focused condition when using either foot. These studies provide evidence that high-level skill execution is harmed when conscious attention is paid to the individual steps of an automatic process. Like golf and soccer skills in an expert, vision is an automatic process. We suspect that visual metacognition is often inaccurate because it is tested in a way that requires conscious access to unconscious automatic processes.

We propose that metacognitive tasks are often inaccurate because they require conscious access to naturally fast, automatic processes and thus produce interference. The amount of interference from conscious analysis of processing may be modulated by factors such as the time course or other properties of the task. Cary and Reder (2002) have proposed that easier tasks are associated with less awareness of metacognitive processes. More difficult tasks may lead to greater awareness because of the greater number of errors or longer time course of execution. The nature of the cognitive processes used by a participant in a problem-solving task, whether reflective, deliberate, or routine (Carlson, 1997), may thus also determine the degree of metacognitive consciousness. For instance, protocol analysis relies on accessing cognitive processing throughout a much longer time course, which allows for greater awareness (Ericsson and Simon, 1998).

Are Perceptual and Conceptual Information Really Different?

Similarities exist between strategy selection and comparison processes. Decisions about when to retrieve versus calculate an answer to a math problem are analogous to decisions about whether to search a complex scene or rely on the information that calls for attention. If the scene appears familiar to us, or if we are not motivated by some external factor, we may not use our limited resources to carefully search the details of the scene. The information that is readily apparent, which draws our attention, is deemed sufficient. The same is true of answering math problems. If the problem seems familiar or the likely benefit from a correct answer seems slight, we may choose to retrieve an answer that may well be not accurate. The resources that would be used to carefully calculate the problem can then be applied elsewhere.

The phenomenon of change blindness is not unlike the cognitive illusion known as the "Moses illusion." Even when warned to be wary of distorted questions, participants answer, "Two," to the question "How many animals of each kind did Moses take on the ark?" (Erickson and Mattson, 1981). The correct answer would be "None," given that Noah, not Moses, was the figure associated with the ark. Participants are extremely bad at detecting these substitutions even when the critical word is capitalized, and it is confirmed that they know the correct answer. Researchers and laypersons alike are amazed at their inability to detect these distortions (Erickson and Mattson, 1981). This is similar to the inability of participants to detect a large change in the visual scene (such as a change in the identity of a conversation partner), although they expect that they would be able to detect such a change (Levin et al., 2000). Of course, this type of "trick question," like the Moses illusion, is not one that would be expected in everyday life. Thus it may be adaptive to avoid wasting resources searching for the identity of the person on the ark when we can simply assume that the question has been posed correctly. We will address this possibility at the end of the chapter.

Given that most research on metacognition has involved verbal and semantic tasks and stimuli, it would be ideal to find evidence to support the hypothesis that these conclusions generalize into the visual realm. Elsewhere, we have proposed that perceptual information is represented and processed analogously to conceptual information in memory (Reder, Donavos, and Erickson, 2002). As we argue in this chapter, the same basic processes operate on perceptual as on cognitive illusions, and the processes that operate on verbal and semantic information do so in an analogous fashion on perceptual information as well, such that metacognitive processes (both verbal and visual) can be assumed to proceed in the same way, using the same principles.

A number of theorists (e.g., Schacter, 1994) have postulated that conceptual information is somehow fundamentally different from perceptual information. For example, Roediger (1990) has proposed that explicit tests of memory, though susceptible to changes in conceptual or semantic elaboration, are not typically sensitive to changes in perceptual or surface features. Likewise, theorists (e.g., Gernsbacher, 1985) have proposed that semantic information has a special status in memory, such that it is less likely to be forgotten than the superficial features of verbal information, such as syntax and modality. These assertions are open to debate. For example, Anderson, Badiu, and Reder (2001) were able to account for a wide variety of the findings traditionally used to argue for different decay rates for semantic versus syntactic information, assuming decay rates do not differ for any one type of information. Likewise, Reder and colleagues (Diana, Peterson, and Reder, 2002; Diana and Reder, 2002; Reder et al., 2002) have argued from the findings of numerous studies that perceptual and conceptual information behave according to the same principles, such that the effects of manipulations on both types of information can be accounted for using the same type of memory representation and the same processing assumptions. In fact, recent research (Arndt and Reder, 2003) has shown that perceptual information does have an impact on recognition judgments when it is linked to semantic information.

Early research by Reder and colleagues (see Reder, 1987) demonstrated that subjects can be made to feel they know the answer to a general knowledge question when terms from the question are primed. Perceptual features of an arithmetic problem can likewise influence one's assessment of whether the answer is known. Reder and Ritter (1992) found that unstudied math problems whose operands had frequently been presented in the same problem, but with a different operator, were likely to get a fast "Know it!" response, whereas studied math problems whose operands had merely been transposed ("B*A" instead of "A*B") were judged as unfamiliar. Although, in the former case, the answer was not known, whereas, in the latter, it was, participants' first impressions were influenced by the perceptual features of the problem.

These results can be interpreted in terms of a source of activation confusion (SAC) model (e.g., Reder and Schunn, 1996; Schunn et al., 1997). SAC models represent perceptual and conceptual information in a unified long-term memory network. If a word encoded at study is presented in a relatively unusual font, the representation for the font information is associated with the encoding episode in the same way that the semantic and orthographic information are. If the same font is used to present the word at test, both the word node and the font node will provide sources of activation to send to the episode node, thereby further raising its activation level and increasing the chances of passing threshold for a recollection response (Reder et al., 2000, Reder, Donavos, and Erickson, 2002). An implication of the SAC theory is that no information is privileged. The only reason certain types of information seem less likely to be forgotten is that conceptual information is more easily elaborated and thus more easily reconstructed. Perceptual information, on the other hand, is more difficult to elaborate and therefore subject to interference from outside information (Anderson and Reder, 1979).

It is worth noting that in Reder, Donavos, and Erickson, 2002, perceptual cues, even those not relevant to the judgment task, were shown to influence the accuracy of a recognition judgment. Lists of words were presented, with some words being shown in unique salient fonts, and others in the same salient font. Participants were significantly more likely to recognize a previously presented word when they saw it in the same font at test as at study. Although the finding that a matching font from study to test aids recognition was not new (see, for example, Graf and Ryan, 1990), Reder and colleagues' varying the number of words that shared a salient font was. With this manipulation, they found that the number of other words presented in the same font at study modulated the effectiveness of re-presenting a word in the same font at test as at study. Or, as Arndt and Reder (2003) have suggested, a font becomes less distinctive and thereby a less effective retrieval cue if shared with many other words. Further, Reder, Donavos, and Erickson, 2002, contradicts the thesis that perceptual information is only influential in implicit memory tasks (see McDermott and Roediger, 1994; Richardson-Klavehn and Bjork, 1988). It also supports the proposal that perceptual and conceptual information are processed in the same way within memory, which it explains in terms of the same memory principles that Reder and colleagues used to explain verbal learning effects such as word frequency.

Source of activation confusion models theorize that any memory trace, whether semantic or perceptual, is subject to the same laws of memory and follows the same principles of decay, strengthening, and elaboration. Modeling efforts have lent support to the thesis that decay processes are the same for both perceptual and semantic information. SAC models generally maintain the same parameters when the equations are used to explain and predict results from various experiments. Cary and Reder (2001) modeled the experiments in Reder, Donavos, and Erickson, 2002, with a simulation that used the same parameter values for the representations of perceptual and semantic information (e.g., for spread of activation, decay, and strengthening). Thus SAC models, can account (qualitatively and quantitatively) for perceptual matching effects within a unified representational system of memory, using the same mechanisms and parameter values for perceptual and conceptual information.

On the other hand, the perceptual representation system (PRS; Tulving and Schachter, 1990), which is believed to have properties qualitatively different from those of semantic memory, predicts that perceptual information has a special area in memory, one separate from the area for semantic and conceptual information—

a predication disputed by the modeling efforts of Cary and Reder. PRS also predicts that the most important variable in memory experiments is that the same processing is required at testing as at encoding. PRS predicts that the distinctiveness of various perceptual features will not have an effect on the degree to which perceptual match affects memory. Clearly, the findings of Reder, Donavos, and Erickson provide a strong challenge to this theory.

Later research (Diana and Reder, 2002; Diana, Peterson, and Reder, forthcoming) showed that not only does perceptual information influence participants to be more likely to recognize a word they have seen before; it also leads them to believe they have seen a stimulus that is novel. In other words, perceptual features of the verbal stimuli influence the likelihood that participants will spuriously recognize that stimulus. This result is especially interesting because it provides evidence that familiar perceptual features, as well as semantic features, can produce false memories. The Deese, Roediger, and McDermott paradigm (see Roediger and McDermott, 1995) shows that when words from a given semantic category are presented, participants are more likely to falsely believe that they have seen another word from that semantic category than one from a separate category, a result that supports the thesis that false memories can result from perceptual influences alone.

Our ongoing studies are investigating the degree to which the same effects can be found within the domain of face recognition memory as within that of perceptual and conceptual information memory. Our preliminary findings (Diana and Reder, 2002) suggest that irrelevant perceptual information also influences one's ability to recognize a face, that there is no need to propose a separate explanation for facial memory representations over verbal memory representations. Source of activation confusion models can make predictions about both visual/facial and verbal memory phenomena simply by assuming that the two types of information are governed by the same principles.

Metacognitive Processes Are Adaptive

Research on metacognition in laboratory tasks has led to the belief that our metacognitions are frequently inaccurate. While the evidence appears to support this belief, it is important to keep in mind that laboratory tasks may create artificial situations that subvert the adaptive character of metacognition. Human cognition is set up to deal with the real world and to conserve resources whenever possible. One major area of resource expenditure is careful and detailed attention to an entire scene, document, or conversation. Visual metacognition is important because it would be impossible to process all of the visual information in a complex scene. People require heuristics to figure out what aspects of a scene or display should receive attention. This is may help to explain change blindness—there are simply not enough resources to continually process all aspects of a scene.

What heuristics do we use to decide whether to direct attention to something? We learn the regularities in the display or scene and we focus our attention on those aspects we have not yet learned are best to ignore (i.e., because they are unchanging or irrelevant). That people learn to anticipate where to look and what to ignore has been demonstrated in low-level attentional tasks (e.g., Chun and Jiang, 1998; Reder, Weber, Shang, and Vanyukov, 2003) and higher-level tasks such as air traffic control or solving algebra equations (e.g., Lee and Anderson, 2001).

This is why change blindness strikes us as so bizarre. In real life, things such as the identity of our conversational partner do not change unexpectedly. When a person we do not know presents us with a task in an experiment, we do not bother to encode the facial features of that person because they are not relevant to the task at hand and because we certainly do not expect the identity of the person to change "before our eyes." Because of the specialization of our system, we are unlikely to miss a change when it is feasible and important, thus we are unlikely to realize that we have missed a change at some later point. We think that we see everything because we have grown to expect stability in certain areas and similar configurations within scenes of the same type. Based on our previous life's experience, we believe that our visual perception is accurate. Thus, when our metacognitions are accessed in answer to the question, "Would you be likely to detect a change in this scene?" we respond based on our experience.

Even if humans had the cognitive capacity to encode all the information in a visual scene, the overwhelming amount of information would take such great lengths of time to process that the human processor would freeze in confusion. The trade-off of occasional mistakes in unlikely situations is preferable to the overload of storing and attempting to use a huge amount of unnecessary information. Processes become routine over time, as the needless steps and processing are weeded out. The predictability of the world allows us to learn and to increase our efficiency, a principle that may be true of all metacognition, both visual and verbal, and one even more necessary in visual metacognition than in semantic metacognition. Visual input is much richer than semantic input and requires a much greater degree of filtering, although, of course, this assumption may also be an illusion. The voice of the speaker, the intonation, the problem of invariance in phonemes, or the font of the typeset are all extra information in semantic processing. We usually take these sources of information for granted and ignore them in our overall processing. Metacognition is the key to deciding where resources should be expended and what information is important.

Conclusions

Metacognition can be explained as part of an integrated cognitive system and does not need to be proposed as a separate one. The role of metacognition in general cognition is to provide a feedback loop by which strategy selection (e.g., memory search versus reasoning an answer; statistical learning) can be accomplished.

Some metacognition can and does occur implicitly when time or resources are constrained. These implicit processes are less likely to cause interference in the task at hand. The inaccuracies commonly found in metacognition may result from attempts to access a system that is normally implicit and automatic. Because we propose that there is no separate system for perceptual versus conceptual information in general cognition, we also believe that the same system exists for perceptual and conceptual metacognitions. Therefore, visual metacognition results from the same mechanisms and obeys the same properties as metacognition in general.

Acknowledgment

Preparation of this chapter was supported by grant 2-R01-MH52808 and by training grant 5-T32-MH19983 from the National Institutes of Mental Health.

References

Anderson, J. R. (1982). Acquisition of cognitive skill. *Psychological Review, 89,* 369–406.

Anderson, J. R., Budiu, R., and Reder, L. M. (2001). A theory of sentence memory as part of a general theory of memory. *Journal of Memory and Language, 45,* 337–367.

Anderson, J. R., and Reder, L. M. (1979). An elaborative processing explanation of depth of processing. In L. S. Cermak and F. I. M. Craik (Eds.), *Levels of processing in human memory* (pp. 385–403). Hillsdale, NJ: Erlbaum.

Arndt, J., and Reder, L. M. (2003). The effect of distinctive visual information on false recognition. *Journal of Memory and Language, 48,* 1–15.

Beilock, S. L., and Carr, T. H. (2001). On the fragility of skilled performance: What governs choking under pressure? *Journal of Experimental Psychology: General, 130,* 701–725.

Beilock, S. L., Carr, T. H., MacMahon, C., and Starkes, J. L. (2002). When paying attention becomes counterproductive: Impact of divided versus skill-focused attention on novice and experienced performance of sensorimotor skills. *Journal of Experimental Psychology: Applied, 8,* 6–16.

Berry, D. C., and Broadbent, D. E. (1984). On the relationship between task performance and associated verbalizable knowledge. *Quarterly Journal of Experimental Psychology, 36A,* 209–231.

Busey, T. A., Tunnicliff, J., Loftus, G. R., and Loftus, E. F. (2000). Accounts of the confidence-accuracy relation in recognition memory. *Psychonomic Bulletin and Review, 7,* 26–48.

Carlson, R. A. (1997). *Experienced cognition.* Mahwah, NJ: Erlbaum.

Cary, M., and Reder, L. M. (2001). Support for a dual-process account of mirror effects in recognition. Paper presented at the Forty-second Annual Meeting of the Psychonomic Society, Orlando.

Cary, M., and Reder, L. M. (2002). Metacognition in strategy selection: Giving consciousness too much credit. In M. Izaute, P. Chambres, and P. J. Marescaux (Eds.), *Metacognition: Process, Function, and Use* (pp. 43–78). New York, NY: Kluwer.

Chun, M. M., and Jiang, Y. (1998). Contextual cueing: Implicit learning and memory of visual context guides spatial attention. *Cognitive Psychology, 36,* 28–71.

Diana, R. A., Peterson, M. J., and Reder, L. M. (Forthcoming). The role of spurious feature familiarity in recognition memory. *Psychonomic Bulletin and Review.*

Diana, R. A., and Reder, L. M. (2002). The effects of identity irrelevant characteristics in face recognition memory. Paper presented at the Kent State Applied Psychology Forum on Visual Metacognition, Kent, Ohio.

Dodson, C. S., Johnson, M. K., and Schooler, J. W. (1997). The verbal overshadowing effect: Why descriptions impair face recognition. *Memory and Cognition, 25,* 129–139.

Erickson, T. D., and Mattson, M. E. (1981). From words to meaning: A semantic illusion. *Journal of Verbal Learning and Verbal Behavior, 20,* 540–551.

Ericsson, K. A., and Simon, H. A. (1998). How to study thinking in everyday life: Contrasting think-aloud protocols with descriptions and explanations of thinking. *Mind, Culture, and Activity, 5,* 178–186.

Gernsbacher, M. A. (1985). Surface information loss in comprehension. *Cognitive Psychology, 17,* 324–363.

Graf, P., and Ryan. (1990). Transfer-appropriate processing for implicit and explicit memory. *Journal of Experimental Psychology: Learning, Memory, and Cognition, 16,* 978–992.

Graham, G., and Neisser, J. (2000). Probing for Relevance: What metacognition tells us about the power of consciousness. *Consciousness and Cognition, 9,* 172–177.

Gruneberg, M. M., Monks, J., and Sykes, R. N. (1977). Some methodological problems with feelings of knowing studies. *Acta Psychologica, 41,* 365–371.

Haines, R. F. (1991). A breakdown in simultaneous information processing. In G. Obrecht and L. Stark (Eds.), *Presbyopia research* (pp. 171–176). New York: Plenum Press.

Kentridge, R. W., and Heywood, C. A. (2000). Metacognition and awareness. *Consciousness and Cognition, 9,* 308–312.

Koriat, A. (2000). The feeling of knowing: Some metatheoretical implications for consciousness and control. *Consciousness and Cognition, 9,* 149–171.

Lee, F. J., and Anderson, J. R. (2001). Does learning a complex task have to be complex?: A study in learning decomposition. *Cognitive Psychology Special Issue, 42,* 267–316.

Lemaire, P., and Reder, L. (1999). What affects strategy selection in arithmetic? The example of parity and five effects on product verification. *Memory and Cognition, 27,* 364–382.

Levin, D. T., Momen, N., Drivdahl, S. B., and Simons, D. J. (2000). Change blindness blindness: The metacognitive error of overestimating change-detection ability. *Visual Cognition, 7,* 397–412.

Lewicki, P., Hill, T., and Bizot, E. (1988). Acquisition of procedural knowledge about a pattern of stimuli that cannot be articulated. *Cognitive Psychology, 20,* 24–37.

Logan, G. D. (1985). Skill and automaticity: Relations, implications, and future directions. *Canadian Journal of Psychology Special Issue: Skill, 39,* 367–386.

Logan, G. D. (1988). Toward an instance theory of automatization. *Psychological Review, 95,* 492–527.

Lovett, M. C., and Anderson, J. R. (1996). History of success and current context in problem solving. *Cognitive Psychology, 31,* 168–217.

MacLeod, C. M., and Dunbar, K. (1988). Training and Stroop-like interference: Evidence for a continuum of automaticity. *Journal of Experimental Psychology: Learning, Memory, and Cognition, 14,* 126–135.

McDermott, K. B., and Roediger, H. L. (1994). Effects of imagery on perceptual implicit memory tests. *Journal of Experimental Psychology: Learning, Memory, and Cognition, 20,* 1379–1390.

Meissner, C. A., and Brigham, J. C. (2001). A meta-analysis of the verbal overshadowing effect in face identification. *Applied Cognitive Psychology, 15,* 603–616.

Metcalfe, J., and Shimamura, A. P. (1994). *Metacognition: Knowing about knowing.* Cambridge, MA: MIT Press.

Miner, A. C., and Reder, L. M. (1994). A new look at feeling of knowing: Its metacognitive role in regulating question answering. In J. Metcalfe and A. P. Shimamura (Eds.), *Metacognition: Knowing about knowing* (pp. 47–70). Cambridge, MA: MIT Press.

Nelson, T. O., Gerler, D., and Narens, L. (1984). Accuracy of feeling-of-knowing judgments for predicting perceptual identification and relearning. *Journal of Experimental Psychology: General, 113,* 282–300.

Reber, A. S. (1989). Implicit learning and tacit knowledge. *Journal of Experimental Psychology: General, 118,* 219–235.

Reder, L. M. (1982). Plausibility judgments versus fact retrieval: Alternative strategies for sentence verification. *Psychological Review, 89*, 250–280.

Reder, L. M. (1987). Strategy selection in question answering. *Cognitive Psychology, 19*, 90–137.

Reder, L. M. (1988). Strategic control of retrieval strategies. In G. Bower (Ed.), *The psychology of learning and motivation*. Vol. 22 (pp. 227–259). New York: Academic Press.

Reder, L. M. (1996). Different research programs on metacognition: Are the boundaries imaginary? *Learning and Individual Differences, 8*, 383–390.

Reder, L. M., Donavos, D. K., and Erickson, M. A. (2002). Perceptual match effects in direct tests of memory: The role of contextual fan. *Memory and Cognition, 30*, 312–323.

Reder, L. M., Nhouyvanisvong, A., Schunn, C. D., Ayers, M. S., Angstadt, P., and Hiraki, K. (2000). A mechanistic account of the mirror effect for word frequency: A computational model of remember/know judgments in a continuous recognition paradigm. *Journal of Experimental Psychology: Learning, Memory, and Cognition, 26*, 294–320.

Reder, L. M., and Ritter, F. (1992). What determines initial feeling of knowing? Familiarity with question terms, not with the answer. *Journal of Experimental Psychology: Learning, Memory, and Cognition, 18*, 435–451.

Reder, L. M., and Schunn, C. D. (1996). Metacognition does not imply awareness: Strategy choice is governed by implicit learning and memory. In L. M. Reder (Ed.), *Implicit memory and metacognition* (pp. 45–77). Mahwah, NJ: Erlbaum.

Reder, L. M., and Weber, K. H. (1997). Spatial habituation and expectancy effects in a negative priming paradigm. Paper presented at the Annual Meeting of the Psychonomics Society, Philadelphia, November.

Reder, L. M., Weber, K. H., Shang, Y., and Vanyukov, P. (2003). The adaptive character of the attentional system: Statistical sensitivity in a target localization task. *Journal of Experimental Psychology: Human Perception and Performance, 29*, 631–649.

Regan, J. E. (1981). Automaticity and learning: Effects of familiarity on naming letters. *Journal of Experimental Psychology: Human Perception and Performance, 7*, 180–195.

Rensink, R. A., O'Regan, J. K., and Clark, J. J. (1997). To see or not to see: The need for attention to perceive changes in scenes. *Psychological Science, 8*, 368–373.

Richardson-Klavehn, A., and Bjork, R. A. (1988). Primary versus secondary rehearsal in an imagined voice: Differential effects on recognition memory and perceptual identification. *Bulletin of the Psychonomic Society, 26*, 187–190.

Roediger, H. L. (1990). Implicit memory: Retention without remembering. *American Psychologist, 45*, 1043–1056.

Roediger, H. L., and McDermott, K. B. (1995). Creating false memories: Remembering words not presented in lists. *Journal of Experimental Psychology: Learning, Memory, and Cognition, 21*, 803–814.

Schacter, D. L. (1994). Priming and multiple memory system: Perceptual mechanisms of implicit memory. In D. L. Schacter and E. Tulving (Eds.), *Memory systems* (pp. 233–268). Cambridge, MA: MIT Press.

Schooler, J. W., and Engstler-Schooler, T. Y. (1990). Verbal overshadowing of visual memories: Some things are better left unsaid. *Cognitive Psychology, 22*, 36–71.

Schunn, C. D., Reder, L. M., Nhouyvanisvong, A., Richards, D. R., and Stroffolino, P. J. (1997). To calculate or not to calculate: A source activation confusion model of problem familiarity's role in strategy selection. *Journal of Experimental Psychology: Learning, Memory, and Cognition, 23*, 3–29.

Simons, D. J., and Levin, D. T. (1998). Failure to detect changes to people during a real-world interaction. *Psychonomic Bulletin and Review, 5*, 644–649.

Smith, E. E., Haviland, S. E., Reder, L. M., Brownell, H., and Adams, N. (1976). When preparation fails: Disruptive effects of prior information on perceptual recognition. *Journal of Experimental Psychology: Human Perception and Performance, 2*, 151–161.

Tulving, E., and Schacter, D. L. (1990). Priming and human memory systems. *Science, 247*, 301–306.

Westerman, D. L., and Larsen, J. D. (1997). Verbal-overshadowing effect: Evidence for a general shift of processing. *American Journal of Psychology, 110*, 417–428.

Winer, G. A., Cottrell, J. E., Karefilaki, K. D., and Chronister, M. (1996a). Conditions affecting beliefs about visual perception among children and adults. *Journal of Experimental Child Psychology, 61*, 93–115.

Winer, G. A., Cottrell, J. E., Karefilaki, K. D., and Gregg, V. R. (1996b). Images, words, and questions: Variables that influence beliefs about vision in children and adults. *Journal of Experimental Child Psychology, 63*, 499–525.

Yzerbyt, V. Y., Lories, G., and Dardenne, B. (1998). *Metacognition: Cognitive and social dimensions.* London: Sage.

Chapter 10

Zoning Out while Reading: Evidence for Dissociations between Experience and Metaconsciousness

Jonathan W. Schooler, Erik D. Reichle, and David V. Halpern

As you begin this chapter, you are probably paying at least some attention to the words you are reading. After a page or two, however, there is a real possibility if not likelihood, that your attention may wander. Should that happen, your eyes may continue moving across the page, the phonology of the words may continue sounding in your head, yet your mind will be elsewhere. This phenomenon of "zoning out" while reading is ubiquitous. Whenever we ask people about it, their response is almost invariably the same: a sheepish grin and the confession "Well, yes, this happens all the time." Although all too common in its occurrence, scientific discussions of the phenomenon of zoning out while reading have been markedly lacking. This oversight is notable for several reasons. From a pragmatic perspective, if people zone out as frequently as informal anecdotes suggest, then we may have overlooked a potentially important reason for reading failures. If one reads without devoting any attention to the text, then it stands to reason that one's comprehension will be compromised. Equally important, however, are the metacognitive implications of zoning out while reading. If, as seems likely, people understand that zoning out is inherently incompatible with successful reading, then their reports of zoning out while reading suggest that people can fundamentally lack an awareness of the contents of their consciousness.

The disassociation between the experience of zoning out while reading and the awareness that one has been zoning out illustrates the value of distinguishing between experiential consciousness, corresponding to the contents of experience, and what we alternatively refer to as "metaconsciousness" or "meta-awareness"[1] (Schooler, 2001, 2002; Schooler, Ariely, and Loewenstein, 2003), corresponding to one's explicit awareness of the contents of consciousness. Accordingly, when people zone out, they are experientially conscious of whatever topic has grabbed their attention, while at the same time lacking metaconsciousness of the fact that they are zoning out. At some point during the reading episode, they suddenly become metaconscious that they have been zoning out and realize that for some time they have been reading without comprehension. In a recent analysis of possible dissociations between consciousness and metaconsciousness, Schooler (2002) refers to such consciousness in the absence of metaconsciousness as a "temporal dissociation." There are many cases where the application of metaconsciousness to the experience may actually interfere with the experience itself, that is, where temporal dissociations between consciousness and metaconsciousness may actually be adaptive, as, for example, when one is in a "flow" state (Csikszentmihalyi, 1990) of deep concentration or when one is engaging in automatic (Baumeister, 1984) or intuitive (Schooler, Ohlsson, and Brooks, 1993; Wilson and Schooler, 1991) processes. Yet there are other cases in which the absence of metaconsciousness can pose a problem. The failure to notice that one's mental reveries have curtailed one's comprehension during reading is a case in point.

In this chapter, we consider how a distinction between experiential consciousness and metaconsciousness can help both to characterize and to explain zoning out during reading. We begin by reviewing two surprisingly scant lines of previous empirical research relevant to zoning out while reading: educational research on comprehension monitoring and cognitive research (both laboratory and clinical) on task-unrelated images and thoughts. Although the findings of both these lines of research have important implications for the phenomenon of zoning out while reading, their oversight in not addressing zoning out directly has gone largely unnoticed. We correct this oversight by describing two recent experiments we conducted to explore the frequency, awareness, and comprehension implications of zoning out while reading. We conclude by considering the implications of our findings for theories of visual ocular motor control associated with reading specifically, and for theoretical conceptualizations of mindless behaviors more generally.

Previous Research Relevant to Zoning Out while Reading

Given the intimate familiarity that most people have with the experience of catching themselves zoning out while reading, it is rather remarkable that so little research has addressed this phenomenon. There are, however, two general lines of research that are clearly relevant. In the domain of reading, there is a large literature on what has variously been referred to as "comprehension monitoring" (e.g., Brown, 1980), "metacomprehension" (e.g., Maki and Berry, 1984), or "self-regulated comprehension" (e.g., Hacker, 1998). This work, although overlooking the possibility that people can fail to notice that they are not attending to the text at all, demonstrates the importance of metacognitive monitoring strategies in the maximization of reading performance. A second relevant literature, on what has somewhat awkwardly been referred to as "task-unrelated images and thoughts" (TUITs; see Giambra, 1995; Singer, 1993, for reviews), has devoted substantial attention to situations in which people's minds wander from the task on which performance is being measured. With several important exceptions, however, this research has explored TUITs associated with nondemanding tasks for which successful performance is not undermined by following an unrelated train of thought. This research thus provides relatively little insight into either the costs of mind wandering or the cases where people may not realize that their minds have wandered. In the following section, we briefly review the respective literatures on comprehension monitoring and on TUITs as these may pertain to the largely unstudied topic of zoning out while reading.

Comprehension Monitoring

In recent years, both researchers and educators have increasingly come to appreciate the importance of comprehension monitoring for successful comprehension performance, that readers who attend to how well they understand what they are reading can better repair misunderstandings than readers who do not. Two general approaches have been devoted to exploring comprehension monitoring: training studies, where readers are taught techniques to increase their comprehension monitoring, and assessment studies, where readers' monitoring performance is assessed and related to their comprehension performance.

Training Comprehension Monitoring   Numerous successful reading enhancement programs have been developed on the premise that encouraging comprehension monitoring will enhance performance. This basic thesis represents the backbone of Palincsar and Brown's "reciprocal teaching" approach (1984), in which the metacognitive monitoring of comprehension is encouraged by engaging students in a dialogue with teachers on applying the four reading comprehension strategies of summarizing, question generating, clarifying, and predicting. Students involved in this training approach become increasingly adept at using these strategies and show significant improvement in their reading comprehension. A similar type of reading enhancement program that also emphasizes the importance of metacognitive monitoring of comprehension, Brown and Pressley's "transactional strategies instruction" (1994), trains students in the use of strategies such as question generating, clarifying, and so on, and engages them in didactic interactions with teachers to enhance the use of these skills. Like reciprocal teaching, transactional strategies instruction has been shown to enhance the effective use of self-regulated strategies (as revealed by think-aloud protocols) and to improve reading comprehension performance (as measured by standardized tests).

The finding that reading comprehension is facilitated by training students to use strategies that enhance comprehension monitoring is consistent with the hypothesis that the metacognitive lapse of zoning out while reading may undermine reading performance. Clearly, readers cannot zone out if and while they are actively engaging in strategies (such as question generating and clarifying) that require comprehension monitoring. Nevertheless, not only have discussions of why strategy use may be effective in enhancing reading comprehension failed to address this metacognitive lapse; many of the techniques used to assess strategy use (e.g., think-aloud protocols) require readers to be "on task." In short, although comprehension-monitoring training may reduce the frequency of zoning out, the types of monitoring failures explicitly envisioned by such programs involve lapses in how deeply readers are thinking about the text, rather than in whether they are thinking about the text at all.

Assessing Comprehension Monitoring   Another approach for establishing the relationship between comprehension monitoring and performance has been, first, to identify dependent measures of comprehension monitoring and, then, to examine their relationship to reading performance. Two general methodologies have been explored: error detection (e.g., Glenberg, Wilkinson, and Epstein, 1982), where participants must detect inconsistencies embedded in text, and comprehension prediction (e.g., Maki and Berry, 1984), where participants read text passages and attempt to predict how well they will perform on a subsequent reading comprehension test. Strikingly, although both purportedly measure the same thing, these two approaches have diverged in their ability to distinguish more versus less successful readers. One possible reason for this divergence is that the two approaches may be differentially sensitive to zoning out.

Research on comprehension prediction has been rather unsuccessful in documenting a clear relationship between comprehension monitoring and performance. In several of the original investigations, readers were found to be at chance in predicting how well they would perform on a subsequent reading comprehension text (e.g., Glenberg and Epstein, 1985). More recent studies (e.g., Maki, 1995) have found that if readers are given a sufficient number of test questions per prediction, then they perform better than chance in their predictions (presumably because this method provides a more sensitive measure). Nevertheless, even when readers are found to be above chance at predicting their comprehension performance, the relationship between readers' skill in making predictions and their reading performance has proved quite equivocal. Although some studies (Glover, 1989; Maki and Berry, 1984) found a strong positive relationship, others have found no relationship (Glenberg and Epstein, 1985; Lovelace, 1984; Maki, Jonas, and Kallod, 1994), and at least one found a negative relationship (Gillstrom and Ronnberg, 1995). One potential reason why prediction studies have failed to find a relationship may be that the prediction activity encourages a level of monitoring that is sufficient to prevent a key type of monitoring lapse (i.e., zoning out). In other words, individual difference measures that require one to attend to the text in order to assess monitoring skill may fail to identify individuals whose monitoring difficulties involve periodically failing to attend to the text altogether.

Research on error detection has been somewhat more successful in documenting a relationship between monitoring performance and comprehension. Studies examining participants' ability to catch inconsistencies in text typically have found that good readers are more likely than poor readers to detect textual inconsistencies (e.g., Garner and Kraus, 1981–82; Garner and Reis, 1981). One of the enigmatic findings in this literature, however, is that even good readers show a surprisingly high capacity to miss textual incoherencies (e.g., Glenberg,

Wilkinson, and Epstein, 1982). In fact, the suggestion that all readers—both good and poor—are occasionally susceptible to zoning out may help to explain this finding, for even the best readers will have difficulty detecting text inconsistencies when they are zoning out. The suggestion that error detection may be sensitive to zoning-out episodes may also help to explain why comprehension-monitoring performance is predictive of reading ability when assessed by error detection measures but not when assessed by comprehension prediction measures. Accordingly, if zoning out is a fundamental type of comprehension-monitoring failure, then measures that are sensitive to zoning out should be more predictive of comprehension performance than measures that are not.

Task-Unrelated Images and Thoughts

Arguably, the research most directly relevant to the general topic of zoning out while reading is that on task-unrelated images and thoughts (TUITs). Pioneered by Jerome Singer (e.g., 1978), John Antrobus (e.g., Antrobus et al., 1970), and more recently pursued by Leonard Giambra (e.g., 1995), this line of research has sought to explore the nature and causes of daydreaming. In the majority of studies on this topic, participants are given a dull vigilance task and are asked to report every time they experience a task-unrelated thought. Over the years, considerable knowledge has been gained regarding the circumstances under which TUITs are most likely to occur. For example, TUITs are particularly likely to happen when individuals are stressed (e.g., Antrobus, Coleman, and Singer, 1967), when the experimenter and participant are of opposite sex (Singer, 1988), when a participant's circadian rhythm is at a relatively high level of arousal (Giambra et al., 1988), or when the task is less demanding (Giambra and Grodsky, 1989). Additional studies have demonstrated reliable individual differences in people who are more versus less likely to experience TUITs. For example, TUIT occurrence tends to be positively correlated with the self-reported frequency of daydreaming (Antrobus, Coleman and Singer, 1967) and with a prior history of attention deficit disorder (Shaw and Giambra, 1993), whereas it tends to be negatively correlated with age (Giambra, 1989).

Generalizing conclusions, however clearly pertinent, from the literature on task-unrelated images and thoughts to the domain of zoning out while reading is complicated because the vast majority of studies have used inherently dull and nondemanding vigilance tasks for which successful performance does not require participants' undivided attention. Given that such tasks are apt to encourage participants to knowingly think about unrelated topics (to "tune out"), much of the research on TUITs cannot speak to the situations in which counterproductive mind-wandering episodes may initially proceed unnoticed.

Although the vast majority of studies on task-unrelated images and thoughts have involved nondemanding tasks, two rarely cited studies (Giambra and Grodsky, 1989; Grodsky and Giambra, 1991) examined the incidence of TUITs in the more demanding task of reading; moreover, they did so by training participants to differentiate between intentional TUITs (i.e., deliberately thinking about something unrelated to the text) and unintentional TUITs (i.e., unintentionally thinking about unrelated thoughts). In Giambra and Grodsky, 1989, participants were required to read multiple passages of text that varied with respect to both interest and difficulty and to report, using a computer response key, every time they experienced a TUIT, whether intentional or unintentional. Even though successful reading would seem to be incompatible with TUIT generation, Giambra and Grodsky, 1989, found that successful readers regularly reported both intentional and unintentional TUITs. It also found that attentional demands were unrelated to TUIT frequency: difficult text was no less likely than easy text to produce TUITs. Not surprisingly, however, dull text was more likely than easy text to lead to TUITs. Using a similar paradigm, Grodsky and Giambra, 1991, replicated these results and found that TUIT frequency on a reading task was correlated with TUIT frequency on a vigilance task.

The Giambra and Grodsky, 1989, findings on task-unrelated images and thoughts—particularly unintentional ones—while reading are consistent with anecdotal reports that people can zone out while reading without initially noticing it. However, strong conclusions regarding the occurrence of unaware zoning out and its impact on reading performance are limited for various reasons. First, Giambra and Grodsky, 1989, focused on individuals' intention to engage in TUITs rather than on their awareness that they were engaging in TUIT's. Although potentially related, there are distinct differences between the intention to do something and the awareness that one is doing something. It is quite plausible that individuals might not intend to think about an unrelated thought, and yet nevertheless immediately notice when they do so. By way of analogy, just because people do not intend to slip does not mean they are not immediately aware of slipping. That individuals reported unintentionally engaging in TUITs thus does not necessarily imply that they were unaware of doing so. Second, people are actually quite poor at assessing their own intentionality, and have been shown to freely take responsibility for initiating actions they could not possibly have intended to undertake (Wegner and Wheatley, 1999). Such findings raise important questions about whether people can effectively discriminate between intentional and unintentional thoughts. A final, and most important, limitation of earlier research on TUITs while reading is that it did not explore the relationship between TUIT occurrence and reading performance. Though consistent with the premise that people may regularly fail to notice that they are zoning out while reading, the work on TUITs and reading allows us neither to know whether such lapses can go undetected nor to assess the potential impact they may have on reading comprehension.

Recent Research on Zoning Out while Reading: A New Paradigm

To correct the oversight of the two lines of previous relevant research, we (Schooler, Reichle, and Halpern, in preparation) developed a new paradigm specifically designed to explore people's awareness of zoning out while reading and the impact of zoning out on reading performance, and we employed that paradigm in two experiments. The paradigm required participants to read what was for many of them a rather dull text (the opening chapters of *War and Peace*) on a computer screen and to indicate with a keypress every time they caught themselves zoning out. The experience of zoning out was defined as a situation in which readers realized they had "no idea what [they] just read" and that they were "not really thinking about the text, but . . . of something else altogether." Consistent with our anecdotal experiences, participants readily understood the concept of zoning out and typically reported that they were intimately familiar with the phenomenon.

Experiment 1   Our first experiment included 45 participants and involved a 2×2 between-subjects design with two variables (1) whether participants received the intermittent zone-out experience-sampling probe; (2) whether the text was presented paragraph by paragraph or page by page. Both variables were included in order to assess the robustness of the procedure to modest task variations. Because neither the introduction of the experience-sampling probes nor the text presentation format had any significant effects on either zoning out or reading comprehension performance, the data reported are collapsed across these variables.

Two separate innovations were introduced in order to explore the hypothesis that individuals can zone out without (at least initially) realizing that they are doing so. First, each time participants reported zoning out, they were simply asked to respond to the question "Were you aware that you were zoning out while you were zoning out?" Second, half of the participants were intermittently probed regarding whether, at that particular moment, they had been zoning out. This experience-sampling procedure (e.g., Hurlburt, 1993) occurred 2–4 min after the initiation of the experiment and then occurred every 2–4 min following a previous zone-out report or probe. We reasoned that if we could catch participants zoning out before they caught themselves, then this would provide evidence that they had not realized that they were in fact zoning out before the probe.

Finally, in order to examine the relationship between zoning out and reading comprehension, we included a forced-choice comprehension test at the end of the experiment. If zoning out represents a form of comprehension-monitoring failure that impacts reading ability, then we should find a relationship between the frequency of zoning out and comprehension performance.

The results of our first experiment demonstrated that it is readily possible to observe zoning out during reading in a controlled laboratory context. On average, participants caught themselves zoning out approximately 5.4 times during the 45 min reading period. Several findings were consistent with the hypothesis that people are often (at least initially) unaware of the fact that they are zoning out. On approximately 67% of zone-out responses, participants specifically indicated they believed they had not been aware that they were zoning out while they were zoning out. In addition, the probe procedure was successfully able to catch people zoning out before they had caught themselves. On average, participants were caught zoning out by the probe 1.6 times per session. Although this may seem like a relatively modest frequency, it is important to note that the participants were only probed on average 6 times per session. Thus the most useful way to conceptualize the probe measure is in terms of the proportion of zone-out probes that actually caught the participants zoning out. This measure, or probe-catch ratio, indicated that nearly 13.2% of the time participants were zoning out, without being sufficiently aware of it to report it.

Analysis of individuals' characterizations of their zoning-out episodes indicated that they were only very rarely (less than 3% of the time) thinking about what they were reading when they reported zoning out. Although they sometimes reported thinking about nothing at all (18%), more often participants reported thinking about specific things, such as school-related topics (27%), fantasies (19%), and themselves (11%). In short, although participants were often unaware of the fact that they were zoning out, their minds were nevertheless being occupied by rich thoughts that were completely unrelated to what they were reading.

A key issue in assessing the importance of readers' zoning-out responses is whether they are predictive of actual reading performance. Although, in this experiment, the frequency of self-caught zone-outs was unrelated to comprehension performance ($r = .07$; n.s.), the probe-catch ratio (i.e., the proportion of probes that caught individuals zoning out) was highly correlated with subsequent recognition performance ($r = -.55$, $p < .05$). This finding suggests that the tendency to zone out without noticing it may be a key source of reading error.

In sum, our first experiment demonstrated that it is relatively easy to catch participants zoning out while reading in a laboratory experiment. Analysis of participants' characterizations of their zone-outs was consistent with the claim that zoning out typically involves thinking about unrelated topics without initially noticing that one is doing so. Additional evidence that readers often fail to notice that they are zoning out comes from the experience-sampling condition in which 13% of the time participants were caught zoning out by the probes before they had caught themselves.

Experiment 2

Although clearly encouraging, one reasonable question about the results of our first experiment arises: How do we know that participants were genuinely zoning out when they reported doing so? One source of evidence that participants were in fact being factual in their reports is the correlation between zoning out and final recognition performance. Given that this result was merely correlational, however, it is possible that other factors (e.g., being low in motivation) may have contributed to both reports of zoning out and poor reading comprehension performance. This concern is particularly salient in that we only observed the correlation between comprehension and zoning out with the experience-sampling measure. Accordingly, it is quite plausible that unmotivated subjects may have both read carelessly and almost never spontaneously reported catching themselves zoning out. Nevertheless, when directly confronted by a probe, these same participants may have characterized their general low involvement by indicating that they were zoning out. Therefore, to more directly validate that participants really are not attending to the text when they report zoning out, it was important to get a more on-line measure of comprehension. Experiment 2 addressed this issue by following every report of zoning out with a text recognition question that queried participants about what they had just been reading. As a baseline control, other participants were randomly probed about the text material without being asked if they had been zoning out. If individuals who report zoning out are genuinely not attending to the text at the time they report zoning out, then their performance on the preceding text should be lower than the baseline performance of participants who are randomly queried with the same questions.

A second potential concern with the procedure introduced in experiment 1 was the potential impact that the various measurements may have had on reading. Although experiment 1 suggested that the inclusion of the intermittent probe measure had no effect on the frequency of self-caught zone-outs, it is quite possible that a reverse effect (i.e., an effect of self-catching zone-outs on the frequency of probe-caught zone-outs) may have occurred. Indeed, having people continuously attend to whether they are zoning out could in principle increase or decrease the incidence of zoning out as revealed by the experience-sampling procedure. Continuously monitoring the occurrence of zoning out might decrease its overall frequency due to increased vigilance. Alternatively, continuous monitoring might increase zoning out because monitoring for unwanted thoughts can—under some situations—increase the likelihood of their occurrence (Wegner, 1994, 1997). To explore the potential reactivity of the various manipulations used in this paradigm, experiment 2 systematically varied the type of interruptions that participants were given during their reading episodes. The resulting design led to 6 conditions. In condition 1, participants simply read the text is a self-paced fashion, and were not provided with any information regarding zoning out. In condition 2, called "zoning out," as in experiment 1, participants were instructed to indicate whether they were zoning out whenever they received a probe. In condition 3, participants were instructed as in condition 2 but, in addition, were asked to indicate whenever they self-caught themselves zoning out, thereby partially replicating the page-by-page, self- and probe-caught condition of experiment 1. As mentioned, however, conditions 1–3 differed from their counterparts in experiment 1 in that, after reporting a zoning-out episode, participants were given a recognition test corresponding to the text they were reading just before they reported zoning out. To test for the impact of this measurement, conditions 4–6 were identical to conditions 1–3, respectively, except that participants were not required to perform this recognition test.

The results of experiment 2 replicated and extended those of experiment 1. As in experiment 1, participants who were asked to self-catch zoning-out regularly caught themselves with an average of 2.9 self-caught zone-outs per session and participants who were probed regarding whether they were zoning out were once again frequently "caught" zoning out, with an average probe-catch ratio of 23%. Experiment 2 also found that the zoning-out paradigm is robust against minor modifications in the procedure. Neither the text recognition probes nor the introduction of self-monitoring instructions influenced the likelihood that participants were caught zoning out by the probes. That the self-monitoring instructions had no appreciable effect on the frequency of probe-caught zone-outs suggests that attending to zoning out neither increases zoning out due to the increased accessibility of suppressed thoughts (Wegner, 1994, 1997) nor decreases it due to increased vigilance.

Of critical interest in experiment 2 was participants' performance on the text recognition probes. A comparison of text recognition performance on those responses where participants indicated they were zoning out revealed markedly lower comprehension levels than the baseline performance of those participants who were randomly given text recognition probes: .54 versus .78, respectively. This finding provides behavioral evidence consistent with the claim that zoning-out episodes are associated with particularly low levels of attention to the text.

Finally, an analysis of the relationship between zoning out and reading comprehension performance on the final test again revealed that a tendency to zone out is associated with generally reduced levels of comprehension. In experiment 2, the relationship between zoning-out frequency and performance on the final comprehension test was observed both with the probe-catch ratio ($r = -.27$) and with the overall frequency of self-caught zone-outs ($r = -.56$). In addition, a relationship was observed between zoning-out frequency and comprehension, as revealed by overall performance on the intermittent recognition tests. Specifically, we observed negative correlations between the performance on the intermittent recognition tests and both the frequency of self-caught zone-outs ($r = -.42$) and the probe-catch ratio ($r = -.32$).

Although a relationship was found between zoning out and comprehension performance, there was no difference in the comprehension performance of participants who monitored their zoning out versus those who did not, nor was there any effect of the intermittent recognition tests on final performance. These findings suggest that the procedures we used to tap the key reading processes did not themselves disrupt them.

Summary

Two experiments demonstrated the viability of laboratory investigations of zoning out while reading. In addition, these studies provided initial support for the claims that (1) participants genuinely are failing to attend to the text when they report zoning out; (2) zoning out happens, at least initially, without meta-awareness that it is occurring; and (3) zoning out is associated with overall poor comprehension of the text being read. Evidence that people really were zoning out when they said they were came from both the observed relationship between frequency of zoning out and comprehension performance, and from the finding that the participants' ability to recognize what they had been reading immediately before their zone-out reports was compromised relative to baseline performance. The participants' initial absence of meta-awareness that they had been zoning out was indicated by their self-reports that they were not aware that they were zoning out when they actually were. An absence of meta-awareness of zoning out was also suggested by the fact that the experience-sampling probes frequently caught people zoning out before they had caught themselves. Finally, evidence that zoning out may significantly impact reading performance came from the finding, in both experiments, that the more often participants were found to be zoning out, the worse their overall reading comprehension. Indeed, in experiment 2, the frequency of zoning out was a better predictor of reading comprehension than one of the best standard measures—general vocabulary. Thus a potentially critical, but heretofore overlooked source of reading comprehension failure appears to be the failure of readers to notice they are not attending to the text.

Theoretical Implications of Zoning Out while Reading

There are a number of important implications for the finding that people regularly fail to notice that they are thinking about something completely unrelated to what they are reading. These implications range from very specific potential predictions regarding the nature of eye movement control associated with zoning out, to more general implications about dissociations between experience and meta-consciousness. We consider these topics in turn.

Implications of Zoning Out for Theories of Eye Movement Control

Although the majority of reading research most directly relevant to zoning out while reading, that is, research on comprehension monitoring, has largely overlooked the potential impact of zoning out while reading, the prospect of mindless reading has been anticipated in discussions of the nature of eye movement control during reading. Observing that "most readers have probably had the experience of moving their eyes across text while at the same time their mind wandered so that nothing was comprehended from the text," Rayner and Fischer (1996, p. 746) suggested that this phenomenon would be interesting to study, but that "this 'daydream' mode would be very difficult to study experimentally." Our experiments are one attempt to do so, and thus speak to the question addressed by Rayner and Fischer: What determines when and where the eyes move while reading?

The issue of eye movement control during reading has been the focus of considerable research and debate because the eye-mind link is central to many cognitive activities, including navigating one's environment, driving, and scene perception (to name just a few; see Rayner, 1998, for review). Now that eye-tracking technology has made it possible to measure precisely the eye movements of subjects while they perform a variety of on-line and ecologically valid tasks (e.g., solving math problems; Salvucci, 2001), this information can be used to make inferences about the cognitive processes underlying their task performance. Of course, the validity of this approach depends on there being a link between the eye movements and cognition. Researchers have therefore expended considerable effort to specify the precise nature of this link, building a variety of computational models that—to varying degrees—account for various aspects of the eyes' behavior, particularly in the context of reading text (see Reichle and Rayner, 2002, for review).

Models of eye movement control during reading span a continuum with regards to how the eye-mind link is conceptualized (Reichle, Rayner, and Pollatsek, forthcoming). At one end of this continuum are the oculomotor models, which hold that the moment-to-moment guidance of the eyes through the text is primarily determined by visual and oculomotor constraints (O'Regan, 1990, 1992; Reilly and O'Regan, 1998; Suppes, 1990, 1994; Yang and McConkie, 2001). On the other end of the continuum are the processing models, which assume that eye movements are guided by the immediate demands of linguistic processing (Just and Carpenter, 1980, 1987; Thibadeau, Just, and Carpenter, 1982; Salvucci, 2000). Other models fall somewhere in between these two extremes, for example, in the E-Z Reader model (Reichle et al., 1998; Reichler, Rayner, and Pollatsek, 1999, forthcoming), lexical processing largely determines the timing of eye movements from one word to the next, whereas visual and oculomotor factors determine where within a given word the eyes actually fixate.

At present, there is ample evidence that eye guidance through text is affected by both cognitive variables, such as word frequency (Altarriba, et al., 2001; Inhoff and Rayner, 1986; Schilling, Rayner, and Chumbley, 1998) and noncognitive variables, such as word length (O'Regan, 1979, 1980; Rayner, 1979; Rayner and Morris, 1992). Thus the "either or" nature of the debate about the cognitive determinants of eye movement control has evolved into an effort to better understand the extent to which different cognitive and noncognitive variables affect eye movements during reading. This is exemplified by recent experiments that examined how a parametric manipulation of the demands imposed by linguistic processing affected both the global patterns of eye movement (e.g., fixation duration, skipping rates, etc.) and the local patterns (e.g., fixation locations, the probability of making a refixation as a function of the initial fixation location, etc.) that were observed (Rayner and Fischer, 1996; Vitu et al., 1995). The subjects in these experiments were instructed (1) to read short passages of text; (2) to read short passages of "text" in which all of the upper- and lowercase letters were replaced, respectively, with upper- and lowercase zs (e.g., "The cat started to . . . became "Zzz zzz zzzzzzz zz . . ."); or (3) to scan short passages of text and indicate the presence of pre-specified targets (e.g., the word *zebra*). The results of these studies revealed notable differences in the patterns of eye movements that were observed in each of the three conditions; as one might expect, the immediate effects of linguistic processing (e.g., word frequency effects) that were present in normal reading were absent in the both the z-reading and target-scanning conditions.

On the basis of the aforementioned results, Rayner and Fischer (1996) concluded that the decision about when to move the eyes is primarily determined by ongoing linguistic processing. Unfortunately, as Rayner and Fischer point out, the fact that the subjects (college undergraduates) had many years of reading experience may have allowed them to move their eyes in a manner that approximated the patterns of eye movements that are observed during normal reading. To the extent that this happened, it would minimize any differences between the patterns of eye movements observed in the normal reading and z-reading conditions, and thus fail to provide an adequate estimate of how much the demands of linguistic processing affect the on-line guidance of the eyes during normal reading. As we suggested earlier, the procedure that was used in our two experiments may offer an alternative means by which to explore this issue; the question simply needs to be reframed: What determines when and where the eyes move when a reader (who is supposed to be reading for comprehension) is zoning out? The answer to this question may shed light on the nature of the eye-mind link.

For example, it is conceivable that word identification (being a largely automatic process in highly skilled readers; Rayner and Pollatsek, 1989) proceeds in the absence of conscious effort (i.e., during zoning out), whereas higher-level linguistic processing does not. If this conjecture is true, then lexical-level variables (e.g., word frequency) should continue to influence when the eyes move, whereas higher-level variables (e.g., word predictability) should not. This would lead to frequency effects in the absence of predictability effects whenever readers are attempting to read for comprehension but are zoning out. Furthermore, one might speculate that any eye movements that are observed during zoning-out episodes might closely resemble those that are predicted by one or more of the eye movement models (e.g., E-Z Reader; Reichle et al., 1998; Reichle Rayner and Pollatsek, 1999, forthcoming) if their parameters are adjusted so as to eliminate any effect that word predictability would otherwise have on the rate of lexical processing. Of course, those models of eye movement control that neither allow for the effects of linguistic processing (i.e., oculomotor models) nor allow for dissociations in this processing at different levels (e.g., lexical versus superlexical) should not—at least in principle—be able to account for the patterns of fixation durations that are observed during zoning-out episodes. Thus such data might prove to be extremely useful in evaluating current models of eye movement control. Reichle and colleagues are currently developing an eye-tracking procedure to collect such data.

Implications for the Relationship between Consciousness and Behavior
That readers were regularly caught zoning out without realizing it and that zoning out appears to undermine reading comprehension performance raises a central question: How can one fail to notice what is occupying one's own mind? In the following discussion, we first briefly outline our account of how a distinction between experiential consciousness and metaconsciousness might address this question—central to understanding the phenomenon of zoning out—and then we contrast our account with other theoretical approaches to mindless behavior that might also apply.

The Experiential Consciousness versus Metaconsciousness Distinction   In a recent discussion of the potential relationship between metaconsciousness and experience, Schooler (2002) argued that, whereas conscious experience and the tacit monitoring of cognitive activities occur continuously throughout our waking hours, only periodically is attention specifically devoted to assessing the contents of experience (see figure 10.1). Within the context of a theory of metaconsciousness, zoning

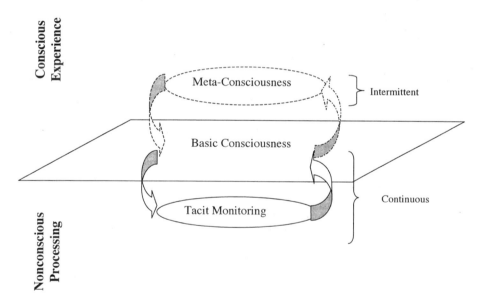

Figure 10.1
Rudimentary characterization of the relationship between metaconsciousness and consciousness. Throughout waking hours individuals continuously experience basic consciousness, including perceptions, feelings, and nonreflective cognition. Basic consciousness is monitored by a tacit system that continuously checks consciousness for certain types of goal failure, unwanted thoughts, and so on. Intermittently, situations arise (e.g., a significant goal failure that requires attention, a strong emotional response, a request to report experience, etc.) in which individuals must explicitly appraise the contents of their experience (metaconsciousness). (After Schooler, 2002)

out can be conceptualized as occurring in those situations where the tacit monitoring system misses a goal failure, so that a correction must await detection by metaconsciousness. Accordingly, as individuals engage in thought, it is likely that they tacitly monitor the coherence of their train of thought, often repairing it seamlessly without even realizing that they have done so. When the mind wanders, however, the tacit monitoring of the conceptual coherence of thought may be thrown off because cognition continues to be coherent. In such situations, the reader is simply not focused on what is being read. Recognizing the fact that one has been zoning-out may therefore require a higher-order form of monitoring (i.e. metaconsciousness) in which one assesses the specific content of thought in relationship to the current goals regarding what one wants to think about. If the intended and actual contents of thought largely overlap, then attention can once again be returned entirely to the train of thought. If, however, a discrepancy arises, then a correction must be initiated. Because metaconscious reflection is resource demanding, it is likely to be curtailed once a correction has been made, thereby setting the stage for another, initially unnoticed, zone-out episode.

Although the above framework is clearly in need of elaboration, it provides a general account of why readers zone out (i.e., their tacit monitoring systems are insensitive to errors of this type) and the process by which zoning out is ultimately caught (i.e., metaconsciousness is eventually directed to the contents of thought). Although simplistic, it is notable that this account provides insights into the phenomenon that seem overlooked by other relevant accounts of mindless behavior.

Other Potentially Applicable Theoretical Approaches   That readers were regularly caught zoning out without realizing that they were failing to attend to a task that demanded their attention raises the genuine possibility that people may routinely zone out without realizing it. Although we investigated this phenomenon in the context of reading, it seems quite plausible—if not likely—that zoning out without realizing it is a ubiquitous phenomenon. If so, then the question arises as to why various theoretical views of the relationship between consciousness and behavior have largely overlooked this phenomenon. The explanation for this oversight seems to stem from the simple observation that most theoretical approaches to mindless behavior fail to distinguish between having an experience (i.e., experiential consciousness) and realizing that one is having an experience (i.e., meta-consciousness).

SITUATION AWARENESS   The theoretical construct of "situation awareness" (see Durso and Gronlund, 1999, for review) is closely related to that of zoning out. Research on situation awareness examines the factors that affect performance in contexts such as air traffic control or piloting "in which the environment is dynamically changing and the operator is responsible for maintaining or achieving particular states or goals" (Durso and Gronlund, 1999, p. 283), where situation awareness is said to occur when people tightly focus their attention on the task at hand. Although considerable research has been devoted to documenting the key cognitive elements of situation awareness, including appropriate allocation of attention and adequate working memory resources (Carretta, Perry, and Ree, 1996), little consideration has been given to the metacognitive component of situation awareness. This point is illustrated by the largely overlooked dissociations between situation awareness and meta-awareness. It is possible to have situation awareness with out meta-awareness. For example, when people are engaging in demanding tasks (as when they are tracking dynamic environments), their performance is often optimal when they are not explicitly reflecting on what they are doing (Csikszentmihalyi, 1990). It is also possible to be metaconscious of the fact that one is currently lacking situation awareness. Drivers who listen to books on tape during long drives knowingly sacrifice situation awareness to the extent that they intentionally direct the focus of their attention away from the road. Thus zoning out can be described as an absence of situation awareness, although research on situation awareness does not offer a theoretical explanation of how people can fail to realize that they are zoning out.

MINDFULNESS   Another theoretical construct that is highly pertinent to the notion of zoning out while reading is "mindfulness" (e.g., Langer, 2000), which entails being "actively engaged in the present, noticing new things and [being] sensitive to context" (Langer, 2000, p. 220). The construct of mindfulness overlaps substantially with situation awareness but is typically discussed in contexts outside of tracking dynamic environments. As in the case of situation awareness, discussions of mindfulness have typically failed to differentiate between the performance failures associated with mindfulness and the metacognitive failures that allow such lapses to occur in the first place. Much research has been devoted to identifying the situations in which performance will be enhanced by encouraging mindfulness. For example, activities that force people to think more deeply about a task (e.g., by framing it in a more ambiguous manner or asking questions about it) enhance mindfulness (Langer, 2000). Indeed, researchers on zoning out while reading have observed that encouraging mindfulness during reading is critical to maximum comprehension (e.g., Pressley et al., 1995); moreover, the example of mindfulness during reading also highlights the distinction between mindfulness and metaconsciousness. Consider the case of readers deeply absorbed in a novel. Such people are extremely mindful of what they are reading, appreciating the language, visualizing the scenes, and often experiencing the emotions of the characters. Yet, at the same time, they may be said to be lacking in metaconsciousness of what it is that they are doing, which is why we refer to such situations as being *"lost"* in a novel." Thus the construct of mindfulness, while useful in characterizing the state of zoning out, fails to offer the metacognitive elements that would be sufficient to explain how people can fail to notice that they are zoning out in the first place.

THE AUTOMATIC VERSUS CONTROLLED PROCESSING DISTINCTION   Central to the notion of zoning out while reading is the observation that people are engaging in a highly complex task without attention. The capacity to perform complex tasks without attention is of course a defining attribute of what is typically referred to as "automatic behaviors" (e.g., Shiffrin and Schneider, 1977). It is relatively straightforward to apply the automatic-controlled processing distinction to the case of zoning out, where whatever process it is that can be described as "reading" (i.e., whatever process allows the eyes to continue moving across the page) presumably involves only automatic processing, which draws on few cognitive resources, whereas the contents of the mind (i.e., whatever thoughts occur during the mind-wandering episode) presumably involve controlled processing, which requires considerable cognitive resources. However, although the automatic versus controlled processing distinction maps onto zoning out while reading, it does not provide a full characterization of the phenomenon for several reason. First, automatic processing is typically characterized as nonconscious, a characterization that does not seem quite accurate in the case of reading while zoning out, where people may be consciously experiencing their eyes moving across the page, and may even experience the phonology of the words sounding in their mind's ear, but nevertheless fail to elaborate on this experience.

More important, the automatic versus controlled processing distinction does not address the metacognitive aspects of the situation. The unintended thought processes associated with zoning out can reasonably be characterized as involving controlled processing: they demand attention, and their resulting products are consciously experienced. Nevertheless, there is a peculiarity to designating the processes associated with zoning out as "controlled processing" because they ultimately reflect a *failure* of control stemming from the fact that people have lost meta-awareness of what they are doing. Thus the case of zoning out while reading illustrates the importance of including discussions of metaconsciousness into analyses of mental control.

THE COGNITION VERSUS METACOGNITION DISTINCTION   On the surface, the distinction between cognitive and metacognitive processes might seem to be the most promising existing approach for conceptualizing zoning out while reading. In introducing the construct of metacognition, Flavell (1979, p. 906) argued that there are two types: metacognitive knowledge corresponding to individuals' general knowledge about what they know, and metacognitive experiences that involve "any conscious cognitive or affective experiences that accompany and pertain to any intellectual enterprise." The experience of suddenly realizing that one has been zoning out certainly represents a metacognitive experience in Flavell's use of the term. Nevertheless, the notion of metacognition in general, and the specific distinction between metacognitive knowledge and metacognitive experience fails to adequately capture the zoning-out phenomenon. As with the other constructs considered above, it is easy to identify dissociations between metacognition and metaconsciousness. For example, one might well have a metacognitive experience, such as a dull sense of confusion, without explicitly being metaconscious of this experience. At some point one realizes (i.e., becomes metaconscious of the fact) that one is experiencing confusion, but this may be the culmination rather than the beginning of the metacognitive experience that led to this realization.

Ultimately, the inadequacy of the cognition versus metacognition distinction for capturing the zoning-out phenomenon is best illustrated by the simple fact that, although researchers have been exploring the metacognition associated with reading for decades, they have entirely overlooked the phenomenon of zoning out. This problem reflects the fact that, while the distinction between cognition and metacognition recognizes that people may vary in their knowledge about what they know, it does not explicitly acknowledge the possibility that people might lack a basic awareness of the contents of their experience. Accordingly, research on the metacognition of reading has considered people's awareness of how well they are comprehending the text they are reading; but has overlooked their varying awareness of whether they are attending to the text at all.

Having reviewed a number of theoretical distinctions that might apply to the case of zoning out while reading, it seems clear that, while each approach might offer useful insights into the phenomenon, they are all limited by their general failure to recognize that people can have experiences without explicitly recognizing that they are having those experiences. Although the claim that one can be unaware of one's current experience, at first blush, sounds almost nonsensical, it ultimately seems to be the only way to explain why people continue to read even though their mind is occupied by completely unrelated thoughts. Thus an appreciation and understanding of such fluctuations in one's awareness of one's conscious experience is substantially enhanced by considering the notion of a metalevel of consciousness.

A Few Unresolved Questions

We have argued that the metacognitive lapses associated with zoning out while reading have important implications for understanding both the specific cognitive and visual processes associated with reading and the more general manner in which consciousness can become dissociated from metaconsciousness. In closing, we mention just a few of the many questions raised by this analysis.

What Triggers Metaconsciousness?

According to the view that we have been promoting, zone-out lapses are caught when consciousness is directed onto itself. The question thus arises as to what initiates this metalevel of reflection. One condition under which metaconsciousness is initiated is quite clear: people attend to their conscious states when they are explicitly directed to do so. But what about cases in which individuals are not explicitly reminded to consider whether they have wandered off task? It may be that there is some type of periodic cycle in which metaconsciousness intermittently (at a rate that may vary as a function of the importance of the task and the likelihood that lapses may occur) assesses whether current goals are being met. Or it may be that the tacit monitoring system is sensitive to at least some cues that are indicative of zoning out. For example, pauses in thought (which in principle should not occur if a person is reading fluently) might trigger metaconscious reflection. Various extrinsic cues may also be important. For example, breaks in the text, the turning of pages, environmental sounds, and perhaps even textual conventions (e.g., boldface or italicized text) may interrupt the flow of internal musings, and thereby encourage a moment of metaconscious scrutiny. Future research might profitably explore the contingencies that induce metaconsciousness. Such investigations might enhance our understanding of this largely unexplored monitoring process, and may provide practical tips on how to write texts in order to minimize zoning-out episodes.

Can Zoning Out Sometimes Be Helpful?

However self-evidently counterproductive zoning out may be in many situations, there are certainly situations where it may be useful. If one is engaged in a dull activity that does not require resources, then clearly the tendency for thoughts to move in a more interesting direction is desirable. Indeed, even when reading, it is often helpful for readers to elaborate on the textual information. As noted at the outset, elaborative reading is often crucial for maximum comprehension. The challenge is to enable such elaborations to take place without undermining attention to the text. This analysis suggests that, while a very dull text may encourage zoning out because other topics of thought become inherently more attractive, a highly interesting text may also encourage zoning out by virtue of its thought-provoking nature. Future research may therefore benefit by examining the relationship between zoning-out experiences, text interest, and comprehension, as well as the intriguing possibility that, for certain types of texts, a high incidence of brief zoning-out experiences may actually be associated with superior comprehension performance.

Can We Find Independent Markers of Both Zoning Out and Metaconsciousness?

Although we believe that the relationship between zoning-out reports and various reading comprehension measures provides an important first step in validating individuals' self-reports of zoning out, it is nevertheless clear that a key limitations to our approach is its reliance on self-report measures. One of the key implications of dissociations between metaconsciousness and experience is that self-reports (which necessarily rely on metaconscious rerepresentation of experience) can provide potentially seriously distorted accounts of actual experience (Schooler, 2002). Thus even partially validated self-reports must be taken with a grain of salt. Moreover, even though we found little evidence of reactivity from our measures, it is clear that asking participants to monitor and report their zone-out experiences must have some effect on the natural occurrence of zone-out experiences. Indeed, it seems quite possible that the introduction of our measures may have reduced the overall frequency of zoning out, thereby providing an underestimation of the frequency with which they naturally occur. It would thus be useful to identify other measures that might provide alternative ways of tracking cases of zoning out. As noted earlier, it seems quite plausible that eye movement during reading may qualitatively change when readers are zoning out. It is also possible that certain electroencephalographic (EEG) measures might be sensitive to fluctuations in coherence (e.g., Klemm, Li, and Hernandez, 2000) depending on whether the information processing associated with what is being read is being integrated with what is being thought about. If such measures revealed signatures of zoning out that corroborated one another and self-reports, then we could have more confidence in self-report measures. Moreover, in principle, it would then be possible to study zoning out without having to rely on self-report measures at all. Such an advance would allow us to investigate a host of intriguing questions such as how often individuals zone out without noticing it, when self-reports and indirect measures are more versus less well calibrated, how long zone-out episodes last, and what situations determine whether a zone-out episode is explicitly caught.

It would also be very informative to explore the neurological markers of meta-consciousness itself. Recent studies, using both event-related potential (ERP) and Functional magnetic resonance imaging (fMRI), have found that the anterior cingulate is especially important in conflict monitoring processes (Carter et al., 1998). There is also some evidence suggesting that the area of the cingulate activated depends on whether the monitoring process is implicit or explicit (van Veen and Carter, 2002). Future imaging research might profitably explore the relationship between activation of the cingulate and both the occurrence of zoning out and the metaconscious realization that one is zoning out. Such an analysis could provide a foundation for a model of cognitive monitoring grounded both in brain activity and in phenomenological experience.

Note

1. What we refer to as "experiential consciousness" has previously been called "phenomenal consciousness" (Block, 2001) and "perceptual consciousness" (Armstrong, 1998). And what we refer to interchangeably as "meta-awareness" or "metaconsciousness" has previously been called "reflexive consciousness" (Farthing, 1992), "introspective consciousness" (Armstrong, 1998), and "reflectivity" (Block, 2001). Although this distinction is clearly more important than the particular terms we use to characterize it, apt, precise terminology helps to ensure accurate communication and to avoid the sleight of hand that can occur when conclusions appropriate to one meaning of a term are inappropriately applied to a different meaning of the same term. We are partial to the terms *meta-awareness* (see also Cicogna and Bosinetti, 2001; Jack and Shallice, 2001; Schooler, 2001) and *metaconsciousness* (Schooler, 2002) for several reasons. First, the notion of metaconsciousness as consciousness of consciousness aptly captures Tarski's "meta" construct (1956, 1985) of "whatever about whatever." Second, the terms *metaconsciousness* and *meta-awareness* highlight the importance

of relating metacognition to consciousness—a fruitful endeavor (see Nelson, 1996) that occurs surprisingly seldom. Finally, although any of the previously used terms could capture the distinction, many bear the burden of multiple connotations. Although the terms *consciousness* and *awareness* also hold multiple meanings, it is their shared meaning that most closely captures the basic concept of consciousness as being the contents of one's subjective experience. Thus applying the "meta" prefix to both "awareness" and "consciousness" may help to ensure that both resulting compounds draw on the common meaning of "consciousness" that the two base terms share.

References

Altarriba, J., Kambe, G., Pollatsek, A., and Rayner, K. (2001). Semantic codes are not used in integrating information across eye fixations in reading: Evidence from fluent Spanish-English bilinguals. *Perception and Psychophysics, 63,* 875–890.

Antrobus, J. S., Coleman, R., and Singer, J. L. (1967). Signal detection performance by subjects differing in predisposition to daydreaming. *Journal of Consulting Psychology, 31,* 487–491.

Antrobus, J. S., Singer, J. L., Goldstein, S., and Fortgang, M. (1970). Mindwandering and cognitive structure. Reprinted from *Transactions of the New York Academy of Sciences, 32,* 242–252.

Armstrong, D. (1998). What is consciousness? In N. Block, O. Flanagan, and G. Guzeldere (Eds.), *The nature of consciousness* (pp. 721–728). Cambridge, MA: MIT Press.

Baumeister, R. F. (1984). Choking under pressure: Self-consciousness and paradoxical effects of incentives on skillful performance. *Journal of Personality and Social Psychology, 46,* 610–620.

Block, N. (2001). Paradox and cross purposes in recent work on consciousness. *Cognition 79,* 197–219.

Brown, A. L. (1980). Metacognitive development and reading. In R. J. Spiro, B. C. Bruce, and W. F. Brewer (Eds.), *Theoretical issues in reading comprehension* (pp. 453–481). Hillsdale, NJ: Lawrence Erlbaum Associates.

Brown, R., and Pressley, M. (1994). Self-regulated reading and getting meaning from text: The transactional strategies instruction model and its ongoing evaluation. In D. Schunk and B. Zimmerman (Eds.), *Self-regulation of learning and performance: Issues and educational applications.* Hillsdale, NJ: Erlbaum.

Carretta, T. R., Perry, D. C., and Ree, M. J. (1996). Prediction of situational awareness in F-15 pilots. *International Journal of Aviation Psychology, 6,* 21–41.

Carter, C. S., Braver, T. S., Barch, D. M., Botvinick, M. M., Noll, D. C., and Cohen, J. D. (1998). Anterior cingulate cortex, error detection, and the online monitoring of performance. *Science, 280,* 747–749.

Cicogna, P. C., and Bosinetti, M. (2001). Consciousness during dreams. *Consciousness and Cognition, 10,* 26–41.

Csikszentmihalyi, M. (1990). *Flow: The psychology of optimal experience.* New York: Harper and Row.

Durso, F. T., and Gronlund, S. D. (1999). Situation awareness. In F. T. Durso, R. S. Nickerson, R. W. Schvaneveldt, S. T. Dumais, D. S. Lindsay, and M. T. H. Chi (Eds.), *Handbook of applied cognition* (pp. 283–314). New York: Wiley.

Farthing, G. W. (1992). *The psychology of consciousness.* Englewood Cliffs, NJ: Prentice Hall.

Flavell, J. H. (1979). Metacognition and cognitive monitoring: A new area of cognitive-developmental inquiry. *American Psychologist, 34,* 906–911.

Garner, R., and Kraus, C. (1981–82). Good and poor comprehenders' differences in knowing and regulating reading behaviors. *Educational Research Quarterly, 6,* 5–12.

Garner, R., and Reis, R. (1981). Monitoring and resolving comprehension obstacles: An investigation of spontaneous text lookbacks among upper grade good and poor comprehenders. *Reading Research Quarterly, 16,* 569–582.

Giambra, L. M. (1989). Task-unrelated thought frequency as a function of age: A laboratory study. *Psychology and Aging, 4,* 136–143.

Giambra, L. M. (1995). A laboratory method for investigating influences on switching attention to task-unrelated imagery and thought, *Consciousness and Cognition, 4*, 1–21.

Giambra, L. M., and Grodsky, A. (1989). Task-unrelated images and thoughts while reading. In J. Shorr, P. Robin, J. A. Connella, and M. Wolpin (Eds.), *Imagery: Current perspectives* (pp. 26–31). New York: Plenum Press.

Giambra, L. M., Rosenberg, E. H., Kasper, S., Yee, W., and Sack, D. A. (1988). A circadian rhythm in the frequency of spontaneous task-unrelated images and thoughts. *Imagination, Cognition, and Personality, 8*, 307–312.

Gillstrom, A., and Ronnberg, J. (1995). Comprehension calibration and recall prediction accuracy of texts: Reading skill, reading strategies, and effort. *Journal of Educational Psychology, 87*, 545–558.

Glenberg, A. M., and Epstein, W. (1985). Calibration of comprehension. *Journal of Experimental Psychology: Learning, Memory and Cognition, 11*, 702–718.

Glenberg, A. M., Wilkinson, A., and Epstein, W. (1982). The illusion of knowing: Failure in the self-assessment of comprehension. *Memory and Cognition, 10*, 597–602.

Glover, J. A. (1989). Reading ability and the calibrator of comprehension. *Educational Research Quarterly, 13*, 7–11.

Grodsky, A., and Giambra, L. M. (1991). The consistency across vigilance and reading tasks of individual differences in the occurrence of task-unrelated and task-related images and thoughts. *Imagination, Cognition, and Personality, 10*, 39–52.

Hacker, D. J. (1998). Self-regulated comprehension during normal reading. In D. J. Hacker, J. Dunlosky, and A. C. Graesser (Eds.), *Metacognition in educational theory and practice* (pp. 165–191). Mahwah, NJ: Erlbaum.

Hurlburt, R. T. (1993). *Sampling inner experience in disturbed affect.* New York: Plenum Press.

Inhoff, A. W., and Rayner, K. (1986). Parafoveal word processing during eye fixations in reading: Effects of word frequency. *Perception and Psychophysics, 40*, 431–439.

Jack, A. I., and Shallice, T. (2001). Introspective physicalism as an approach to the science of consciousness. *Cognition, 79*, 161–196.

Just, M. A., and Carpenter, P. A. (1980). A theory of reading: From eye fixations to comprehension. *Psychological Review, 87*, 329–354.

Just, M. A., and Carpenter, P. A. (1987). *The psychology of reading and language comprehension.* Boston: Allyn and Bacon.

Klemm, W. R., Li, T. H., and Hernandez, J. L. (2000). Coherent EEG indicators of cognitive binding during ambiguous figure tasks. *Consciousness and Cognition, 9*, 66–85.

Langer, E. J. (2000). Mindful learning. *Current Directions in Psychological Science, 9*, 220–225.

Lovelace, E. A. (1984). Metamemory: Monitoring future recallability during study. *Journal of Experimental Psychology: Learning, Memory, and Cognition, 10*, 756–766.

Maki, R. H. (1995). Accuracy of metacomprehension judgments for questions of varying importance levels. *American Journal of Psychology, 108*, 327–344.

Maki, R. H., and Berry, S. (1984). Metacomprehension of text material. *Journal of Experimental Psychology: Learning, Memory, and Cognition, 10*, 663–679.

Maki, R. H., Jonas, D., and Kallod, M. (1994). The relationship between comprehension and metacomprehension ability. *Psychonomic Bulletin and Review, 1*, 126–129.

Nelson, T. O. (1996). Consciousness and metacognition. *American Psycologist, 97*, 19–35.

O'Regan, J. K. (1979). Eye guidance in reading: Evidence for linguistic control hypothesis. *Perception and Psychophysics, 25*, 501–509.

O'Regan, J. K. (1980). The control of saccade size and fixation duration in reading: The limits of linguistic control. *Perception and Psychophysics, 28*, 112–117.

O'Regan, J. K. (1990). Eye movements in reading. In E. Kowler (Ed.), *Eye movements and their role in visual and cognitive processes* (pp. 395–453). Amsterdam: Elsevier.

O'Regan, J. K. (1992). Optimal viewing position in words and the strategy-tactics theory of eye movements in reading. In K. Rayner (Ed.), *Eye movements in visual cognition: Scene perception and reading* (pp. 333–354). New York: Springer-Verlag.

Palincsar, A. S., and Brown, A. L. (1984). Reciprocal teaching of comprehension-fostering and comprehension-monitoring activities. *Cognition and Instruction, 1,* 117–175.

Pressley, M., Brown, R., Beard El-Dinary, P., and Afflerback, P. (1995). The comprehension instruction that students need: Instruction fostering constructively responsive reading. *Learning Disabilities Research and Practice, 10,* 215–224.

Rayner, K. (1979). Eye guidance in reading: Fixation locations within words. *Perception, 8,* 21–30.

Rayner, K. (1998). Eye movements in reading and information processing: Twenty years of research. *Psychological Bulletin, 124,* 372–422.

Rayner, K., and Fischer, M. H. (1996). Mindless reading revisited: Eye movements during reading and scanning are different. *Perception and Psychophysics, 58,* 734–747.

Rayner, K., and Morris, R. K. (1992). Eye movement control in reading: Evidence against semantic preprocessing. *Journal of Experimental Psychology: Human Perception and Performance, 18,* 163–172.

Rayner, K., and Pollatsek, A. (1989). *The psychology of reading.* Englewood Cliffs, NJ: Prentice Hall.

Reichle, E. D., Pollatsek, A., Fisher, D. L., and Rayner, K. (1998). Toward a model of eye-movement control in reading. *Psychological Review, 105,* 125–157.

Reichle, E. D., and Rayner, K. (2002). Cognitive processes and models of reading. In G. Hung and K. Ciuffreda (Eds.), *Models of the visual system* (pp. 565–604). New York: Plenum Press.

Reichle, E. D., Rayner, K., and Pollatsek, A. (1999). Eye movement control in reading: Accounting for initial fixation locations and refixations with the E-Z Reader model. *Vision Research, 39,* 4403–4411.

Reichle, E. D., Rayner, K., and Pollatsek, A. (Forthcoming). *Behavioral and Brain Sciences.*

Reilly, R., and O'Regan, K. J. (1998). Eye movement control in reading: A simulation of some word-targeting strategies. *Vision Research, 38,* 303–317.

Salvucci, D. D. (2000). An interactive model-based environment for eye-movement protocol visualization and analysis. In *Proceedings of the Eye Tracking Research and Applications Symposium* (pp. 57–63). New York: ACM Press.

Salvucci, D. D. (2001). Automated eye-movement protocol analysis. *Human Computer Interaction, 16,* 39–86.

Schilling, H. E. H., Rayner, K., and Chumbley, J. I. (1998). Comparing naming, lexical decision, and eye-fixation times: Word frequency effects and individual differences. *Memory and Cognition, 26,* 1270–1281.

Schooler, J. W. (2001). Discovering memories in the light of meta-awareness. *Journal of Aggression, Maltreatment and Trauma, 4,* 105–136.

Schooler, J. W. (2002). Representing consciousness: Dissociations between consciousness and meta-consciousness. *Trends in Cognitive Science, 6,* 339–344.

Schooler, J. W., Ariely, D., and Loewenstein, G. (2003). The explicit pursuit and monitoring of happiness can be self-defeating. J. Carrillo and I. Brocas (Eds.), *Psychology and economics.* (pp. 41–70). Oxford: Oxford University Press.

Schooler, J. W., Ohlsson, S., and Brooks, K. (1993). Thoughts beyond words: When language overshadows insight. *Journal of Experimental Psychology: General, 122,* 166–183.

Schooler, J. W., Reichle, E., and Halpern, D. (In preparation). Lost out of a novel: Zoning out and lapses of metaconsciousness during reading.

Shaw, G. A., and Giambra, L. M. (1993). Task-unrelated-thoughts of college students diagnosed as hyperactive in childhood. *Developmental Neuropsychology, 9,* 17–30.

Shiffrin, R. M., and Schneider, W. (1977). Controlled and automatic human information processing: 2. Perceptual learning, automatic attending, and a general theory. *Psychological Review, 84,* 127–190.

Singer, J. L. (1978). Experimental studies of daydreaming and the stream of thought. In K. S. Pope and J. L. Singer, *The stream of consciousness: Scientific investigations into the flow of human experience* (pp. 187–223). New York: Plenum Press.

Singer, J. L. (1988). Sampling ongoing consciousness and emotional experience: Implications for health. In M. J. Horowitz (Ed.), *Psychodynamics and cognition* (pp. 297–346). Chicago: University of Chicago Press.

Singer, J. L. (1993). Experimental studies of ongoing conscious experience. In *Experimental and theoretical studies of consciousness* (pp. 100–122). Ciba Foundation Symposium 174. Chichester England: Wiley.

Suppes, P. (1990). Eye-movement models for arithmetic and reading performance. In E. Kowler (Ed.), *Eye movements and their role in visual and cognitive processes* (pp. 455–477). Amsterdam: Elsevier.

Suppes, P. (1994). Stochastic models of reading. In J. Ygge and G. Lennerstrand (Eds.), *Eye movements in reading* (pp. 349–364). Oxford: Pergamon Press.

Tarski, A. (1956). The concept of truth in formalized languages. In A. Tarski (Ed.), *Logic, semantics, mathematics* (pp. 152–178). Oxford: Alarendon Press.

Tarski, A. (1985). The semantic conception of truth. In A. P. Martinich (Ed.), *The philosophy of language* (pp. 48–71). Oxford: Oxford University Press.

Thibadeau, R., Just, M. A., and Carpenter, P. A. (1982). A model of the time course and content of reading. *Cognitive Science, 6*, 157–203.

van Veen, V., and Carter, C. S. (2002). The timing of action-monitoring processes in the anterior cingulate cortex. *Journal of Cognitive Neuroscience, 14*, 593–602.

Vitu, F., O'Regan, J. K., Inhoff, A. W., and Topolski, R. (1995). Mindless reading: Eye movement characteristics are similar in scanning letter strings and reading text. *Perception and Psychophysics, 57*, 352–364.

Wegner, D. M. (1994). Ironic processes of mental control. *Psychological Review, 101*, 34–52.

Wegner, D. M. (1997). Why the mind wanders. In J. D. Cohen and J. W. Schooler (Eds.), *Scientific approaches to consciousness* (pp. 295–315). Mahway, NJ: Erlbaum.

Wegner, D. M., and Wheatley, T. (1999). Apparent mental causation: Sources of the experience of will. *American Psychologist, 54*, 480–492.

Wilson, T. D., and Schooler, J. W. (1991). Thinking too much: Introspection can reduce the quality of preferences and decisions? *Journal of Personality and Social Psychology, 60*, 181–192.

Yang, S. N., and McConkie, G. W. (2001). Eye movements during reading: A theory of saccade initiation time. *Vision Research, 41*, 3567–3585.

Chapter 11

What Lies Beneath? Understanding the Limits of Understanding

Frank C. Keil, Leonid Rozenblit, and Candice M. Mills

At one time or another, virtually every one of us has launched into an explanation in answer to a "why" question, only to founder halfway through. At such times, we are often surprised at our inability to explain something that seemed beautifully clear a moment before. The experience is a common one, not only for parents of young children, but also for teachers and for expository writers, indeed, for all persons who daily confront their inability to explain.

A major part of our intellectual lives is concerned with understanding the causal structure of the world around us. We ask "why" questions frequently, about topics as diverse as interpersonal relationships, the weather, the stock market, fax machines, and earthquakes. Moreover, this search for causal explanations emerges early in development. Almost as soon as they can talk, children start to ask, "Why?" The very first attempts may very well be just a communication ritual, but shortly thereafter, such questions represent a genuine effort to understand the causes that give rise to salient phenomena.

The desire to know why, however, must be driven at least in part by dissatisfaction with one's existing understanding. One must realize that one does not fully grasp a phenomenon to feel that one needs to learn more. Thus, to seek an explanation, one must first assess one's own knowledge.

Such a self-assessment might seem to be a quintessential example of metacognition—the conscious self-examination of one's internal mental states. Yet the emergence of "why" and "how" questions so early in development is puzzling. How can we reconcile the pursuit of explanations by preschoolers with the extensive evidence that these children's metacognitive skills are severely limited?

In this chapter, we argue that the key to solving this puzzle is understanding that our intuitive epistemology is misleading: we are misled by a mistaken intuition about the completeness of our explanatory knowledge. The true source of our frequent sense of causal insight is far different from what it seems to be, not just in children, but also throughout life. Furthermore, certain properties of explanatory understanding distinguish self-assessments of explanatory knowledge from those of other sorts of knowledge, such as how well we understand procedures, narratives, or simple facts.

Our argument reflects a new research focus. Although considerable work has been done on the ability to assess how well one has understood new information (e.g., Glenberg, Wilkinson, and Epstein, 1982; Glenberg and Epstein, 1985; Markman, 1977, 1979), far less work has been done on the ability to assess knowledge one has gradually accumulated over the years, and almost none on systematically comparing different forms of such long-term knowledge.

We suggest here that adults and children alike are under the sway of the "illusion of explanatory depth" (IOED): they feel they understand the world in far greater depth and detail than they actually do (Rozenblit and Keil, 2002). In striking ways, being blind to the shallowness of one's understanding of causal structure parallels being blind to the highly incomplete ways we seem to represent information in visual scenes—"change blindness blindness" (CBB; Levin, et al., 2000; see also Levin and Beck, chapter 6, this volume). Does this striking surface similarity reflect a more profound connection? Are there, perhaps, common processes involved in producing both kinds of impressions of fine-grained representations when in fact much coarser ones are really at work? We will consider the parallels and differences between the IOED and CBB in a separate section near the end of this chapter.

To make a convincing case for a similarity of mechanism between the illusion of explanatory depth and change blindness blindness, we should first attempt to deal with one widely held motivational explanation for the IOED, namely, that it arises from the need to mask our cognitive limitations and, ultimately, from the need to preserve our self-esteem. Such explanations have been quite common in discussions in the social psychological literature and are also commonly invoked to account for greater estimates of one's own abilities than of others' (see Bjork, 1998; Fischhoff, 1982; Lin and Zabrucky, 1998, for reviews; see also Lichtenstein and Fischhoff, 1977, Yates, Lee, and Bush, 1997; Yates, Lee, and Shinotsuka, 1996). A motivated self-serving bias is unlikely to be involved in change blindness blindness, however: people have been shown to overestimate the change detection abilities of others as well as of themselves (Levin et al., 2000).

Although self-serving biases may contribute to the illusion of explanatory depth, we contend that it is not its predominant cause. Indeed, we argue that the illusion may instead be an adaptive way of dealing with a world of indefinitely deep causal complexity, that the false sense of knowing why and how with depth and detail may be a by-product of a genuine insight, although at a level and of a kind far different from what our lay intuitions first suggest. It is our claim that the sense of insight in the IOED indicates a glimpse, not into the mechanism underlying a particular phenomenon, but into the skeletal causal patterns that constrain an explanatory domain that are plausible for a class of phenomena (e.g., knowing that mechanical causation involves contiguous interacting parts). These skeletal patterns may be quite sparse, but they are nevertheless essential to real-time causal interpretations. They may also be involved in intuitions about where true expertise resides (i.e., knowing which experts know which sorts of things), and in judging the quality of explanations. Our implicit detection of these causal patterns in a particular domain produces a flash of insight that we mistake for having a detailed mechanistic understanding of a particular phenomenon.

The adaptive sense of the illusion provides a conceptual bridge between adult and child metacognition. As we argue at the end of the chapter, there is a surprising continuity between children's and adults' self-assessment of explanatory knowledge. The continuity is less surprising if we understand the illusion as a by-product of an adaptive search for genuine, but sparse, causal patterns.

The Illusion of Explanatory Depth

Most of the ways we understand the world around us are not neatly and explicitly presented to us just before we have to self-assess them. Our understanding of biological reproduction, weather, friendships, or how our car works usually reflects knowledge we have accumulated slowly and implicitly, often over several years. We may, for example, understand how friendships are formed and maintained through a set of implicit hypotheses we have never been taught. Perhaps an occasional admonition that we "shouldn't do that" influences our views of how to form and maintain friendships, but explicit instruction of any sort is rarely involved.

Explanatory understanding, of course, is not the only form of knowledge that is acquired in this implicit, long-term manner. Knowledge of the spatial layout of one's neighborhood or of the intricacies of a department of motor vehicles office may also be slowly acquired and largely implicit. Even factual databases that are occasionally subjects of explicit instruction may, in reality, be learned through gradual exposure. Consider that one may have been taught the capitals of various countries quite explicitly, yet most of us tend to learn their names through the news media or, if we are fortunate, through travel.

Given that much explanatory knowledge builds up over long periods of time, how do we measure self-calibration for estimates of explanatory understanding—that is, the correlation between estimates of explanatory understanding and actual understanding—in a laboratory setting? In our research, we have used a method that usually involves five steps

> 1. Training. Through a series of examples, we train our participants in using a scale of seven levels to rate understanding. Thus, for a crossbow, an annotated diagram showing all the important causal relationships for the device represents level-7 (complete) understanding, whereas an annotated diagram showing only general information about the overall shape and function of the crossbow represents level-1 (very shallow) understanding. We train our participants on the use of this scale both with a relatively simple device, such as a crossbow, and a relatively complex one, such as a global positioning system (GPS) receiver.

2. First rating (T1). Having been trained to use the rating scale, participants are then asked to evaluate their own understanding of various devices and phenomena, such as how helicopters fly, why the tides occur, or how a flush toilet works. In most of our studies, participants give first ratings to a large list of such items.

3. Second rating (T2). When all the first ratings of knowledge are given, participants are then asked to give as complete explanations as they can for a subset of the original list. Because it takes quite some time to give a complete explanation, a subset typically consists of only four or five items. Participants are then asked to rerate their original understanding of each explained item in light of the explanations they have just produced. The second round of ratings allows us to measure whether actually providing the explanation corroborated participants' original ratings or showed them to be too pessimistic or too optimistic.

4. Third rating (T3). After participants have given explanations and have rerated their understanding, they are then asked a "diagnostic question," which probes their grasp of a particularly important aspect of a good understanding of a device or phenomenon. For example, participants giving high ratings to their understanding of how a helicopter flies would be asked how a helicopter files forward from a stationary hovering position. After giving their best answer to the diagnostic question, participants are again asked to rerate their original understanding on the same scale.

5. Fourth and fifth ratings (T4 and T5). Finally, participants are presented with an expert explanation, compiled from expert sources, and are once again asked to rate their original understanding in light of reading that explanation.

In some studies, we also include an additional step in which participants are asked to evaluate their own understanding as a result of having read the expert explanation. This final rating is a manipulation check. Presumably, participants who were following experimental instructions should increase their ratings at least somewhat as a result of having learned new information. The manipulation check also allowed us to establish two important points. First, if the final ratings increased, we could conclude that participants' confidence was not so globally shaken by our procedure that they could no longer ascribe themselves a high level of understanding. Second, we could show that the expert explanations were comprehensible and that laypeople felt that they could gain genuine insight by reading them.

Figure 11.1 shows a summary of how ratings of one's own explanatory understanding changed over the series of self-assessments (adapted from Rozenblit and Keil, 2002). Across the several studies summarized in Rozenblit and Keil, 2002, we consistently found a large drop after the initial attempt at explanation, a second drop after answering the diagnostic question, and no further change after seeing

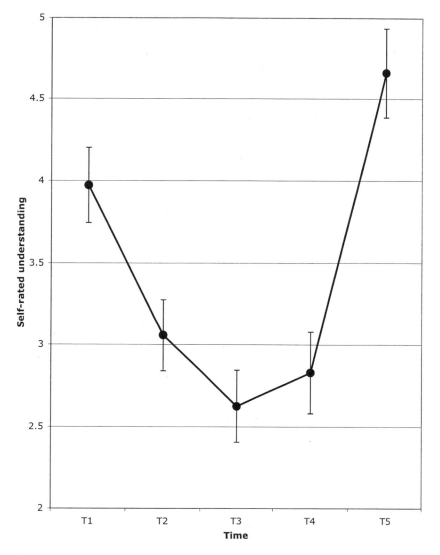

Figure 11.1
Self-ratings of knowledge averaged across all items and subjects for all explanations studies (devices and natural phenomena). The *x*-axis shows the sequence of self-ratings from time 1 to time 5. T1 is the initial self-rating, prior to any attempt to produce an explanation. T2 is the rating immediately after the first effort to explain. T3 is the rating after an attempt to answer a diagnostic question. T4 is the rerating of one's initial knowledge provided after reading an expert explanation. T5 is the rating of one's current knowledge acquired as a result of reading an expert explanation, and is essentially a manipulation check. Self-ratings of knowledge decrease as the result of efforts to explain. (Adapted from Rozenblit and Keil, 2002)

the expert explanation. In those cases where participants were also asked to evaluate their new understanding in light of reading the expert explanation, there was always a large rise.

Some other patterns across the studies are also relevant here. First, follow-up studies showed that participants were not inflating their initial estimates merely because they though it was socially desirable to know certain explanations. When another group of participants was asked to rate which explanatory knowledge "it would be most embarrassing" not to know, their ratings were not related to the strength of the illusion of explanatory depth across items. The illusion seems to be created by other factors. Second, the illusion is not a reflection of overconfidence bred by attending selective universities, by having had high levels of success in the academic arena, or by having had many years of advanced education. In fact, if anything, our studies suggest an opposite trend: lower academic achievement is associated with a stronger IOED. One interpretation of this trend is that the less one understands a domain, the larger the mismatch between what one thinks one knows and what one really knows. That is, ignorance has the paradoxical effect of producing overconfidence about one's knowledge. Conversely, the more one knows about a field, the more accurately tuned one's metacognitive awareness about one's knowledge seems to be. This interpretation would be consistent with the "dual burden of incompetence" argument made by Kruger and Dunning (1999), who suggest that those not competent in a domain are especially overconfident in their abilities. Finally, it is important to note that the IOED holds even when participants are explicitly warned, before giving any ratings, that they will be challenged on their knowledge by a series of probing questions. Although such instructions do make participants more conservative, they still show significant drops over successive episodes of rerating.

The Illusion of Explanatory Depth versus Other Self-Evaluations of Knowledge

A critical part of our account is our claim that the illusion of explanatory depth is more powerful than many other kinds of illusions of knowing. That is, we predict that comparisons across knowledge types will illustrate a greater overconfidence for knowledge of causal explanations than for other types of knowledge. We make this claim because we see several factors uniquely converging to create an especially strong illusion for explanations. To evaluate this claim, we need to examine the nature of knowledge representation across different domains.

Even confining our analysis to long-term knowledge that people bring to the experimental setting leaves many possible types of knowledge representations to consider: for example, those involved in knowledge of facts, such as the capitals of countries or the past winners of the World Series in baseball; in knowledge of procedures, such as how to make an international telephone call or ride a unicycle; or in knowledge of narratives, fictional and nonfictional accounts of various agents' actions over time. Still other representations might be involved in knowledge of songs, languages, rules of etiquette, and settings. To the extent that these different types of knowledge involve different representations, and invoke different naive epistemic theories, we would expect variance in calibration across domains.

If the claim that calibration of knowledge assessment should vary systematically across domains seems self-evident, consider that a vast branch of judgment and decision-making (JDM) literature on overconfidence has acted as if the opposite were true. A large number of studies on "overconfidence about general knowledge" seem to proceed on the assumption that calibration is independent of the types of representation involved (e.g., Griffin and Buehler, 1999; Griffin and Tversky, 1992; Fischhoff, Slovic, and Lichtenstein, 1977; Lichtenstein and Fischhoff, 1977, Yates, Lee, and Bush, 1997; see Bjork, 1998; Lin and Zabrucky, 1998, for reviews). Here, by contrast, we suggest that the nature of the knowledge type can have large effects on the quality of self-assessments.

We do not argue, by the way, that the universe of "knowledge types" is well defined, or that the dimensions we identify have universal significance. To test our claims, we have attempted to select knowledge types that contrast in clearly definable ways with explanatory knowledge. We have focused on other cases of knowledge that are not heavily perceptual or motor in nature, namely knowledge of facts, nonmotor procedures, and narratives. Each of these contrasts with explanatory knowledge in different ways.

Explanations versus Facts
Factual knowledge seems to be potentially the type most different from explanatory knowledge. Facts tend to be brief statements of a property or relation without much internal structure, whereas explanations have a good deal of internal structure, which can produce misplaced feelings of confidence in a number of ways. One of the most powerful ways it does this is through the confusion of information that is internally represented with information that is recoverable or constructible in real time when the device or phenomenon is present for inspection. It is quite easy to convince oneself that one fully knows how a device such as stapler works because one has successfully deciphered its mechanism when it was at hand and open for inspection. The structural relations of parts are often laid out in such a manner that most observers can figure out the roles of all the parts in making the device work. That ability, however, is far different from actually mentally representing all the parts of stapler and their causal relationships— the mechanism by which structure produces function. People tend to confuse the two, however, mistaking their strong sense of being able to understand a device or system when it is at hand, with its structure and function exposed to view, for their having an equally detailed representation clearly in mind. Compare, in this regard, explanatory knowledge with factual knowledge. If one were asked to estimate how well one knows the capital of, say, Australia, one is unlikely to be misled into a false sense of knowing by the recollection of having

visited Australia or of having studied a political map of the continent. In either case, the sense that one knows the capital of Australia is likely to coincide with one's actual knowledge.

A related difference is that people can self-test factual knowledge quickly and easily. You can, for example, ask yourself whether you know the capital of Australia and, if you recover "Canberra" with great confidence, you will rate your knowledge with the same confidence; if you recover both "Canberra" and "Sydney," feeling uncertain which is correct, you will respond almost as quickly and easily, but with corresponding uncertainty. On the other hand, if asked how a helicopter flies, you cannot quickly self-test your explanatory knowledge: a full explanation, even for an expert, takes time to generate and assess.

Moreover, the parameters of a successful explanation are much less clear. It is much more difficult, for example, to tell when an explanation is complete. If a name strongly comes to mind with respect to knowledge of a capital, you can be fairly confident that you have adequate information to answer the question. But with explanations, even vivid recall of some parts of an explanation is no guarantee that you can produce the full account (or even that you will know what constitutes a full account).

In our research, one factor made comparing facts with explanations easier. We found that participants exhibited the same overall initial confidence levels with facts as with explanations of devices and natural phenomena. Because they were often not sure about which of two or more cities was the capital of a country, their initial ratings were often in the middle of the scale, as they were for judgments of explanatory understandings of devices and natural phenomena. But when asked to produce the capital and rerate their knowledge, participants showed very little drop in ratings, far less than with explanations. Similarly, providing them with an "expert" answer did not change their ratings any further (see figure 11.2).

Facts, however, are a special case because they represent simple, usually unstructured, kernels of knowledge altogether different from the complex structure of most explanations. Perhaps the illusion of knowing will be equally compelling for all complex knowledge structures. On the other hand, several differences persist between explanatory structures and other knowledge structures that might continue to make the illusion stronger for explanatory understanding.

Explanations versus Procedures

Consider knowledge of procedures. For many procedures, the presence of the objects that are used in the procedure may not serve to help one know the procedure itself. The presence, for example, of a telephone, will not help one know how to make an international telephone call, nor the presence of a flag, how to fold it in a military fashion. One is therefore less likely to confuse what one has mentally represented with what one is able to do when in the presence of the objects associated with the procedure.

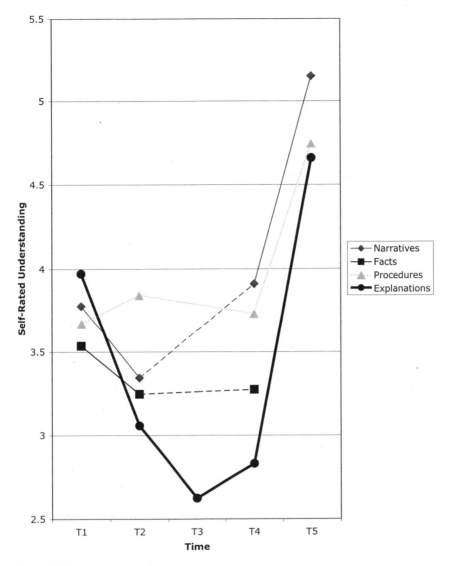

Figure 11.2
Self-ratings of knowledge averaged across all items and subjects for explanations (devices and natural phenomena) facts (capital of countries), procedures (e.g., how to bake chocolate chip cookies from scratch), and narratives (plots of movies). The axes are the same as in figure 11.1. (Adapted from Rozenblit and Keil, 2002)

Procedures also differ in that there is less of an opportunity to confuse higher-level functional relations with lower-level, more mechanistic ones. Procedures are usually considered fully known if one knows the steps to execute to reach a desired goal. There is no sense of a limited understanding if one cannot decompose a step into smaller ones so long as one can perform it. One tends to encode action at certain macro level of analysis that is adequate to then reproduce an effective version of the action.

Finally, the criteria for successfully performing a procedure are usually quite clear-cut making it much easier to self-test one's knowledge of the procedure. One can ask if one has successfully made an international telephone call or folded a flag military style and use goal attainment as a reliable indicator of having the knowledge. Because we rarely give explanations, however, and because the criteria for giving a good explanation are less clear-cut, explanatory knowledge is much more difficult to self-test.

Taking all these factors together, we predicted that people would be much better calibrated in their estimates of their own procedural knowledge. In a task modeled closely on the illusion of explanatory depth task, we trained participants to use a scale with examples of knowing how to fold a flag military style at different levels of completeness. Participants were then asked to rate their self-knowledge for a large set of procedures and to write down in detail all they knew about how to do a subset of those procedures; they rerated their knowledge in light of having written out the procedure; they were given an expert, full description of the procedure and asked to rerate their initial knowledge in light of that expert description. The results were strikingly different from those found for the knowledge of explanations: instead of a significant drop in ratings, we saw a slight (nonsignificant) increase (see figure 11.2).

Explanations versus Narratives
Theories are sometimes considered to be, in essence, stories about how or why things are they way they are. Thus one of the strongest tests of the potential specificity of the illusion of explanatory depth might involve people's estimates of their narrative knowledge and a comparison of those estimates to those for intuitive theories and explanatory understanding, although we predicted that people would be much better calibrated for narratives than for explanations. There is less opportunity for confusion between levels of description in narratives than in explanations. Narratives are also usually undertaken without physical tokens as part of the process, hence having little potential for confusing what is represented with what is decipherable in real time with the phenomenon present. Moreover, people often tell stories of past events, thus having a good deal of experience with how well or poorly they recall narratives. Finally, narratives tend to describe the paths of individuals over time, whereas explanations tend to describe timeless causal cycles. Encoding the paths of individuals is certainly phenomenologically different from encoding explanations of causal relationships within a complex system.

In a narrative self-assessment task, again analogous to the original IOED task, we had participants rate how well they thought they knew the plots of well-known movies; they were then asked to write out the plots for a subset of those movies they had seen and to rerate their original knowledge; finally, participants read summaries of the movie plots from a movie review database and again rerated their original knowledge. (The summaries were brief—less than one page in length—and came from the same database as the plot summaries used in training examples. Thus participants had a consistent sense of how to match level of detail to the rating scale throughout the experiment.) However, unlike with explanations, there was no significant drop of ratings over time (see figure 11.2).

In short, over a wide variety of other knowledge domains, we find little or no drop in ratings of the quality of one's knowledge after being asked to provide the knowledge and then being given a detailed "expert" description. Figure 11.2 shows a summary across all these follow-up studies and a comparison to the original IOED summary. The large differences imply that a distinctive set of factors converge to create an especially large metacognitive error with explanatory knowledge.

Developmental Issues

We began this chapter with the idea that knowing how well we understand causal structure in the world around us may underpin our drive to seek out explanations and to expand our understandings. We have shown that the estimates of understanding are systematically miscalibrated—the illusion of explanatory depth makes us think we understand more than we do, leading us to be satisfied well before we reach "full understanding." This finding raises two questions. First, why should shallow understanding feel satisfactory? Second, how does the ability to assess one's understanding change over time? We will start with the second question in this section, and address the first question in the following section.

How does an ability to assess one's understanding emerge during development? Young children seem to be globally overconfident about their knowledge, and thus it might seem that they would not show a specific illusion for explanatory knowledge. Instead, it seems they show homogeneous and extensive overconfidence for *all* kinds of knowledge, and only later, as their metacognitive skills improve, does the illusion gradually narrow down to explanations. There is an extensive body of work on children's metacognitive errors, including persuasive demonstrations of overconfidence in estimates about one's knowledge and memory, with especially large overconfidence for younger children. For example, in a classic study in the field, young elementary school children were presented with a series of pictures to remember. Pictures were presented serially, then covered, and children were asked if they could remember the covered items. Quite a few of the younger children would assure the experimenter that they could still remember all the covered items even when that number might include fifteen or so items (Flavell, Freidrichs, and Hoyt, 1970); yet when asked to actually recall the pictures, they often could only recall one or two.

These much larger errors of self-knowledge estimates in younger children raise the question of whether the specificity of the illusion of explanatory depth does not hold for younger ages. Perhaps an overall effect of overconfidence trumps younger children's sensitivity to the type of knowledge. However, one consideration that leads us to suspect developmental continuity of the IOED (an explanation-specific overconfidence) is this: the factors that converge to create a strong specificity of the illusion in adults might be at work in quite young children as well. The levels of analysis confusion and the represented versus decipherable confusion, for example, might influence the knowledge judgments of young children. A critical issue is whether those factors require mediation through a form of metacognitive awareness that is unavailable to young children.

Additional work in our laboratory has explored the presence of the illusion of explanatory depth and its possible specificity in children as young as five years of age. In those studies (Mills and Keil, 2004), an extensive training regime was needed to ensure that children understood the scales for self-ratings. Children who successfully passed the scale training then were given a task modeled after the adult IOED task except that simple devices and phenomena were used, and oral explanations instead of written ones were taken as data and then transcribed. In accord with previous metacognitive work, we found that the younger the children, the higher the average self-ratings of knowing a set of explanations. Beyond that effect, however, we found clear evidence for the IOED in children as young as 7: children dropped their ratings after an effort to explain, and this drop was independent from the effect of overconfidence. In fact, there was a suggestion of the same pattern even in 5-year-olds, but the effect was not significant, presumably due to the higher variance in responses. These results suggested that the presence of the IOED was quite different from a general developmental effect of greater overconfidence in younger ages.

To test the specificity of the illusion of explanatory depth more explicitly, we used a simplified methodology to explore young childrens' knowledge of procedures. As with adults, we found no drop in the successive ratings of their original knowledge after they expressed it orally or after hearing an expert account. This was in sharp contrast to the drops found with explanations. Again there was a generally higher level of confidence in younger children, but that effect, which is closer to the classic studies on metacognitive errors, is different from the within-subject decrease in self-ratings found with explanations (see figure 11.3).

We strongly suspect that the specificity of the illusion of explanatory depth to explanatory knowledge will also hold in children when the IOED is tested with respect to their knowledge of narratives and of facts as well. If so, then the special nature of explanatory knowledge and its unique relations to metacognitive abilities may emerge very early. It seems implausible that it would be present in

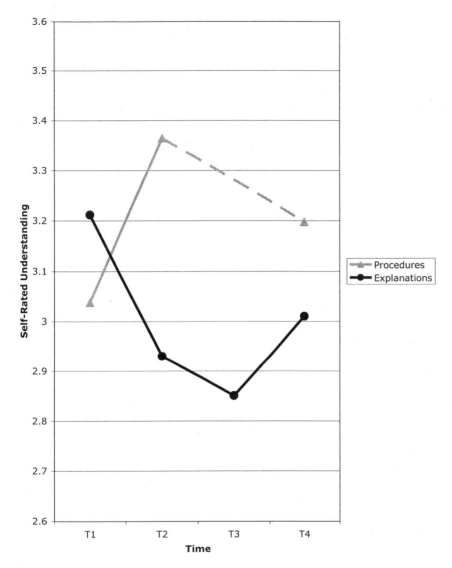

Figure 11.3
Self-ratings of knowledge averaged across all items and grades (K, 2, and 4) for explanations and procedures. The y-axis shows the children's average ratings on a 5-star scale (as opposed to the 7-level one used for adult studies). The x-axis is the same as in previous figures. (Adapted from Mills and Keil, 2004)

infants, but it may well start to emerge in the preschool years. This early emergence leads us to suspect that the effect will also be found in most cross-cultural comparisons.

Indirect Evidence for a Misleading Intuitive Epistemology

One way to get a sense of people's limitations is to consider how much they underestimate the work involved in construction and design of everyday devices. Even something as simple as a hammer or a snow shovel contains information about relative weights and torques that make for efficient and reliable use (e.g., Norman, 1989, pp. 141–151). This error is vividly demonstrated by the popularity of various novels about people transported back in time (or to a primitive planet) who then proceed to re-create much of the technology of their own civilization in situ. The original instance of this plot device, quite familiar to readers of the science fiction genre, can be found in Mark Twain's classic novel *A Connecticut Yankee in King Arthur's Court*. These stories of individuals single-handedly rebuilding high technology are engaging, but they are almost always utterly implausible to anyone who has a sense of the intense division of labor (including cognitive labor) on which a technological civilization depends. The history of technological progress and the individual experience of those of us who have tried their hand at design show that development from concept to prototype takes an enormous amount of trial and error.

Consider gunpowder, for example. How likely is it that an average citizen of 2004, thrust into a low-technology world, would be able to reinvent gunpowder as a propellant for cannon balls? The process of making gunpowder itself seems easy enough on the surface. Many of us have learned in high school chemistry that it is made by mixing carbon, sulfur, and saltpeter in the right proportions. Even if we do not remember the correct proportions for rapid-burning black powder (75% saltpeter; 14% carbon; and 11% sulfur), the ratios seem easy enough to derive through some elementary experimentation. Ignore, for the moment, any difficulties we might have in figuring out how to obtain the ingredients (how many of us know what saltpeter is, let alone where we might find it?). Also ignore the considerable problems of constructing cannon barrels strong enough to contain an explosion, of devising a reliable firing mechanism, and of making cannon balls of the appropiate size, weight, and composition. Consider only the problems of making gunpowder function as a propellant for cannon balls.

History gives some clues as to how difficult the problem really is. The formula, though well known to the Chinese since at least the tenth century, did not arrive in Europe until the early fourteenth century. The first cannons, however, were quite ineffective as siege devices (their primary use for the next 300 years), compared to the advanced trebuchet catapults of the period, and were even less effective on the battlefield. Indeed, gunpowder-propelled cannon balls would not become central to European warfare until the early sixteenth century (Hall, 1997; LeBlond, 1746).

Obviously, knowing the formula for gunpowder does not translate into a decisive military advantage in any direct sense. One problem is that simply mixing the components of the high school chemistry gunpowder formula produces an inefficient and unpredictable propellant, "serpentine" black powder, which tends to separate into its constituent parts during transportation. Worse, the burn rate of the powder—a critical factor to efficient propulsion of projectiles—is strongly influenced by small changes in compression. Tamp the powder too much and it burns too slowly; tamp it too little and it burns too quickly, with possibly disastrous results for the cannoneers.

Nearly 200 years of development passed before gunpowder became a sufficiently effective propellant for cannons to compete with catapults. A key insight was that wetting the gunpowder, then drying it into cakes, which were then granulated, produced several desirable properties. Granulated or "corned" gunpowder is much more stable and produces a substantially more powerful propulsive force. More importantly, by controlling the size of the granules, the manufacturer could control the burn rate, and produce different powder for different-sized cannons (Hall, 1997; LeBlond, 1746; to get a better sense of the complexity of the gunpowder manufacturing process, see Chambers, 1881).

Granulated gunpowder powder, when combined with advances in cannon manufacturing (e.g., the development of blast furnaces permitted casting of iron cannons) enabled artillery to destroy standing walls, thus changing the face of European warfare at the very end of the fifteenth century (Volkman, 2002). Further advances in cannon design made gunpowder the central force on the battlefield by the early sixteenth century (Hall, 1997). But how many time travelers, armed with the high school chemistry formula, would be able to re-create the 200 years of research and development in their lifetimes? Given that wetting one's gunpowder is not an especially intuitive step (until the invention of "corning," getting powder wet was considered a sure form of spoilage), we would venture, "Not many."

A Functional Account of the Illusion of Explanatory Depth

The "illusion" in the illusion of explanatory depth implies that the IOED is an error. However, as with other "errors" in reasoning, it may be misleading to think of the IOED as usually putting people at a disadvantage (see, for example, Gigerenzer, Hoffrage, and Kleinboelting, 1991; Gigerenzer, 1996). In many ways the IOED may be an adaptive and useful way of guiding our search for understanding. In particular, it may help us track causal patterns in the world at a grain of resolution that is just coarse enough to allow us to make headway in several domains of cognition without being swamped by the details of mechanism in any one domain.

The causal complexity of many natural and artificial systems is potentially unbounded in two senses. First, one can unpack causes into other causes almost without end. Ask most people how an electric motor works and they may refer to "magnetic forces" and "rotors." Ask them, further, how these forces work, and most "explainers" will founder as on the complexities of atomic and subatomic physics. The problem is even more evident in explaining biological phenomena such as how the heart beats. After first explaining the heart in terms of functional relations between anatomical units such as chambers and valves, most people will founder on the physiological and biochemical complexities of how the living tissues in those units work.

The problems of fully explaining anything are hardly new—science certainly gets along fine without "going all the way down" with causal explanations (Kitcher, 1993)—but they illustrate how, even in the sciences, we make considerable sense of the world with only partial explanations. Often we proceed by taking for granted certain sets of background assumptions that we unquestioningly use in our accounts. We might, for example, assume magnets have poles and fields with characteristic shapes without ever needing to know why those poles and field shapes exist.

This difficulty with complete explanations is not the only source of the illusion of explanatory depth, however. Much of the IOED effect seems to arise from omissions of detail at a surprisingly high level of explanation. People who overestimate their ability to explain how a helicopter flies are not overestimating their understanding of the particle physics of gases and airfoils. Instead, they are missing key details of the mechanics of rotors and blades. Similarly, the ignorance people confront in explaining flush toilets, zippers, and can openers is all at the level of mechanics. Even when they confuse having insights at one level with knowing the mechanisms of subassemblies, those subassemblies are often still explainable using principles of the same sort, such as physical mechanics. For example, if I do know that a bicycle derailleur moves the chain in and out so as to change gears, I may confuse having insight into that high level mechanical action with knowing the details of how that movement takes place.

By demonstrating that our representations of causal systems are not nearly as deep as we believe, the illusion of explanatory depth helps us constrain the nature of lay theories. Fully complete theories (of the sort that scientist strive for) are unlikely to be the common currency of everyday cognition. Most of us only hold deep, detailed understandings in relatively narrow areas of expertise. Yet we are often quite satisfied with learning a few bits here and there. A small thing, like understanding that the size of gunpowder granules determines the burn rate by controlling the amount combustible surface exposed to air, triggers a sense of comprehension.

Why should the feeling of insight come to us so early, at so little cost? We argue that the feeling of insight into causal systems indicates, not the sort of complete comprehension we intuitively assume, but rather the successful acquisition of a representation of a wholly different sort than a complete causal diagram.

The adaptive value of the illusion of explanatory depth may center around the ways it gives us tacit insight into various causal patterns, enabling us to make good guesses on how to seek out appropriate experts for further information. You may not know how a helicopter works in detail, for example, but you may have a sense of what sorts of causal patterns are relevant and who is likely to know more about those patterns. In addition, if you hear two competing explanations, you may be able to choose between them because you have some sense of what a decent mechanical explanation is likely to look like. Similarly, when you have the object in front of you, your coarse coding of causal relations may help guide your search for additional mechanistic details.

Put differently, the illusion of explanatory depth may reflect a genuine knowledge of high-level causal patterns and relations that are typically associated with broad domains such as mechanics, adaptive biology, chemistry, and social interactions. For example, much of mechanics is governed by immediate consequences of actions with monotonic relations between the force of a cause and the effect. For social interactions, altogether different parameters are more typical. The IOED may serve to tell us that we know enough to be able to judge explanations given by others, seek out appropriate experts, or guide ourselves profitably when we encounter an object or a phenomenon again. Thus the IOED is not, as is often assumed about general overconfidence, a false comfort in the face of ignorance, but rather a by-product of an accurate sense of knowing something more general, and more difficult to articulate: the implicit skeletal patterns of a device or phenomenon. The illusion occurs when we mistake having insight into the pattern of the sketch with knowing the mechanistic details.

Parallels with Change Blindness Blindness

There is now a well-documented illusion of knowing for visual scenes known as "change blindness blindness" (CBB; Levin, et al., 2000). People are grossly miscalibrated about what they think they can remember from recently viewed scenes; they seem to assume they have something like a video recording of a visually experienced event when their actual representation is much closer to a primitive sketch. The sketch captures overall layout of the terrain and some larger objects fairly well, but lacks details concerning the properties of objects such as color, shape, and even kind and presence. Although we are agnostic on the current debate about the role of eye movements in encoding object properties, and whether some trace of object properties is always encoded (e.g., Hollingworth and Henderson, 2002), regardless of the outcome of that particular debate, there is clearly a large mismatch between what people think they can report from experiencing a visual scene and what they can actually report.

To what extent is the miscalibration of change blindness blindness related to the illusion of explanatory depth? In both CBB and the IOED, individuals appear to hold misleading intuitive epistemologies. But, at higher resolution, the relationship may seem more remote. Most CBB tasks involve recall of information presented in an experiment as opposed to gradually acquired, longstanding knowledge of the sort used in the IOED tasks. In addition, CBB tasks seem to involve visual, apparently nonpropositional memories, whereas the IOED seems very much involved with propositional knowledge. We think these differences are consequential and that CBB and the IOED are different, but the parallels are intriguing and may illuminate important issues in both lines of research. First, we see no reason why a kind of scene blindness might not exist for much longer-term sorts of scene knowledge than the sort tested in the usual paradigm. Take, for example, errors of recall of the details of a highly familiar object such as a penny or a building that people have entered hundreds of times (Nickerson and Adams, 1979; Norman and Rumelart, 1975). A classroom demonstration that coauthor Rozenblit has used successfully also comes to mind. Cover your wristwatch without glancing at it first. Now, try to describe what the numerals on the face look like. Are they Roman or Arabic? What color are they? What is the shape of the hands? Most people are quite surprised by how little they recall of an object they have looked at thousands of times.

Although errors in recalling the details of familiar objects have traditionally been considered examples of schema abstraction, we think it highly likely that people's estimates of what they would know about such objects are severely at odds with what they actually know. We predict that similar errors would exist in people's judgments of how well they know features of their cars, their homes, or various national landmarks. We make this prediction because we believe visual recall to be another instance of misleading intuitive epistemology producing a systematic and gross metacognitive error.

A second point of convergence for change blindness blindness and the illusion of explanatory depth is a shared confusion between internally represented information and information that is recoverable in real time. Indeed, this has been an important claim in the CBB literature. A number of authors have suggested that the "out there" versus "in the head" confusion contributes to CBB; some have further argued that it is often more adaptive not to try to internally represent all the information in a scene when it easily recoverable as needed with additional glances (e.g., O'Reagan, 1992; Rensink, 2000). We have made a parallel argument for the adaptive nature of the IOED earlier.

The format of information remembered from scenes may also not differ as much from explanations as it seems. Indeed, propositional or verbal encoding of features seems to be an especially important way of increasing accuracy of recall of properties and relations from scenes (Simons, 1996). In addition, a sense of the perceptual properties of complex systems may play an important role in contributing to the illusion of explanatory depth. Our evidence for the last claim comes from exploring the magnitude of the illusion for explanations of different devices. When we looked at the differences between various explanations, we found that the strongest predictor of an especially large IOED is the proportion of visible components or processes (Rozenblit and Keil, 2002). For example, the larger the proportion of visible to nonvisible parts in a device, the stronger the initial confidence and overconfidence. It appears that having visual access to mechanism information increases the sense of understanding, often falsely. This finding also confirms our suspicion that confusion between represented information and information decipherable in real time contributes to the IOED: it is considerably easier to decipher systems with a higher ratio of visible parts.

If we are right in arguing that both the illusion of explanatory depth and change blindness blindness result in part from misleading intuitive epistemic theories, then the systematic differences in the magnitude of the IOED across different types of knowledge raises questions about the stability of CBB across different kinds of scenes. For example, having to identify objects in a heavily cluttered scene may make viewers more conservative about their abilities in much the same way that having to explain objects with mostly nonvisible parts would (for results suggesting that this prediction will hold, see Levin, 2002).

One difference between the illusion of explanatory depth and change blindness blindness may involve animation. Static visual arrays may not fully capture the perceptual factors that contribute to the IOED, one of whose sources may be people's ability to perform vivid mental animations of some simple causal relations, leading them to mistake successful animations with more complete understanding. For example, when asked to explain a simple mechanical device like a can opener, most of us have no trouble mentally animating some of the components, like the handle turning and the blade cutting into the lid. The vivid mental movie may be enough to give a false sense of understanding the whole system. Many of us would be surprised at not being able to describe, step by step, why the blade is cutting into the lid, or how the handle's turning makes the blade move forward rather than just spin in place. If we are right, we might analogously predict a stronger CBB for highly constrained animated scenes than for static ones.

Our basic point here is that understanding the relationship between the illusion of explanatory depth and change blindness blindness highlights the inaccurate (though possibly adaptive) naive epistemic theories most of us hold. The comparison also suggests an intriguing program of research that explores the content of those theories in more detail.

Future Directions

There are several lines of research that follow from the studies conducted thus far on how people assess the quality of their explanatory knowledge. One line follows from suggestions in our studies that expertise should be negatively correlated with overconfidence. We would like to test this explicitly. The most obvious test is to more systematically vary expertise in a domain and see how it varies with estimates of the details of one's understanding. Assuming the expert calibration effect is found within a domain, the question then arises as to whether expertise in a given domain immunizes one against overconfidence in neighboring domains. Does being an expert chemist, for example, make one appropriately cautious about one's understanding of physics? Does that caution extend to all disciplines or does it gradually diminish as a function of taxonomic distance? If a gradient for expert caution can be demonstrated, it might, in turn, be used as a measure of people's intuitive notions of the theoretical distances between domains.

A further question asks whether "expert explainers" are less subject to the illusion across domains. Teachers and expository writers face explanatory difficulties daily. If any group should show conservative estimates of their ability to explain, it is these expert explainers. Thus high-level experts who are not normally burdened with having to explain their work to outsiders might have a larger IOED than those who are.

Ideally, these issues should be explored under experimental conditions that manipulate the level of explanatory expertise. One such method could involve giving an experimental group hands-on training in how to explain complex concepts to an audience and how to assess their understanding. A control group would spend an equivalent amount of time in workshops, but would not get direct practice in explaining and in assessing comprehension. We predict that direct experience with providing explanations and getting audience feedback will, for a time, reduce the IOED. A follow-up study would explore how rapidly the inoculation against the IOED fades over time.

A different issue concerns the evaluation of one's own knowledge, as opposed to others'. Because self-assessment is involved, the observed overconfidence may be enhanced by a self-serving bias of the sort commonly noticed in several areas of social psychology. Our studies demonstrating differences in overconfidence across knowledge domains help make the self-serving bias account less likely. However, a more direct way to rule out the entire class of explanations that have to do with the drive to think positively of oneself would be to examine whether the IOED occurs with respect to others' knowledge. If the IOED is the result of an intuitive epistemology systematically misleading people into thinking their representations of complex systems are richer than they actually are, then the illusion should hold for others as well as for oneself. The target of the estimate (self versus other) did not matter with CBB (Levin et al., 2000), and if analogous factors are at work, it should not matter with the IOED either.

We are currently running a series of studies that asks people to predict how much others will know about various phenomena, and measures whether they are surprised by another person's inability to explain. We give the participants the same training on the same 7-level scale used in our earlier studies. Then we ask them to rate how well they think an average Yale undergraduate would be able to explain various devices or natural phenomena. We then show the participants actual explanations produced by actual Yale undergraduates (we have a large database of such explanations from our previous studies), and ask them to rate those explanations. Although data collection is not complete, the pilot results show a clear pattern. For both devices and natural phenomena, people appear just as overconfident about the explanatory understanding of others as they are about their own.

A question that intersects especially well with visual metacognition asks whether the perceptual salience of components contributes to the illusion. We can test whether perceptually salient components add to an illusion of understanding by (1) asking participants to visualize and mentally animate mechanical systems before rating their initial knowledge and (2) showing the same systems in both a "perceptually salient" condition (e.g., transparent casing, which shows the shows the working of internal parts) and a normal condition.

The principles governing the illusion of explanatory depth should also be used to predict instances of *under*confidence about knowledge. In general, we expect underconfidence when explanations are highly, but not obviously, constrained. Topics that can be taught using the Socratic method may be especially suitable because that method relies on the discovery of latent knowledge that one implicitly brings to the situation. For example, basic theorems of geometry and number theory, explanations of evolved social institutions (e.g., what does it take to create a common-law marriage?), and specific applications of general principles of justice should all produce minimal overconfidence, if not underconfidence.

Finally, to come full circle and return to visual metacognition, it would be interesting to explore how change blindness blindness for complex causal systems, such as intricate devices, relates to the illusion of explanatory depth. To what extent are ill-founded notions of having a vivid image of a device related to thinking one understands how it works?

Conclusion

We began by arguing that even a simple act of asking questions requires sophisticated metacognitive abilities. One needs to know that one does not know—to have some intuitive impressions of the limits of one's own knowledge. Metacognition has a profound impact on how we learn new information and understand new relationships. We need a better understanding of how people form metacognitive judgments about what they know. We began to explore how people assess their understanding with a particularly striking instance of miscalibration: the illusion of explanatory depth. We showed how the miscalibration for explanatory knowledge contrasted with relatively accurate calibration for procedures, narratives, and facts. We have further argued that the difference in calibration can be understood by exposing differences in domain-specific representations, and their interaction with people's naive epistemic theories.

The magnitude of the systematic metacognitive error with explanations suggests our intuitive epistemologies are misleading in predictable ways. A more thorough grasp of the illusion of explanatory depth will help us with the more general problem: understanding how people seek out new information and assess the quality of what they know. At the same time, the IOED may point to an important feature of lay theories. The functional account of the IOED we have proposed suggests nonexpert representations of causal systems should be sparse. The IOED may have an important role in enabling us to get the gist of key relations in a domain without being swamped by details. The benefits of getting by on lean cognitive representations of the causal relations around us may well outweigh the costs of being under an illusion of explanatory depth.

Acknowledgments

We would like to thank Paul Bloom, David Armor, Marcia Johnson, and Daniel Levin for their insightful comments and helpful suggestions. The preparation of this chapter was supported by National Institutes of Health grant R37-HD23922 to Frank Keil and a National Science Foundation Graduate Research Fellowship to Candice Mills.

References

Bjork, R. A. (1998). Assessing our own competence: Heuristics and illusions. In D. Gopher and A. Koriat (Eds.), *Attention and performance XVII: Cognitive regulation of performance: Interaction of theory and application* (pp. 435–459). Cambridge, Mass.: MIT Press.

Chambers, E. (1881). *Library of universal knowledge.* Edinburgh. Reprint, New York: American Book Exchange, 1728. (Reprint of last edition of Chambers's *Cyclopaedia,* with copious additions by American editors.)

Fischhoff, B. (1982). Debiasing. In D. Kahneman, P. Slovic, and A. Tversky (Eds.), *Judgement under uncertainty: Heuristics and biases* (pp. 422–444). Cambridge: Cambridge University Press.

Fischhoff, B., Slovic, P., and Lichtenstein, S. (1977). Knowing with certainty: The appropriateness of extreme confidence. *Journal of Experimental Psychology: Human Perception and Performance, 3,* 552–564.

Flavell, J. H., Freidrichs, A. G., and Hoyt, J. D. (1970). Developmental changes in memorization processes. *Cognitive Psychology, 1,* 324–340.

Gigerenzer, G. (1996). On narrow norms and vague heuristics: A reply to Kahneman and Tversky. *Psychological Review, 103,* 592–596.

Gigerenzer, G., Hoffrage, U., and Kleinboelting, H. (1991). Probabilistic mental models: A Brunswikian theory of confidence. *Psychological Review, 98,* 506–528.

Glenberg, A. M., and Epstein, W. (1985). Calibration of comprehension. *Journal of Experimental Psychology: Learning, Memory, and Cognition, 11,* 702–718.

Glenberg, A. M., Wilkinson, A. C., and Epstein, W. (1982). The illusion of knowing: Failure in the self-assessment of comprehension. *Memory and Cognition, 10,* 597–602.

Griffin, D., and Buehler, R. (1999). Frequency, probability, and prediction: Easy solutions to cognitive illusions? *Cognitive Psychology, 38,* 48–78.

Griffin, D., and Tversky, A. (1992). The weighting of evidence and the determinants of confidence. *Cognitive Psychology, 24,* 411–435.

Hall, B. S. (1997). *Weapons and warfare in Renaissance Europe.* Baltimore: Johns Hopkins University Press.

Hollingworth, A., and Henderson, J. M. (2002). Accurate visual memory for previously attended objects in natural scenes. *Journal of Experimental Psychology: Human Perception and Performance, 28,* 113–136.

Kitcher, P. (1993). *The advancement of science.* Oxford: Oxford University Press.

Kruger, J., and Dunning, D. (1999). Unskilled and unaware of it: How difficulties in recognizing one's own incompetence lead to inflated self-assessments. *Journal of Personality and Social Psychology, 77,* 1121–1134.

LeBlond, G. (1746). *A treatise of artillery: or, Of the arms and machines used in war since the invention of gunpowder.* London: E. Cave. (Available on the Internet at http://www.napoleonic-literature. com/Book_17/001-Title_Page.html.)

Levin, D. T. (2002). Change blindness blindness as visual metacognition. *Journal of Consciousness Studies, 9,* 111–130.

Levin, D. T., Momen, N., Drivdahl, S. B., and Simons, D. J. (2000). Change blindness blindness: The metacognitive error of overestimating change-detection ability. *Visual Cognition, 7,* 397–412.

Lichtenstein, S., and Fischhoff, B. (1977). Do those who know more also know more about how much they know? *Organizational Behavior and Human Decision Processes, 20,* 159–183.

Lin, L. M., and Zabrucky, K. M. (1998). Calibration of comprehension: Research and implications for education and instruction. *Contemporary Educational Psychology, 23,* 345–391.

Markman, E. M. (1977). Realizing that you don't understand: A preliminary investigation. *Child Development, 48,* 986–992.

Markman, E. M. (1979). Realizing that you don't understand: Elementary school children's awareness of inconsistencies. *Child Development, 50,* 643–655.

Mills, C. M., and Keil, F. C. (2004). Knowing the limits of one's understanding: The development of an awareness of an illusion of explanatory depth. *Journal of Experimental Child Psychology, 87,* 1–32.

Nickerson, R. S., and Adams, M. J. (1979). Long-term memory for a common object. *Cognitive Psychology, 11,* 287–307.

Norman, D. A. (1990). *The design of everyday things.* New York: Doubleday.

Norman, D. A., and Rumelhart, D. E. (1975). *Memory and knowledge.* In D. A. Norman, D. E. Rumelhart, and LNR Research Group (Eds.), *Explorations in cognition* (pp. 3–32). San Francisco: Freeman.

O'Regan, J. K. (1992). Solving the "real" mysteries of visual perception: The world as an outside memory. *Canadian Journal of Psychology, 46,* 461–488.

Rensink, R. A. (2000). The dynamic representation of scenes. *Visual Cognition, 7,* 17–42.

Rozenblit, L., and Keil, F. C. (2002). The misunderstood limits of folk science: An illusion of explanatory depth. *Cognitive Science, 26,* 521–562.

Simons, D. J. (1996). In sight, out of mind: When object representations fail. *Psychological Science, 7,* 301–305.

Volkman, E. (2002). *Science goes to War.* New York: Wiley.

Yates, J. F., Lee, J. W., and Bush, J. G. (1997). General knowledge overconfidence: Cross-national variations, response style, and "reality." *Organizational Behavior and Human Decision Processes, 70,* 87–94.

Yates, J. F., Lee, J. W., and Shinotsuka, H. (1996). Beliefs about overconfidence, including its cross-national variation. *Organizational Behavior and Human Decision Processes, 65,* 138–147.

Chapter 12

Misunderstanding Ability, Misallocating Responsibility

Jeffrey J. Rachlinski

Allocating responsibility for accidents is one of the law's primary functions. A default principle of accident (or tort) law in the Anglo-American legal tradition is that harm must "lie where it falls" (Holmes, 1881, at pp. 144). When harm results from conduct that the law considers negligent, however, then the law imposes the costs of the harm on the negligent party. Defining negligent conduct and administering this definition properly are therefore critical to determining who bears the cost of accidents.

Although the courts have adopted numerous formulations of negligence, all revolve around the reasonableness of a party's behavior. As the influential *Restatement (Second) of Torts* (ALI, 1965, sec. 283) puts it, "the standard of conduct to . . . avoid being negligent is that of a reasonable man under like circumstances." Even though virtually all activities create a risk of injury to others, tort law is not meant to convert everyone into insurers whenever they undertake some action (Henderson, 1976). But when conduct is unreasonable, liability attaches.

In turn, the determination of reasonableness can only be made with reference to the underlying purposes of tort law. Scholars and courts disagree somewhat as to the primary purpose of tort law, but there is substantial agreement on a number of basic principles (Dobbs, 2000). The two purposes scholars and courts most commonly cite for tort law are to encourage efforts to minimize the cost of accidents (the deterrence function; see Polinsky, 1989) and to make careless parties compensate their innocent victims (the corrective justice function; see Weinrib, 1992). In general, when people do not account for the risk of harm to others that their activities pose, courts will consider their conduct unreasonable. Holding people responsible for their conduct when the likelihood or degree of harm it poses is high, or when the harm is easy to avoid furthers the goal of deterring socially undesirable conduct by forcing those who engage in such conduct to pay for the harm it causes (Landes and Posner, 1987). Liability also furthers corrective justice goals by forcing those who engage in destructive behavior to compensate the victims of their actions (Fletcher, 1972).

In determining what constitutes reasonable conduct, however, the courts might have inadvertently set unattainable standards. On its face, the law demands nothing more than that people perform as well as their physical abilities allow.

People are only required to apply such skill and care in avoiding accidents as a reasonable person would under the circumstances (ALI, 1965, sec. 289). To determine whether a party's conduct was reasonable, courts inevitably must examine the circumstances surrounding an accident and judge whether a reasonable person could have avoided the accident. If the reasonable person, using ordinary attention, memory, and perceptual abilities, could have avoided an accident, then the fact that an accident occurred implies that the party was engaged in some unreasonable conduct. Thus, determining whether a reasonable person could have avoided an accident requires endowing the hypothetical reasonable person with cognitive abilities.

As discussed elsewhere in this volume, recent advances in metacognition suggest that the tort law's seemingly sensible reasonable person test holds people to a standard that they cannot achieve. The law's hypothetical reasonable person possesses those mnemonic and perceptual abilities consistent with the lay intuition of a judge or jury. If lay intuition suggests people can see things that most people actually fail to see, hear sounds that most people actually cannot hear, attend to stimuli that most people actually miss, and remember events that most people actually forget, then the reasonable person is a kind of superhero; ordinary people cannot conform their conduct to the entity endowed with these abilities. By comparing the conduct of ordinary people to an idealized superhero, the law allocates fault where none exists and labels reasonable conduct as unreasonable. Because recent research suggests that people commonly overestimate cognitive abilities, the application of the reasonable person test might undermine deterrence and produce results wholly inconsistent with ordinary notions of fairness and justice.

This chapter explores the question of whether the law's reliance on an intuitively based standard creates a kind of strict liability for accidents and identifies the consequences of this system. Unlike some of the cognitive impediments to sound legal judgment (Rachlinski, 1998), courts have never really considered the possibility that they systematically overstate people's cognitive abilities. Consequently, it is hard to place this metacognitive difficulty into a legal analysis. Nevertheless, this chapter attempts to do so, first by defining the reasonable person standard in greater detail and assessing whether this standard is excessive in light of recent research on metacognition, and then by describing the consequences of an excessive standard. Even though the standard appears too high, other factors suggest that perhaps an excessive, idealized standard is not so disastrous to the system as to warrant significant reform.

The Reasonable Person and the Real Person

It is well understood that tort law's reasonable person represents an idealized standard to which no one conforms all of the time (Keeton, 1984). People commonly take risky shortcuts and attention often lapses in the face of monotonous tasks: such is the stuff of negligence. Even though the standard is defined in terms of idealized rather than actual behavior, the reasonable person is intended to describe an ideal to which all can, if they try, conform. When people choose to take shortcuts or let their minds wander, then the law requires only that they pay for the harm that this choice produces. If the hypothetical reasonable person possesses abilities that exceed those of most real people, however, then the courts are holding people liable for innocent conduct.

Who Is the Reasonable Person?

The definition of the reasonable person must incorporate the purposes underlying the tort system: deterring socially undesirable conduct and compensating the victims of such conduct. In an effort to further these goals, however, the tort system has, somewhat intentionally, created a standard to which no one conforms all of the time. In effect, the system signals acceptable and unacceptable behavior. Everyone sometimes behaves in a socially unacceptable manner and the obligation that the reasonable person test creates is simply to pay for the consequences of such conduct. The reasonable person test is meant to create an administratively workable scheme for identifying inappropriate choices that people make.

The Reasonable Person and the Purpose of Tort Law   The reasonable person is a fiction, a "creature of the law's imagination" (Harper and James, 1956, at pp. 902). Courts and legal scholars have made numerous efforts to define the reasonable person precisely, but its meaning remains elusive. Inevitably definitions of the reasonable person are intertwined with tort law's diverse and sometimes conflicting purposes. Many scholars agree that the purpose of the tort system is to vindicate the rights of aggrieved parties and to compensate them, on the one hand, and to deter people from engaging in excessively risky conduct, on the other (Henderson, Pearson, and Siliciano, 1999). This view is by no means universal, however. Many law-and-economics scholars contend that deterrence is the primary goal of tort law (Posner, 1981). They worry that without the prospect of tort liability, people will take little or no account of the harm that their activities can impose on others (Calebrasi, 1970; Landes and Posner, 1987). For these scholars, tort law is a way of encouraging people to take cost-effective measures to reduce the cost of accidents. Other scholars deny that the tort system is meant to deter economically inefficient activity, arguing that it serves primarily to vindicate the rights of those who have been wrongfully injured (Coleman, 1992; Weinrib, 1992). These scholars argue that people have a right to be free from carelessly caused injuries, and tort law is a way of vindicating that right. This latter notion requires some definition of the rights that tort law will vindicate, but there is general agreement that community standards of conduct determine which risks are unacceptable risks (Coleman, 1992).

Despite some conflicts, the two basic purposes of tort law coincide often enough that the courts rarely find it necessary to delineate tort law's purposes with greater precision (Posner, 1981). Consider a hypothetical to illustrate why. Suppose a salesman driving to a business meeting is running late and wants to speed in order to arrive on time. Assume that, if he is late for the meeting, there is a 1 in 10 chance that his client will be so angry at his tardiness that he will suffer $5,000 in lost sales. Also assume that if he drives fast, he will make the meeting, but if he drives at a normal speed, he will miss it. Further assume that at a normal speed, he incurs a 1 in 100,000 chance of hitting (and seriously injuring) a pedestrian, whereas if he drives fast, that risk increases to 1 in 1,000. Suppose that the accident will impose $1,000,000 in costs on the pedestrian (in terms of lost wages, hospitalization, and some monetary quantification of the pedestrian's pain and suffering). Under these circumstances, the social costs of driving fast are $990 ($1,000,000 × [1/1000 − 1/100,000]) and the social benefits are $500 ($5,000 × [1/10]). Without liability for negligence, the driver faces incentives to drive fast, even though the net social costs outweigh the benefits, because he will realize only the benefits. A liability rule that imposes the full social costs of driving too fast on the driver, however, eliminates this incentive. Thus, according to a deterrence-oriented analysis, driving fast to make the meeting imposes unreasonable risks. An analysis under a corrective justice theory produces a similar result. To expose unwitting strangers to great risks of bodily injury for the sake of a business relationship violates their rights to safety, and a reasonable member of the community would not engage in such conduct.

Both deterrence and corrective justice concerns identify the degree of risk imposed as a critical factor in the negligence calculus (Posner, 1981). Under a deterrence theory, if driving fast only slightly increases the risk of hitting a pedestrian, say to 1 in 10,000, then the social costs of driving fast are relatively small (only $99). In such a case, the decision to drive fast is reasonable, inasmuch as it averts a $500 loss at a cost of only $99. If a business loss seems too trivial to compare to a physical injury, one can change the hypothetical to suppose that the driver is, say, an ambulance driver rushing to an accident, so as to make the type of loss consistent in importance with the type of injury, but, so long as physical injuries can be quantified, this change is not important. Even though the decision to drive fast imposes costs on the pedestrian, the law would consider such costs a necessary part of ordinary life. Likewise, under a corrective justice theory, people are entitled to drive, even though doing so places others at risk. Pedestrians are entitled only to be free from careless driving that needlessly places them at risk of injury. Walking the streets necessarily entails some risks. So long as those risks are not excessive or are not undertaken without regard to the pedestrian's interests, then they lie where they fall. Thus the competing theories underlying tort law often complement rather than compete with each other.

In some instances, however, the principles underlying tort produce different outcomes. Scholars argue, for example, that in many circumstances, even if the private benefits of an activity outweigh the social cost, a reasonable person might refrain from engaging in the activity (Keating, 1996). To see this, consider how the rush of a salesman to a business meeting might be treated differently from the rush of an ambulance driver to an accident. A deterrence theorist might argue that a reasonable person does not rush to a business meeting, but does to a medical emergency, because the stakes in the latter case are higher. Under this analysis, a reasonable person would speed to a business meeting if the stakes were high enough to justify the social costs associated with potential accidents that speeding would cause. A corrective justice theorist might, by contrast, condemn certain activities as inconsistent with social norms and, therefore, unacceptable. Hence speeding to any business meeting, regardless of the stakes, might be considered unacceptable ("unreasonable"), even as an ambulance driver's rushing to an accident might be considered acceptable ("reasonable").

Even with the mix of potentially competing concerns, the courts have settled on a generally accepted definition of the reasonable person. This definition incorporates corrective justice concerns: "The words 'reasonable man' denote a person exercising those qualities of attention, knowledge, intelligence, and judgment which society requires of its members for the protection of their own interests and the interests of others" (ALI, 1965, sec. 283 comment b). The definition also addresses deterrence concerns: the reasonable person determines whether "magnitude of the risk outweighs the value the law attaches to the conduct which involves it [requiring the actor to give] an impartial consideration to the harm likely to be done the interest of the other as compared with the advantages likely to accrue to his own interests, free from the natural tendency of the actor . . . to prefer his own interests to those of others" (ALI, 1965, sec. 283, comment e). In other words, the reasonable person factors the risk of harm to others into decisions about what activities to undertake and how to undertake them (deterrence model); in so doing, the reasonable person takes account of the value society places both on the risk and on the activities (corrective justice model).

Conformity with the Reasonable Person Standard
Whatever the definition, the idealized aspects of the "reasonable person" have long made it a subject of mockery. As one scholar put it, "this excellent but odious character stands like a monument in our Courts of Justice, vainly appealing to his fellow-citizens to order their lives after his own example" (Herbert, 1930, p. 12). According to this influential description, the reasonable person:

> invariably looks where he is going and is careful to examine the immediate foreground before he executes a leap or bound; neither star-gazes nor is lost in meditation when approaching trapdoors or the margin of a dock; never mounts a moving omnibus and does not alight from any car while the train is in motion; will inform himself of the history and habits of a dog before administering a caress; never drives his ball until those in front of him have definitely vacated the putting-green; never swears, gambles, or loses his temper; [and] uses nothing except in moderation. (Herbert, 1930, p. 12)

This tongue-in-cheek description is intended to persuade the reader that everyone engages in conduct that falls short of the requirements of the reasonable person. Although each of the examples above arises from actual cases in which a court held some conduct to be unreasonable, we easily recognize ourselves in at least some of these cases. Only the hypothetical reasonable person is free from negligence all of the time; the rest of us commit negligent acts.

Identifying the characteristics of the reasonable person also reveals the two common ways in which negligence occurs. First, people choose to undertake excessive risk in their activities. They take shortcuts, hurry along at an unreasonable pace, or simply choose to engage in conduct that entails greater risk than is socially sensible. Because the tort system forces people to bear the cost of such decisions, it removes any economic incentives for such conduct. Nevertheless, people might irrationally hope that their choices will not result in harm, or might rationally recognize that, in some circumstances, an injured party is unlikely to bring a successful tort action against them. People often might not even consider the risks to others that their actions create, but tort law holds them responsible for failing to do so. Second, people's attention often lapses in the face of monotonous, albeit dangerous tasks. Despite the law's admonitions, it is difficult to maintain focus on a repetitive task. Failing to pay as much attention to a task as the reasonable person would may not be a conscious choice, but it is still negligence and doubtless a common source of accidents.

The reasonable person, of course, never engages in either folly: She never makes choices that create socially unacceptable risks and never fails to pay attention when undertaking monotonous, dangerous activities. This is not to say the reasonable person does not impose some risks on others, only that those risks are low enough to be socially acceptable.

Why Rely on the Reasonable Person Standard?

Of course, no one conforms to the reasonable person standard all the time. The attributes that courts ascribe to the reasonable actor are true of no one. All of us have, at one time or another, leapt before we looked. Some have called for the elimination of the reasonable person test on these grounds. "If [the reasonable person] is truly an inadequate, unrealistic, and unmanageable creation and cannot readily be transformed into something more satisfactory, perhaps we should admit failure in our attempts to make fault a requisite to negligence liability (Reynolds, 1970, p. 410).

Why does the law rely on a standard to which not even saints conform? The use of a legal fiction to identify unreasonable conduct is a deliberate choice meant to solve a difficult problem of identifying culpable conduct (Keeton, 1984). Identifying when conduct imposes a socially inappropriate degree of risk is no easy task. Risk is an essential part of social life that innocent pedestrians and bystanders are obliged to recognize. At the same time, it is wrong to impose excessive risk on the innocent or impose it for no good reason. So long as the law attempts to sort reasonable risks from unreasonable risks, it is in need of some means of sorting the reasonable from the unreasonable. The courts have developed the hypothetical reasonable person in an effort to make the task tractable.

The administrative challenge of sorting reasonable from unreasonable conduct is complicated by the necessity of incorporating the underlying purposes of tort law into the sorting process. Simply describing the purposes of the system to the decision maker would not provide the decision maker with enough guidance without further elaboration. Identifying the deterrent goal of the system would provide some guidance as to what constitutes unreasonable conduct, but this is clearly inadequate on its own. Rarely will the full numeric estimates needed to impose an appropriate cost-benefit calculus be available. Similarly, identifying the imposition of community norms as the standard is similarly unhelpful without identifying what those norms or standards, are or at least determining how to identify and ascertain them. The only available cost-benefit calculus and sense of community standards are apt to be impressionistic at best.

The reasonable person converts the esoteric and intractable distinction between reasonable and unreasonable risks into a comprehensible, intuitive inquiry. People commonly judge conduct of others in their ordinary lives. Sorting people into those whom we would hire, befriend, or date requires judging the conduct of potential employees, friends, or lovers and assessing it as acceptable or unacceptable. In making such choices, we inevitably judge the conduct of others against an idealized, hypothetical standard. An employee that performs below expectations might get fired; we might reduce contact with a friend who mistreats us; and a disappointing first date might easily be the last date. In all three examples, we must judge the gap between what we expect out of a potential employee, friend, or lover and what we observe. It is only natural that the law should borrow the same judgmental skills for identifying unreasonable conduct. Rather than conduct an open-ended inquiry with no meaning, or a detailed cost-benefit assessment that requires information unlikely to be available, tort law asks only that the fact finder assess the actor's conduct against an idealized norm, just as we tend to do for our acquaintances.

Continuing with the hypothetical of the salesman driver who is late for a meeting, the law asks the fact finder to ask whether a reasonable person, under the same circumstances, would drive fast. A detailed cost-benefit calculation is not available, but an intuitive one is. The risks associated with speeding are well known (or can be identified and articulated during the trial) even though they cannot be quantified precisely. Likewise, most people understand the benefits of getting to a meeting in time. The court can judge, intuitively, whether driving fast is too risky by guessing whether a reasonable person who weighs the risks and benefits and considers community standards would engage in the conduct. If not, then the conduct is unreasonable, negligent, and creates the potential for liability.

The reasonable person inquiry thus performs the basic task of tort law—assignment of responsibility—in a way that relies on familiar cognitive processes.

Just as tort law is attempting to attribute harm either to blameless conduct, where risks are unavoidable or to blameworthy conduct by one or more legal actors, so, too, do ordinary people attribute conduct either to stable personality traits or to the vagaries of a situation in which people find themselves. Even as friends, employees, and lovers sometimes disappoint our expectations, all people inevitably fall short of the reasonable person standard from time to time. Reliance on this test makes the law's inquiry intuitive and tractable.

The use of the reasonable person test has other virtues beyond the familiarity of its methodology. It is also intended to avoid blaming the actor for accidents attributable to inalterable physical abilities (Keeton, 1984). Ascribing liability to someone for physical deficiencies would be inconsistent with both the deterrence and the corrective justice theories of tort law. The question for tort law is not whether a stronger, faster, or taller person would have avoided the accident, but whether a person with the abilities of the actor facing the situation the actor encountered could have avoided the accident. The reasonable person test easily incorporates these concern by formulating its test in terms of whether a reasonable person with the actor's physical characteristics could have avoided the harm (Dobbs, 2000).

Finally, the reasonable person test largely maintains an objective standard for liability (Dobbs, 2000). The test is not whether a person did his or her best to avoid harm, given the person's own personality, concerns, and interests, but whether a reasonable person would have been able to do so. As Justice Holmes put it (1881, p. 108): "When men live in a society, a certain average of conduct, a sacrifice of individual peculiarities going beyond a certain point is necessary to the general welfare. If, for example, a man is born hasty and awkward, is always having accidents and hurting himself or his neighbors, no doubt his congenital defects will be allowed for the courts of Heaven, but his slips are no less troublesome to his neighbors than if they sprang from guilty neglect." The standard of care is that of society at large and not that of the individual. The standard can thus also easily accommodate changes in community norms or even changes in the goals of tort law itself (Dobbs, 2000). Courts can also mold the reasonable person standard to support the underlying purposes of tort law. Under a deterrence analysis, the reasonable person is expected to make choices that maximize social utility. Under a corrective justice analysis, the reasonable person conforms to a community standard of conduct. Should society change what it views as a goal or change how it values certain activities, the reasonable person standard changes with it. In effect, the reasonable person is aware of how the community views certain activities and certain risks and incorporates these views into decision making.

The reasonable person test is thus "a child or certain social necessity" (Collins, 1970). It is designed to provide a means of identifying when it is not appropriate to take a shortcut or to allow oneself to get distracted. If a reasonable person would take the shortcut or get distracted, then doing so poses unavoidable risks and does not entail liability. If not, then doing so poses avoidable risks and entails liability for any harm that results. The exact contours and nature of the risks a reasonable person avoids are defined largely by a collective intuition about appropriate behavior. This makes the standard tractable, properly focuses attention on choices that could have been made, and facilitates change in community norms about behavior.

Beyond these attributes, the persistence of the reasonable person test in tort law also may result from the mild individualistic, almost libertarian, flavor it carries. In the American legal tradition, people are free to let their attentions wander or lapse, just as they are free to trespass or to break contracts, so long as they pay for the consequences of this conduct. Tort law sets a standard intended to guide people's conduct, to identify right and wrong. The obligation tort law creates is merely to pay for the consequences of these lapses, not necessarily to avoid them at all costs. After all, this is tort, not criminal, law. People can avoid liability by paying more attention, avoiding shortcuts, making appropriate inquiry into their surroundings, and generally behaving like the reasonable person.

In creating the hypothetical reasonable person, the law borrows heavily from the intuitive attribution process familiar to social psychologists. Social psychologists have argued that one of the fundamental cognitive tasks people face in social life is determining whether people's conduct results from their personality or from the vagaries of the situation in which they find themselves (Nisbett and Ross, 1980). Although errors can creep into this process, people generally rely on a set of rational heuristics to make such attributions. People attend to whether they observe the same behaviors in different situations and to whether other people behave the same way in the same situation (Kelley, 1968). These observations allow people to assess whether a behavior is the product of a stable, internal characteristic of the actor or whether it is a transient behavior attributable to the features of a situation. The reasonable person inquiry is meant to incorporate these well-developed abilities into the assessment of negligence. If the conduct of even an idealized reasonable person would replicate the adverse outcome that the actor in question produced, then blame for the adverse outcome does not lie with the actor. In such a case, blame is more sensibly ascribed to other actors or to the unavoidable risks of living in a complex industrial society.

The goal of the test is to harness the familiar process of social attribution to the task of identifying when a person should have behaved differently so as to avoid harm to others. The system is designed to avoid making people pay for physical limitations or for harms that result from unavoidably risky situations. Injuries that cannot be avoided cannot be deterred and also do not justify compensation. Thus, the focus of the reasonable person test is on choice and lapses, not on the circumstances or the physical or cognitive deficiencies of the actor.

The Role of Human Abilities in Assessing Reasonableness   The analysis of the reasonable person could end at this point in a tidy conclusion: people are free to make choices about the risk their activities pose to others so long as they pay for any consequences; the reasonable person test is meant to allow the fact finder to distinguish between accidents attributable to avoidable lapses in attention and to avoidable bad decisions from those accidents attributable to unfortunate, but unavoidable, situations or to a lack of physical ability. But such a conclusion overlooks an important consideration. If judges and juries endow the reasonable person with abilities greater than those most people possess, then close attention and good judgment may not be enough to avoid liability. If judges and juries overstate people's physical or cognitive abilities, then accidents that are really attributable to unavoidable risks will be judged avoidable, and reasonable conduct will be considered negligent.

To see this, reconsider the hypothetical, where a salesman driver faces a choice to drive moderately (and risk missing a business meeting) or quickly (and risk hitting a pedestrian). Suppose this driver hits a pedestrian, a woman, say, and the pedestrian sues him. If the accident was caused by negligent haste, then he is liable; if it was the result of ordinary misfortune, then he is not liable. To defend himself, the driver must claim that he was proceeding at a reasonable speed. In some cases, the legal fact finder (judge or jury) might have objective indications of this choice: the length of any skid marks could indicate the driver's speed, or an eyewitness could provide direct information on the reasonableness of the driver's conduct. Commonly, however, such indications are unavailable. Instead, the fact finder must make an inference about the driver's conduct from the circumstances. The question in many cases thus becomes whether a driver proceeding at a reasonable speed would have been able to avoid hitting the pedestrian. If so, then the only logical inference is that the driver was not proceeding at a reasonable speed.

This analysis reveals the important role that lay intuition about cognitive abilities plays in law. The inquiry requires that the fact finder mentally simulate the circumstances surrounding the accident with the hypothetical reasonable person at the wheel. The fact finder must visualize these circumstances, imagine the driver to be a reasonable person traveling at a reasonable speed, and then determine whether this fictitious person could have avoided the accident. This hypothetical driver must have some cognitive abilities in order for the fact finder to ascertain whether the situation would result in an accident.

To make the hypothetical more specific, suppose that the female pedestrian the driver struck had darted out into an intersection. Further suppose that the pedestrian claims that a driver traveling at a reasonably safe speed should have been able to stop or swerve in time to avoid hitting her. The driver denies this claim and asserts that he was traveling at a reasonably safe speed. Unless the trial produces other evidence of the driver's speed, the fact finder will have to infer his speed from the situation. In such a case, the reaction time imputed to a hypothetical reasonable driver could determine the outcome of the case.

Suppose that 25 mph is the speed limit and would be considered a reasonable speed. Further suppose that expert testimony reveals that after the brakes were applied, the driver's car would travel 37.5 feet if the driver were travelling at 25 mph. The fact finder must also impute a perception time (time needed to see the pedestrian and identify her as a hazard requiring full braking) and a reaction time (time needed to get the foot to brake) to the driver. If the fact finder assesses both the perception and the reaction time at 0.5 sec, the fact finder will arrive at a total stopping distance for the car of 74 feet if the driver was traveling at 25 mph (36.5 feet [36.5 fps for 1 sec] plus 37.5 feet of braking). If it can be determined that the pedestrian entered the intersection when the driver was more than 74 feet away, then the fact finder can conclude that the driver was driving too fast. The comparison of the outcome obtained by the driver to the outcome that would have been obtained by a "reasonable person" allows the fact finder to assess whether the driver's conduct was reasonable or unreasonable.

But what if the fact finder has overestimated both the perception and the reaction time of the "reasonable person"? Suppose that most people under these circumstances would actually have taken 0.75 sec to perceive the pedestrian and identify her as a hazard, and 0.75 sec to react. The total stopping distance for the true reasonable actor would therefore be 92.5 feet at 25 mph (55 feet before braking [36.5 fps for 1.5 sec] plus 37.5 feet of braking). Thus, if the driver was actually driving at the reasonably safe speed of 25 mph and the fact finder determines that the driver was 80 feet from the pedestrian when she entered the intersection, then the fact finder will mistakenly find that the driver was negligent.

The problem gets worse as conditions that might impair cognitive ability enter in. Even if a fact finder has a good appreciation of the abilities of the average person under good conditions, the fact finder might fail to appreciate the effects of darkness, unexpected situations, or distractions. In effect, a court cannot easily cure misperception by adopting a uniform standard for human reaction times—they depend too much on conditions. So long as a fact finder overestimates people's abilities or underestimates the effect of adverse condition on those abilities, the fact finder will infer that people are negligent when their behavior was reasonable.

A similar analysis can be applied to lapses of attention. For example, suppose that a woman is walking along a sidewalk under repair. Suppose that just as she approaches a break in the sidewalk that should sensibly be circumvented, she hears screeching brakes and a car sounding its horn in a nearby intersection. Although distracted, she continues walking and catches her heel on the break in the sidewalk. She falls and is seriously injured. Is she negligent? (Note that if she is, she may be unable to recover compensation for her injury from the municipality for failing to repair the sidewalk; but if she is not, then it is possible that she can recover.) The answer turns on whether a reasonable person would have been so distracted under the circumstance as to have failed to notice a break in the sidewalk. If not, then the fact finder must attribute the accident to a negligent lapse in attention; the court must conclude that a reasonable person would not have been so distracted as to be unable to avoid an avoidable hazard.

Thus, although the legal system's goal is to encourage people to make reasonable decisions, the assessment of their conduct commonly turns on an assessment of human abilities. Because of the importance of human abilities, the courts have made efforts to define the cognitive abilities of the reasonable person (Dobbs, 2000). Indeed, an assessment of the reasonable person's cognitive abilities plays an important role in the definition of negligence included in the *Restatement (Second) of Torts* (ALI, 1965, sec. 289), which requires that people use "such attention, perception of the circumstances, memory, knowledge of pertinent matters, intelligence, and judgment as a reasonable man would have." Hence the focus on reasonable behavior quickly turns to an assessment of whether an actor would have avoided causing harm if the actor had behaved reasonably.

At this point, the law provides little further guidance. The courts rely heavily on intuition to define human abilities. They assume only that ordinary people remember things a reasonable person would remember, attend to things a reasonable person would attend to, and see things a reasonable person would see. The courts have assumed that judges and juries have accurate knowledge about ordinary human cognitive abilities. This assumption, however, might be deeply flawed.

The Abilities of the Real Person
Recent research on people's beliefs about cognitive processes indicates that intuition about cognitive process is indeed inaccurate. Although people underestimate some cognitive abilities, such the ability to recognize pictures, research has documented two important circumstances in which people overestimate their abilities: inattention blindness and change blindness blindness (Levin and Beck, chapter 6, this volume). Both are critical to the kinds of tasks that jurors and judges must perform in the legal system and can contribute to misidentifying reasonable behavior as negligent.

First, people show a marked inattention blindness (Mack and Rock, 1998). That is, people over-estimate their ability to detect peripheral stimuli when concentrating on a particular task. In one compelling demonstration, 50% of the subjects concentrating on the complex cognitive task of tracking the movements of three basketballs among six people failed to notice the appearance of a person dressed in a gorilla suit among the basketball players, even though virtually all subjects predicted that they would notice the appearance of such unusual stimuli (Simons and Chabris, 1999). This and several similar demonstrations suggest that people underestimate the dramatic effects of concentrating on a particular task to the exclusion of peripheral events (Levin and Beck, chapter 6, this volume).

Second, people also display an ignorance of change blindness. That is, people fail to appreciate how difficult it is to detect changes in the perceptual environment (Levin et al., 2000). For example, in one study, subjects failed to notice changes in the environment that occurred between cuts in a video portraying a conversation between two women, even though they predicted they would notice such changes (Levin et al., 2000). Even though 76% of the subjects predicted they would notice a change in the color of dinner plates in the video, no subject watching the video actually noticed such a change. Other studies, in which two scenes that differ only slightly were presented in succession, reveal that subjects looking for the change took much longer to identify the change than they predicted they would take (Resnick et al., 1997). People's intuition about vision and attention told them that they would notice these changes right before their eyes, thereby discounting how cognitively difficult it is to recognize many changes.

Both inattention blindness and change blindness blindness have the potential to mislead courts as to the reasonableness of a legal actor's conduct. Drivers who fail to notice a stop sign, bicyclist, or construction worker might not be acting unreasonably. A fact finder might infer that the failure to detect hazards was the result of excess speed or failure to pay adequate attention to the task, even if the appropriate inference is that the hazard presented a particularly difficult detection profile. Similarly, underestimating the length of time that detecting a change in the visual environment takes in an ordinary person can distort the inferences people make about the circumstances surrounding an accident. As noted in the hypothetical, if a fact finder underestimates the length of time perception takes, the fact finder will infer that a driver was traveling faster than was actually the case. These two phenomena suggest that reliance on intuition about cognitive processes will lead courts astray.

The studies of inattention blindness and change blindness blindness arguably fail to reflect natural conditions. People in gorilla suits rarely pop into basketball games and even more rarely are they the cause of accidents. Likewise, the kinds of changes in the change blindness studies often involve unlikely or even impossible changes in the environment. Outside the psychologist's laboratory, plates do not magically change color, nor do scarves magically appear and disappear. By using exotic or outlandish changes, researchers may be exaggerating the existence of such an effect in two ways. First, an impossible change in the environment is necessarily an unexpected change. If people's expectations influence the ease with which they can detect changes, then impossible changes should be among the hardest to detect because they fail to track people's lifetime of experience with the real world. Second, impossible changes seem so outrageous and exotic that once identified, it becomes harder to see how they were missed than more ordinary or mundane changes. To be sure, some of the studies involve changes in meaningless symbols in which no expectations can be said to be present (Mack and Rock, 1998) and others involve impossible, but fairly mundane changes (Levin et al., 2000). Nevertheless, the size of the effects seen in the studies thus far might be far in excess of the size of the effects present in the real world. The underlying processes that produce inattention blindness and change blindness blindness might be, not a generic overstatement of cognitive abilities, but rather a failure to appreciate how sensitive the perceptual system is to distractions and expectations. If so, then the research thus far might be exaggerating the effect.

On the other hand, the subject matter of lawsuits does not consist of a random sample of the experiences people have in the real world. Tort suits occur only when accidents occur, and even then, only when there is some chance that the accident is attributable to the carelessness of someone other than the injured party. If many accidents occur precisely because of unusual or unexpected circumstances, then the research findings on inattention blindness and change blindness blindness may have more external validity than it might otherwise seem. People's sense of the cognitive abilities in many cases keeps them safe. Drivers understand that a complex visual horizon filled with cars, bicycles, pedestrians, construction workers, and complex traffic signs requires them to slow down to process potential hazards properly. If people fail to appreciate the importance of certain kinds of less familiar distractions, however, then they will fail to take precautions against the kinds of change blindness and inattention that lead to accidents. Likewise, the same failure to appreciate change blindness and inattention that caused the accident will influence the fact finder. Thus, courts will necessarily be reviewing behavior in those settings in which inattention blindness and change blindness blindness have the biggest effects. Even if the psychological studies seem a bit artificial, they may actually be identifying the circumstances in which the effects are the most important both to identifying the causes of accidents and to assigning responsibility for accidents.

One final link is also missing to connect the erroneous intuitions about cognitive abilities to the process of assigning blame in the courtroom—there is no direct empirical evidence on the issue. Although psychologists have conducted numerous experiments to identify misperceptions about cognitive abilities convincingly, there is no clear demonstration that these misperceptions lead to mistaken assignments of blame. It may be that the legal context adds safeguards that prevent the kinds of mistaken attributions that might arise form misperception of cognitive ability. A reluctance to blame people who otherwise seem to have tried their best to avoid accidents might make judges and juries skeptical enough to overcome their misunderstanding of cognitive abilities. Nevertheless, in the context of eyewitness identification, psychologists have convincingly demonstrated that mistaken beliefs about cognition can and do lead to wrongful criminal convictions (Findley, 2002). Because assignment of blame in a tort suit is generally much less serious than assignment of guilt in a criminal case, the influence of misperception of cognitive abilities might be even more pronounced in this setting. Indeed, all available evidence supports the intuition that overestimation of cognitive abilities has an enormous bearing on the accuracy of judgments in tort suits.

Consequences of the Mismatch between the Reasonable and the Real Person

A mismatch between people's actual abilities and those of the law's reasonable person seems, at least superficially, to be a legal disaster. Although the effect of the mismatch would vary somewhat in different circumstances, overstating people's ability to avoid accidents would generally lead judges and juries to brand reasonable conduct as negligent. It is easy to overstate the adverse consequences of this mismatch, however. A closer analysis suggests that courts do not completely trust the somewhat ad hoc reasonable person test. Several legal doctrines have evolved that reduce the influence of the reasonable person test and thereby ameliorate, to some extent, the impact of the mismatch. Nevertheless, because these doctrines are designed to address other concerns, including a sense that the reasonable person test is so vague as to be unreliable, they are ill suited to address the intuitive misunderstanding of cognitive abilities.

Strict Liability in the Guise of Negligence

If judges and juries persistently overstate the cognitive abilities of legal actors, then the system of negligence might, in practice, more closely resemble a system of strict liability. When a legal fact finder mistakenly assumes that a reasonable person could have avoided an accident, the fact finder will mistakenly attribute the accident to some unreasonable conduct, rather than to misfortune. Thus, people who are acting reasonably will seem unreasonable, when judged with a standard that misstates human abilities. Although the system purports to hold people liable only when their conduct is negligent, in practice, people will be found liable even when their behavior conforms to that of the reasonable person. The unwitting conversion of de jure negligence into de facto strict liability creates certain adverse incentives with respect to the corrective justice goal of tort law.

Adverse Incentives   Although, intuitively, it would seem that such a conversion would have profound effects on the incentive structure of tort law, the effects are apt to be much more subtle. It is well understood in the legal literature that neither a strict liability nor a negligence regime creates undesirable incentives with respect to the level of care actors might take (Shavell, 1980); under either regime, actors face incentives to take reasonable precautions against causing harm. Under negligence, actors who take all reasonable precautions against causing injury save money by avoiding liability, and any extra safety measures they may take beyond reasonable care simply impose extra costs on them, without conferring extra benefits. Under strict liability, actors are liable for all harm their activities cause, whether they take reasonable precautions or not; they minimize the total costs they face by taking all reasonable, but no further, precautions. So long as courts define reasonableness as minimizing total social costs, then both negligence and strict liability create the same incentives as to how much care to take when engaging in an activity. Both systems encourage people to behave as the reasonable person (Shavell, 1980).

Strict liability even has several advantages. Because the strict liability rule is a comparatively simple one—actors pay for all harm they cause—strict liability is a cheaper system to administer; it does not create complicated and expensive litigation over what constitutes reasonable behavior under a given set of circumstances (Landes and Posner, 1987). Although litigation over whether the actor has actually caused harm can still occur, issues of causation are also litigated under a negligence system. By removing the reasonableness issue from the litigation process, however, strict liability makes the system run more cheaply. Furthermore, strict liability gives actors the incentive to make the best choice with no need for their conduct to be judged afterward by the court. By contrast, because of the uncertainty associated with the reasonableness test, a negligence regime creates incentives to take an excess of care (Calfee and Craswell, 1984; Rachlinski, 1998). This occurs because potential tort defendants may recognize that, if they take a slight excess of care, they might manage to avoid any possibility of being found liable, thereby incurring a significant reduction in the likely costs that they would face.

Strict liability does have problems, however, particularly when it is unintended. Most notably, it raises the cost of the underlying activity (Polinsky, 1989). As can be seen from the hypothetical, it is more expensive to drive under a strict liability than under a negligence regime. By "taxing" an activity, strict liability can inefficiently shift people's behavior from one activity to another. Perhaps more people would walk if driving were governed by strict liability, which might be undesirable (Polinsky, 1989). Therein lies the economic danger of administering a negligence system in a way that unwittingly converts it into a strict liability system. Courts adopted a negligence system deliberately to allow people to drive or walk as they wish, without the costs associated with strict liability.

Also, a strict liability system that results from a metacognitive bias in the negligence determination has other undesirable effects. Inasmuch as it is not straightforward strict liability, it still requires that a court assess reasonableness. Thus, a metacognitively biased negligence system produces costs similar to those for strict liability, but without the litigation cost savings of straightforward strict liability.

What is more troublesome, however, is that such a biased negligence system is also likely to produce incentives to take an excess of care beyond that required by reasonableness alone (Rachlinski, 1998). Because the system is not true strict liability, it holds out the possibility that an actor can undertake such an excess of care that when accidents happen, even with a biased inquiry, the courts would not find the actor's conduct unreasonable. The savings an actor realizes from avoiding liability with the excess precautions encourages the actor to take an excess of precautions. This incentive does not occur with true strict liability because there is no chance the actor will ever avoid liability in the event that harm results.

Consider how this might work with our hypothetical. The fact finder would find the salesman driver driving at the reasonable speed of 25 mph liable because of a mistaken belief that the perception and reaction time of the reasonable person is 1 sec. Suppose, however, the driver drives more slowly, say at 20 mph, even though a reasonable person would take 1.5 sec. If so, then his actual total stopping distance is now 68 feet (44 feet before braking [29.5 fps for 1.5 sec]) plus 24 feet of braking). This means that any accident that occurs would have to have resulted from the pedestrian appearing in front of the driver at 68 feet or less (otherwise the driver would have stopped in time). With its biased assessment of perception and reaction time, the jury would assume that a reasonable person traveling at the "reasonable" speed of 25 mph would have been able to stop within 74 feet (as calculated before); any accident occurring at less than that distance would not be attributed to the driver. Thus, by overcomplying with the reasonable person test, the driver can be sure to avoid liability. This excess compliance will cost the driver in terms of lost time; but that loss is offset by avoiding the risk of liability and might be worth the price to the driver, even though it is inefficient overall.

Although it might seem perfectly sensible for the system to produce incentives to undertake a slight excess of safety, excess safety has hidden costs. Often safety precautions are so cumbersome they make the underlying activity worthless. Consider, for example, police safety vests: they can be made to have open sides or to completely wrap around the user. The latter are safer, but they make it difficult for the user to move, so much so that they create other risks. Similarly, if all drivers slow down, they might reduce the overall speed of traffic, thereby costing other drivers time or creating traffic jams that cause pollution. An excess of safety has costs and might pose hidden risks (Sunstein, 1996).

Corrective Justice   Whatever the economics, strict liability seems unjust. Only law professors and economists are truly sanguine about the label of negligence. Most people regard a legal judgment of negligence as a kind of stigma, not as bad as being judged criminally culpable, but certainly not something that is either desirable or even neutral. As a matter of justice, if the courts have deliberately adopted a system of liability for negligence, then finding people negligent who actually took due care is wrong. It mislabels an innocent party as a wrongdoer and compensates those who have no real entitlement to compensation.

Furthermore, in a case in which the actor only seems negligent because of a biased adjudication process, actor and victim are equally blameless. The victim of the accident did nothing to deserve the injury, but if the actor who caused the injury behaved reasonably then the actor is not at fault either. After all, the actor obeyed society's command to behave reasonably. Such circumstances do not justify charging the actor with the cost of the injury and branding the actor a wrongdoer, nor do they justify giving the injured party compensation. The law's basic maxim to "let the harm lie where it falls" trumps any desire to compensate the injured victim. Unless the actor actually failed to comply with social norms, then neither the cost nor the label can be properly justified. Biased negligence processes thereby undermine the very morality of the tort system.

On the other hand, whatever the label, this misbranding is perhaps not such a serious injustice. Most drivers, for example, know that the act of driving exposes them to liability. They know that even if they are careful, they might find themselves the target of a lawsuit, which they might even lose. Most people insure against serious loss and live with the consequences of a system that might occasionally mislabel one's conduct. Furthermore, after an accident has occurred, the defendant also reviews his own conduct in light of the metacognitive biases that psychologists have identified. If the driver is uncertain about what speed he was traveling, then he might make the same inference that the legal fact finder might make. Oddly enough, even if the process is unjust, the actor himself, suffering from the same cognitive biases as the fact finder, might fail to notice the injustice (Rachlinski, 1998).

Furthermore, there is a global sense in which some of the biases in cognitive metacognition are intuitive. A lifetime of experience teaches people that, when their attention is focused on one task, they often miss distractions. Indeed, the ability to avoid processing distractions is the essence of concentration. In the driving example, it is not so much that the salesman driver was traveling too fast that makes him a danger to pedestrians. Rather, it is the dangerous attentional focus that being late creates. The pressure of having to drive quickly can easily lead the driver to miss important aspects of their environment. The mistake lies in failing to arrange one's time properly so as to avoid having to drive while in a hurry. Arguably, inasmuch as everyone seems to suffer from metacognitive biases, this mistake does not represent negligent behavior; rather, it is a by-product of how reasonable people think about their cognitive abilities. Nevertheless, it is a mistake. In the end, people might get roughly what they deserve: they put others at risk because they overestimate their abilities, and they are held liable because a fact finder also overestimates their abilities.

The Effect of Conflicting Metacognitive Biases   If people overstate their ordinary cognitive abilities, then they might also overestimate their ability to perform various skilled tasks safely. In at least one study, 86% of automobile drivers stated that they drive more safely than the average driver (Svenson, 1981). If people constantly see other drivers failing to react as quickly as they predict they would be able to react, people experience a world filled with unreasonable drivers who are less safe than they are.

Legal scholars have noted that such optimistic overconfidence might lead people to engage in conduct that seems safe to them, but is in fact negligent or even reckless (Jolls, Sunstein, and Thaler, 1998; Korobkin and Ulen, 2000). People who believe that they can easily avoid an accident might not worry much about their risk of causing an accident or the legal liability they might face if they do cause an accident. Overconfidence can thus undermine the ability of the legal system to induce people to undertake reasonable care. People who engage in unreasonable conduct while believing their conduct to be reasonable cannot easily be deterred by the prospects of tort liability.

An excess of optimism can induce people to undertake excessively risky activities, but it can also induce people to undertake excessive precautions (Posner, 2003). Optimism can produce an excess of care if people overestimate the benefits of precautions that they consider taking. For example, if drivers believe that undertaking a single precaution (perhaps driving 5 mph under the speed limit) would reduce the possibility of an accident to zero, then they would undertake that precaution, even if it is not a cost-effective measure to undertake. It is unclear whether an excess of optimism arising from misperception of cognitive abilities would operate in this way. Overestimating one's cognitive abilities seems intuitively like a prescription for inducing dangerous conduct. In particular, overestimation of one's abilities might keep drivers from slowing down when they face a complicated or distracting array of stimuli. If such overestimation also produces a tendency to overestimate one's ability to avoid an accident with just a little excess of care, however, it might produce an excess of care.

If overestimation of cognitive abilities produces excessively risky conduct, then it has a doubly pernicious effect on the legal system. It may be that we have a system in which people unwittingly drive negligently (they drive in a manner they mistakenly feel is safe), while at the same time they are held to a standard that they cannot meet (legal fact finders assume the reasonable person can drive more safely than people really drive). Even though the legal system is actually creating incentives for drivers to drive too slowly, drivers, overconfident in their abilities, fail to recognize or disregard these incentives and go on driving in a dangerous fashion.

Overestimation of cognitive abilities on the part of both potential tortfeasors and legal fact finders thus combine to produce an odd system. Potential tortfeasors overestimate their abilities, thereby failing to undertake reasonable precautions against causing harm. At the same time, the system holds potential tortfeasors as accountable as if the tortfeasors had the abilities that they believed that they possessed. In effect, people behave as if they possess heroic cognitive abilities and are held accountable as if they had such abilities. Although it is possible that tortfeasors recognize that they will be held to a high standard if they are found liable and adjust, it does not seem altogether very likely that this doubly biased system is altogether a sensible arrangement.

Legal Doctrines That Blunt the Effect of Misjudgment

Several developments in the common law over the past century have served to blunt the effect of the mismatch between the reasonable person and the real person. Indeed, if the mismatch were as widespread as the psychological research suggests, it would be surprising if centuries of common-law development had not, in some way, accounted for these misperceptions. Judges, as intuitive psychologists are unlikely to have uncovered the same phenomena that required careful research to document, but they might have observed difficulties with the reasonable person test as it evolved. Biased application of the reasonable person test might produce undesirable or unreliable sets of verdicts over time that astute courts, or even legislatures, might have noticed and attempted to correct. Identification of such problems might be one reason that courts developed alternative means of identifying negligence.

Bright Line Rules   In fact, courts avoid the ad hoc implementation of the reasonable person test if possible. Several bright-line rules of conduct have emerged. Most notably, for accident law, the violation of a safety rule or regulation provides per se evidence of negligence (Dobbs, 2000). For example, driving at a speed in excess of the speed limit is, without excuse or justification (as might be the case for a life-threatening emergency), enough evidence to support a determination that the driver was negligent. In effect, neither are drivers entitled to rely on their own judgment about what would constitute a safe speed nor may a judge or jury substitute their judgment. The law provides a safe maximum speed, and exceeding it is negligence, even if it seems as if a reasonable person would do so.

To be sure, bright-line rules are incomplete; moreover, they tend to be asymmetric. Although exceeding a speed limit provides conclusive evidence that the driver was traveling at a negligent speed, driving within the posted speed limit does not provide per se evidence that a driver was traveling at a reasonable speed (Dobbs, 2000). This leaves plenty of room for judges and juries to make their judgment as to the safety of a driver who does not cross a bright line and might nevertheless be negligent.

Comparative Negligence   Probably the most dramatic shift in negligence law in the last half century has been the nearly universal adoption of shared liability systems (Dobbs, 2000). The common law developed under a fairly absolute system in which the courts attributed liability completely to the plaintiff or the defendant. Defendants found to be negligent could expect to pay for the full extent of harm their negligence caused unless they could show that the plaintiff was also negligent, in which case they would pay nothing. This system, known as "contributory negligence," however, survives only in a handful of American jurisdictions (Dobbs, 2000). Comparative negligence regimes, in which liability is shared between the two negligent parties, are now the dominant norm.

Comparative negligence blunts the effect of any metacognitive biases in the process. Just as a jury that overestimates the defendant's abilities is apt to find even a reasonable defendant's conduct culpable, the jury might do the same to the plaintiff. For example, taking our salesman driver as defendant and our female pedestrian as plaintiff, the jury that believes that a driver who was driving reasonably would have seen a pedestrian in time to have avoided the pedestrian might just as likely believe that a reasonable pedestrian would have seen the driver in time to have leapt out of the way. Under a comparative negligence system, even if both the driver and pedestrian are, in reality, not at fault, both will be held responsible. Although, ideally, if the defendant was not really at fault, he should not have to pay anything, the comparative negligence regime at least ensures that the defendant will pay less than he otherwise would, thereby blunting the effect of metacognitive biases. Likewise, even though the plaintiff might be blameless (hence perhaps entitled to a full recovery), the jury might find her negligent. Under a comparative negligence system, her recovery, though reduced because of metacognitive biases, would not be eliminated, as it would be under a contributory negligence system.

Misperceptions of cognitive abilities help explain the attraction of a comparative negligence system. Although the attraction of a comparative negligence system might seem obvious—in that it apportions liability between the parties in a way commensurate with their relative fault—the system also has a significant downside. Even as it does nothing to make incentives more efficient, it entails substantial litigation costs (Landes and Posner, 1987). Economics aside, comparative negligence also seems to blunt many of the sharp distinctions the law makes between degrees and types of misconduct. Some misconduct is so pernicious that the liability it creates should not be reduced by the good fortune to have been directed at someone who may have been slightly negligent. The overall advantage of a comparative negligence system becomes more apparent, however, once the courts recognize that the negligence analysis they have created contains significant potential for inaccuracy. If the reasonable person test is truly unreliable, then it might make little sense to rely on it as if it were a perfect indicator of reasonable and unreasonable conduct. In effect, the comparative negligence scheme is a less confident approach to liability that softens unnaturally sharp divisions the law might otherwise make. Although the courts' lack of confidence in the reasonable person test can be justified in many different ways, clearly, if fact finders lack a good understanding of human cognitive abilities, their assessments of reasonableness will commonly be inaccurate.

The Adverse Consequences of Comparative Negligence   One interesting aspect of the switch to comparative negligence is that it undermined the development of legal doctrines that could have further reduced the effect of metacognitive biases on the courts. For example, the courts were at one time developing a "legal distraction" doctrine (Keeton, 1984), which holds, as a matter of law, that certain distractions common to modern life were so prevalent, uncontrollable, and pernicious that they constitute a complete defense to a claim of negligence. For example, in one case, a woman tripped on a break in a sidewalk while being distracted by the sound of a nearby car horn (*Knapp v. City of Bradford*, 1968). She claimed that she failed to notice the break in the sidewalk because of the distraction. The court held that such a distraction would have diverted the attention of any reasonable person hence the woman's momentary inattention could not be said to be negligent.

The legal distraction doctrine developed in response to a comment in the *Restatement* defining the skills and abilities of the reasonable person (ALI, 1965, sec. 289, comment b). The comment contends that unavoidable distractions might be said to undo a finding of negligence that would otherwise attach to a lapse in attention. It also identifies examples of avoidable distractions. For example, driving while also trying to quiet a screaming child might still be found negligent, inasmuch as the reasonable driver should pull over. Other, more sudden distractions that would divert most people's attention and were beyond the actor's control, however, should preclude a finding of negligence for inattention.

In developing this "legal distraction" doctrine, the courts were, of course, relying on their own intuition about what a reasonable person would find distracting. In effect, they were substituting their own judgment about the effect of distractions on attention for that of a jury, yet there is no reason to assume that such judgments are any better informed than the ad hoc judgments about cognitive abilities juries are asked to make. Nevertheless, the development of such a doctrine reflects an attempt to reach a consensus on human ability that might at least in part be informed by empirical findings and expert evidence.

The legal distraction doctrine which, like its more influential cousin, the "last clear chance" doctrine, once gained ground as a means of softening the apparent harshness of contributory negligence, is now in retreat, arguably because of the shift to comparative negligence. That a plaintiff driver who would otherwise recover from a clearly negligent defendant driver could lose entirely, under contributory negligence, if the plaintiff's attention had lapsed somewhat seemed to courts an unjust result if the lapse in attention was not really the plaintiff's fault. Hence the courts needed a doctrine to address such circumstances. By contrast, under a comparative negligence regime, they simply place the conduct of each party into evidence and let the fact finder compare fault under the circumstances. Courts have, in effect, taken the easy way out by forcing legal fact finders to weigh the relative fault of each party case by case.

Under a comparative negligence system, the effects of metacognitive biases are uncertain. Both plaintiff and defendant will seem more culpable than they actually are. In practice, the effects of such biases on the two parties are unlikely to cancel each other out; instead, depending on the role that cognitive abilities play in the assessment of each party, one or the other party may gain some unwarranted advantage. Because it is hard to determine whether overestimation of human abilities generally favors plaintiffs or defendants, one cannot come to any clear conclusions about the effects of metacognitive biases under such a system.

The Plaintiff in Products Liability   One area of law where the courts do seem concerned with the overstatement of human abilities is products liability law. If courts overstate people's ability to avoid injuries, then the users of many products might find themselves unable to recover from manufacturers who sell products that fail to protect users against foreseeable lapses in attention or ability. That is, users will often erroneously be found negligent for failing to pay enough attention while using a product or for using the product in an unreasonable fashion. If such findings consistently exonerated manufacturers, they would fail to undertake safeguards against such avoidable injuries. To avoid this problem, courts charge manufacturers with saving plaintiffs from their own negligence, so long as such negligence is foreseeable (Dobbs, 2000).

For example, again consider the hypothetical, where the salesman driver traveling at a reasonable speed is judged unreasonable because the fact finder overestimates his ordinary human ability to react to road hazards. Suppose that, instead of hitting a pedestrian, the driver hits a large rock in the road, causing him to lose control of his vehicle. If a fact finder determines that a reasonable person could have seen the rock sooner or reacted to it more quickly than a real person actually could, the fact finder will identify the driver's negligence as a primary cause of his injuries. If a products liability system recognizes driver negligence as a defense to any claim by the driver that the automobile manufacturer failed to install available, cost-effective safety devices into the car, then the manufacturer will face fewer incentives to install such devices. Misperceptions of cognitive abilities might make negligence determinations against users so common and so erroneous as to dramatically undermine incentives for the manufacturer to make a car crashworthy. Recognizing this, the courts limit findings of negligence when such negligence is foreseeable.

This analysis is even more compelling for lapses in attention. A plaintiff who has mangled a finger while using a meat grinder can still recover from the grinder's manufacturer, even if the plaintiff was negligently distracted while using the product (Dobbs, 2000). The logic underlying this outcome is that manufacturers of such devices know that, given ordinary human cognitive abilities, users will get distracted at one time or another. If, in the face of such knowledge, manufacturers fail to install cost-effective safeguards to protect the users from their own negligent inattention, then the manufacturers will be held liable.

In developing modern products liability law, courts seem to have recognized the inevitability that users will take shortcuts and get distracted. By adopting this position in products liability cases, courts are effectively avoiding ad hoc, case-by-case judgments about users' abilities. The manufacturer, with a wealth of knowledge about the product and the likely lapses in users' attention or abilities, is in a much better position to avoid harm than a user (Dobbs, 2000). Furthermore manufacturers effectively control many of the circumstances determining how their products get used: whether these products will invite distraction, present overly complicated arrays of stimuli, or encourage haste. Manufacturers' design choices are closely analogous to driver's decisions about the circumstances as to when and under what conditions to drive. Like ordinary drivers, manufacturers might also suffer from misunderstandings of cognitive abilities. But, unlike ordinary drivers, manufacturers have the capacity to employ human factors experts and rely on aggregate data on the effects of product design to guide their choices.

Ignorance of human cognitive abilities might constitute a sensible defense for an ordinary automobile driver, but not for an automobile manufacturer.

Hence manufacturers remain accountable, even though it may appear that users are negligent. Although courts will still consider the apparent negligence of user plaintiffs, they will not preclude recovery. In effect, courts do not trust their own judgments about users' negligence, instead forcing manufacturers to guard against foreseeable negligence by users. Thus, even if courts overstate users' abilities, this overstatement does not adversely affect the products liability system.

Expert Testimony on Human Performance and Perception of Human Performance

Perhaps the most straightforward means of correcting erroneous beliefs about cognitive abilities is with expert testimony. Under prevailing standards for admissibility in the federal (and also many state) courts, expert testimony is admissible if it is reliable and would prove helpful to the jury (*Daubert v. Merrell Dow Pharmaceuticals*, 1993). Reliability requires that courts delve into the scientific process, but the standard that courts are using would clearly favor admissibility of the psychological research on both cognitive abilities and metacognition. Virtually all such research is reported in peer-reviewed journals, a consideration courts treat as important; moreover, none of it has been prepared specifically for litigation, a problem for certain types of testimony. Such testimony faces other obstacles, however.

First, some judges might not consider expert testimony on human cognitive abilities to be helpful to the fact finder. To the extent that judges believe that intuition about human cognitive abilities is reasonably sound and universally shared, they will see no need for such testimony. Such reasoning clearly treats psychology as a second-class science, although scholars have identified such treatment in other contexts (Saks and Baron, 1980). A serious review of the research on cognitive beliefs should convince objective observers that there is much about human cognitive abilities that is not intuitive. In essence, the recent metacognitive work should pave the way for admissibility of research on cognitive abilities.

The metacognitive work itself, however, encounters a second problem with admissibility. It is one thing to convince a court that laypersons do not have a firm understanding of intuitive abilities, but metacognitive work goes further, undermining reliance on the reasonable person test altogether. If a court were to accept the validity of testimony on metacognitive biases, it might well conclude that the reasonable person test cannot be administered properly. Indeed, the metacognitive literature has, as yet, found no evidence that erroneous beliefs can be corrected sufficiently to make the reasonable person test workable. Consequently, expert metacognitive testimony indicating that lay intuition overstates cognitive beliefs is more a point of law and policy than of fact, which might dispose of a specific case. As such, this testimony is best addressed toward legal reform rather than case-specific inquiry. Courts will therefore be reluctant to admit it because expert testimony is supposed to help the fact finder to determine what happened, not help the court determine what rules to apply.

Conclusion

The findings of cognitive psychologists who study what people know about cognitive abilities identify a deeply troubling aspect of the reasonable person test. To help the fact finder identify reasonable and unreasonable conduct, the reasonable person must be endowed with cognitive abilities. If these hypothetical abilities exceed those of most people, then the system will improperly identify reasonable conduct as unreasonable. Although some legal doctrines soften the effects of this error, they are not intended to remedy metacognitive biases and so cannot correct for them adequately. Neither can expert testimony be expected to meaningfully correct the problem. In the end, because of the great utility and long tradition associated with the reasonable person test, the courts will likely have to live with the problems that metacognitive biases create.

Realistically, the research on visual metacognition is unlikely to affect the widespread reliance on the reasonable person test as it now exists and is implemented. First, the test has a long history behind it. Second, the intuitive aspects of the test are at the heart of its virtues. The intuitively based aspect of the test is designed precisely to make the negligence inquiry tractable. Tractability at the expense of accuracy is hard to tolerate, but the degree of inaccuracy would have to outweigh the virtues of tractability. Third, as the research now stands, the influence of metacognitive biases on real behavior and real negligence determinations is uncertain. It may be that in the real world, other aspects of cognitive processes allow people to muddle through well enough (see Flavell, chapter 1, this volume). It may be that metacognitive errors lead us astray only in unusual or novel circumstances (see Levin and Beak, chapter 6, this volume).

Despite these limitations, the research on metacognitive biases has serious implications for the legal system that should not be ignored. Even a venerable judicial institution should not be immune from progress in the social sciences. To the extent that the heavy reliance on mistaken intuitive beliefs about cognitive biases creates mistakes, the courts should entertain some remedy.

References

ALI (American Law Institute; 1965). *Restatement (second) of torts*. Philadelphia: American Law Institute.

Calebrasi, G. (1970). *The cost of accidents*. New Haven, CT: Yale University Press.

Calfee, J. E., and Craswell, R. (1984). Some effect of uncertainty on compliance with legal standards. *Virginia Law Review*, 70, 965.

Coleman, J. L. (1992). *Risks and wrongs*. New York: Cambridge University Press.

Collins, R. K. L. (1970). Language, history, and the legal process: A profile of the "reasonable man." *Rutgers-Camden Law Review*, 8, 311.

Daubert v. Merrell Dow Pharmaceuticals, 509 U.S. 579 (1993).

Dobbs, D. B. (2000). *The law of torts.* Saint Paul, MN: West.

Findley, K. A. (2002). Learning from our mistakes: A criminal justice commission to study wrongful convictions. *California Western Law Review, 38,* 333.

Fletcher, G. P. (1972). Fairness and utility in tort theory. *Harvard Law Review, 85,* 537.

Harper, F. V., and James, F. (1956). *The law of torts.* Boston: Little, Brown.

Henderson, J. A. (1976). Expanding the negligence concept: Retreat from the rule of law. *Indiana Law Journal, 51,* 467.

Henderson J. A., Pearson, R. N., and Siliciano, J. A. (1999). *The torts process.* 5th ed. Gaithersburg, NY: Aspen Law and Business.

Herbert, A. P. (1930). *Misleading cases in the common law.* Putnam: New York.

Holmes, O. W. (1881). *The common law.* Reprint, Cambridge, MA: Harvard University Press, 1963.

Jolls, C., Sunstein, C. R., and Thaler, R. T. (1998). A behavioral approach to law and economics. *Stanford Law Review, 50,* 1471.

Keating, G. C. (1996). Reasonableness and rationality in negligence theory. *Stanford Law Review, 48,* 311.

Keeton, W. P. (1984). *Prosser and Keeton on the law of torts.* 5th ed. Saint Paul, MN: West.

Kelley, H. H. (1968). Attribution theory in social psychology. In D. Levin (Ed.), *Nebraska Symposium on Motivation.* Vol. 15. Lincoln: University of Nebraska Press.

Knapp v. City of Bradford, 432 Pa. 172, 247 A.2d 575 (1968).

Korobkin, R. B., and Ulen, T. A. (2000). Law and behavioral science: Removing the rationality assumption from law and economics. *California Law Review, 88,* 1051.

Landes, W. M., and Posner, R. A. (1987). *The economic structure of tort law.* Cambridge, MA: Harvard University Press.

Levin, D. T., Momen, N, Drivdahl, S. B., and Simons, D. J. (2000). Change blindness blindness: The metacognitive error of over-estimating change-detection ability. *Visual Cognition, 7,* 397–412.

Mack, A., and Rock, I. (1998). *Inattention blindness.* Cambridge, MA: MIT Press.

Nisbett, R., and Ross, L. (1980). *Human inference: Strategies and shortcomings of social judgment.* Englewood, NJ: Prentice-Hall.

Polinsky, A. M. (1989). *An introduction to law and economics.* 2nd ed. Boston: Little Brown.

Posner, E. A. (2003). Probability errors: Some positive and normative implications for tort and contract law. Unpublished manuscript.

Posner, R. A. (1981). The concept of corrective justice in recent theories of tort law. *Journal of Legal Studies, 10,* 187.

Rachlinski, J. J. (1998). A positive psychological theory of judging in hindsight. *University of Chicago Law Review, 65,* 571.

Resnick, R. A. et al. (1997). To see or not to see: The need for attention to perceive changes in scenes. *Psychological Science, 8,* 368–379.

Reynolds, O. M. (1970). The reasonable man of negligence law: A Heath report on the odious creature. *Oklahoma Law Review, 23,* 410.

Saks, M. J., and Baron, C. H, Eds. (1980). *The use/nonuse/misuse of applied social research in the courts.* Cambridge, MA: Abt Books.

Shavell, S. (1980). Strict liability versus negligence. *Journal of Legal Studies, 9,* 1.

Simons, D. J., and Chabris, C. F. (1999). Gorilla in our midst: Sustained inattentional blindness for dynamic events. *Perception, 28,* 1059.

Sunstein, C. R. (1996). Health-health tradeoffs. *University of Chicago Law Review, 63,* 1533.

Svenson, O. (1981). Are we all less risky and more skillful than our fellow drivers? *Acta Psychologica, 47,* 143.

Weinrib, E. (1992). Corrective justice. *Iowa Law Review, 77,* 403.

About the Contributors

Dare A. Baldwin is a professor of psychology at the University of Oregon. She received her Ph.D. in psychology from Stanford University. She investigates mechanisms that promote knowledge aquisition, focusing in particular on the acquisition of word meaning and the acquisition of skills for discerning others' goals and intentions.

Melissa R. Beck is a postdoctoral research Associate at George Mason University. She received her PhD in 2003 at Kent State University working with Daniel T. Levin. She studies visual perception, attention, and metacognition and is currently investigating the role of endogenous attention in change detection.

Jane E. Cottrell is a psychology researcher and an author of numerous articles and several books on French, Italian, and Romanian languages and literatures. She received her B.S. in journalism and her M.A. in French literature from Northwestern University and her Ph.D. in psychology from Ohio State University. Her research has focused on children's thinking and on people's understanding of visual perception.

Rachel A. Diana is a graduate student at Carnegie Mellon University working with Lynne Reder. She received her B.S. in psychology with honors from Presbyterian College. Her research on memory includes both verbal and visual domains, as well as the effects of irrelevant perceptual information on memory, with a focus on computational models of recognition memory.

John H. Flavell is a professor emeritus of psychology at Stanford University and a member of the National Academy of Sciences. He is best known for his book *The Developmental Psychology of Jean Piaget* and for his research on the development of communication, memory strategies, metacognition, and theory of mind. He has received several awards and honorary degrees for his cognitive science research.

Carl E. Granrud is an associate professor of psychology at the University of Northern Colorado. He received his B.A. from Luther College and his Ph.D. in developmental psychology from the University of Minnesota. His research focuses on the development of visual perception.

David V. Halpern is a graduate student at the University of Pittsburgh working with Jonathan W. Schooler. He received his B.A. in psychology from Emory University, graduating magna cum laude and as a member of Phi Beta Kappa. In addition to the relationship between metaconsciousness and "zoning out," his research has investigated the various processes that may lead to distortions in autobiographical memory.

David E. Irwin is a professor of psychology at the University of Illinois at Urbana-Champaign and in the Beckman Institute for Advanced Science and Technology. He received his Ph.D. in psychology from the University of Michigan. He taught at Cornell University, the Massachusetts Institute of Technology, and Michigan State University before moving to Illinois in 1991. He does research on eye movements and visual cognition.

Frank C. Keil is professor of psychology and linguistics at Yale University. His research focuses on how children and adults construe the world as being organized into theorylike domains, even though their explicit knowledge of such theories is highly skeletal and fragmentary. It has led him to consider more specific questions about illusions of explanatory understanding, the nature of conceptual change, and notions of the division of cognitive labor.

Arthur F. Kramer is a professor of psychology at the University of Illinois at Urbana-Champaign, in the Campus Neuroscience Program, and at the Institute of Aviation, and is a full-time faculty member of the Beckman Institute Human Perception and Performance Group. He received his Ph.D. in psychology from Illinois. His fields of professional interest are perceptual organization and visual attention, acquisition and utilization of perceptual and cognitive skills, cognition and aging, and cognitive neuroscience.

Daniel T. Levin is an associate professor of psychology at Vanderbilt University. He received his B.A. from Reed College in 1990, and his Ph.D. in psychology from at Cornell University in 1997. His research explores the interface between cognition and perception. One area of research focuses on the role of social categories in constraining face perception. A second area explores the phenomenon of change blindness using a variety of experimental paradigms.

John M. Marazita is an associate professor of psychology at Ohio Dominican University. He received his Ph.D. in experimental psychology from Kent State University. His research focuses on children's word learning and metacogntiion.

William E. Merriman is a professor of psychology at Kent State University. He received his Ph.D. in child psychology from the University of Minnesota. His research focuses on word learning and metacognition in early childhood.

Candice M. Mills is a graduate student at Yale University working with Frank C. Keil and Paul Bloom. She received her B.S. in cognitive neuroscience from the University of Florida. Her research on cognitive development focuses on children's understanding of their own knowledge as well as others'.

Heather L. Pringle is a major in the Air Force and an assistant professor of psychology at the United States Air Force Academy. She received her Ph.D. in psychology from the University of Illinois at Urbana-Champaign. Her research interests include the role of eye movements in scene representation and the relationship between driving performance and change detection. Her recent work examining the presentation of critical information (of varying reliability) and its relationship with eye movements is supported by an augmented cognition grant from the Defense Advanced Research Projects Agency.

Jeffrey J. Rachlinski is a professor of law at Cornell University, where he has taught civil procedure, administrative law, environmental law, natural resources law, and social and cognitive psychology for lawyers. He received his B.A. and M.A. in psychology from the Johns Hopkins University, and his J.D. and his Ph.D. in psychology from Stanford University. He was a National Science Foundation Graduate Fellow in psychology at Stanford University from 1989 to 1993. After graduating from Stanford Law School in 1993, he worked as an associate in the litigation department at Wilson, Sonsini, Goodrich, and Rosati in Palo Alto, California. He has conducted cognitive science research and published several articles documenting the decision-making processes of judges, juries, and litigants.

Lynne M. Reder is a professor of psychology at Carnegie Mellon University. She received her B.S. from Stanford University, graduating with honors and as a member of Phi Beta Kappa, and her Ph.D. in psychology from the University of Michigan. She did postdoctoral training at Yale University until 1978, when she joined the faculty at Carnegie Mellon. Her research aspires to understand and explain a broad range of cognitive phenomena, from strategic adaptivity, attention, and cognitive illusions to how individual differences in working memory capacity can account for performance differences in complex tasks such as air traffic control. Her work involves developing a general model of implicit and explicit memory, as well as building computer-implemented cognitive models of complex tasks. She has published more than eighty works and has recently edited a volume entitled *Implicit Memory and Metacognition.*

Erik D. Reichle is an assistant professor of cognitive psychology at the University of Pittsburgh, a research scientist at the Learning Research and Development Center, and an active member of the Center for the Neural Basis of Cognition. He received his B.S. from University of Massachusetts at Amherst and his Ph.D. in psychology from Carnegie Mellon University, where his postdoctoral training includes three years of fMRI research. His research has focused on understanding how word identification, attention, and visual and oculomotor constraints jointly determine when and where the eyes move during reading. He has most recently used computational modeling, behavioral and eye-tracking experiments, and cognitive neuroscience methods (e.g., ERP) to evaluate theoretical assumptions about reading processes (e.g., visual word identification).

Leonid Rozenblit is a postdoctoral student at the Yale University Department of Psychology. He received a his B.A. from the State University of New York at Buffalo, his J.D. from Louisiana State University, and his Ph.D. in psychology from Yale. His recent work has focused on exploring how intuitive epistemologies guide expectations about what we ourselves and others know.

Megan M. Saylor is currently an assistant professor of psychology at Vanderbilt University. She received her Ph.D. in psychology from the University of Oregon. Her research focuses on the emergence of language and intentional understanding in infants and young children.

Brian J. Scholl is an assistant professor of psychology at Yale University, director of the Yale Perception and Cognition Laboratory, and an associate editor of the journal *Cognition*. He received his Ph.D. in psychology from Rutgers University and completed a postdoctoral fellowship at Harvard University. His recent research, supported by the National Science Foundation and the National Institutes of Mental Health, has focused on the nature of visual attention and awareness, the nature of persisting object representations in the visual system, the perception of causality and animacy, and the infant's object concept.

Jonathan W. Schooler is a professor of psychology at the University of Pittsburgh and an associate editor for the journal *Cognitive Technology*. He received his Ph.D. in psychology from the University of Washington in Seattle. His research interests include long-term memory for natural situations, disruptive effects of verbalization on memory, insight, judgment and decision making, and the relationship between language, thought and consciousness. He was an Osher fellow at the Exploratorium Science Museum in San Francisco.

Daniel J. Simons is an associate professor at the University of Illinois at Urbana-Champaign and an affiliate of the Beckman Institute for Advanced Science and Technology. He received his Ph.D. in psychology from Cornell University. He was a John L. Loeb associate professor of psychology at Harvard University before joining the faculty at Illinois in the summer of 2002. His cognitive science research has been supported by the National Science Foundation, the National Institutes of Mental Health, and the Alfred P. Sloan Foundation.

Gerald A. Winer is a professor of psychology at Ohio State University. He received his B.A. from Trinity College and his Ph.D. in developmental psychology from Clark University. Whereas his early work examined children's performance on Piagetian problems, his more recent research has examined children's and adults' understanding of perception.

Index